Communicative Structures and Psychic Structures

THE DOWNSTATE SERIES OF
RESEARCH IN PSYCHIATRY AND PSYCHOLOGY

Volume 1: COMMUNICATIVE STRUCTURES AND PSYCHIC STRUCTURES
Edited by Norbert Freedman and Stanley Grand

Communicative Structures and Psychic Structures

A PSYCHOANALYTIC INTERPRETATION
OF COMMUNICATION

Edited by

NORBERT FREEDMAN
and **STANLEY GRAND**

Downstate Medical Center
Brooklyn, New York

PLENUM PRESS • NEW YORK AND LONDON

Library of Congress Cataloging in Publication Data

Conference on Research Concerning the Psychoanalytic Interpretation of Communication,
    Downstate Medical Center, 1976.
    Communicative structures and psychic structures.

    (The Downstate series of research in psychiatry and psychology; v. 1)
    "Held at the Downstate Medical Center, State University of New York, Brooklyn, New
York, January 15-17, 1976."
    Bibliography: p.
    Includes index.
    1. Interpersonal communication—Congresses. 2. Psychoanalysis—Congresses. 3. Psycholo-
gy, Pathological—Congresses. I. Freedman, Norbert. II. Grand, Stanley. III. New York
(State). Downstate Medical Center, New York. IV. Title. V. Series.
BF637.C45C67 1976   158'.2   77-9574
ISBN 0-306-34361-4

Proceedings of the Conference on Research Concerning the Psychoanalytic
Interpretation of Communication held at the Downstate Medical Center,
State University of New York, Brooklyn, New York, January 15—17, 1976

© 1977 Plenum Press, New York
A Division of Plenum Publishing Corporation
227 West 17th Street, New York, N.Y. 10011

Printed in the United States of America

FOREWORD

The publication of this volume represents the first in a planned series of special publications on topics of major interest to workers in the fields of psychiatry and psychology. The series will be entitled The Downstate Series of Research in Psychiatry and Psychology and is the outcome of a series of discussions among several senior members of the Department of Psychiatry held about four years ago. Included in this group, were Drs. Benjamin Kissin, Henri Begleiter, Leonard Rosenblum, Herbert Pardes, Norbert Freedman, and myself. The talks were initiated by Dr. Pardes, now Chairman of the Department of Psychiatry at the University of Colorado, and the resultant decision was to hold three day symposia, hopefully of such excellence that the published papers of each symposium would represent a significant contribution to some particular aspect of human psychology. This decision necessitated the choice of suitable topics and distinguished speakers who would present original work coordinated into an integrated framework based upon a selected topic.

We all realized the difficulties inherent in the plan and unanimously selected Dr. Norbert Freedman to arrange the first symposium and its later publication. Many topics were discussed before the present one was chosen. We believe the topic to be timely and important and deserving of being put before the scientific public. Many people worked long and hard on both the symposium and the volume. The contributors provided work of significance and scope, but I wish to single out Dr. Freedman and Dr. Stanley Grand for the dedication they displayed in bringing the entire task to a successful conclusion. They worked long and hard, and chose brilliantly. The mix of basic scientists and psychoanalytic clinicians all contributing to the unifying theme is in itself innovative and unusually instructive. It is my hope that all who read this volume will not only be edified, but that they will also enjoy the presentation.

Special note must be made of the fact that Dr. Ferruccio DiCori was kind enough to secure the funding of this first effort through the generosity of Mr. Lowell Fink.

Robert Dickes
Professor and Chairman
Department of Psychiatry
Downstate Medical Center
Brooklyn, New York

PREFACE

"The Downstate Series of Research in Psychiatry" is a continuing
series devoted to the thematic presentation of behavioral research
around issues of clinical relevance. This is the first volume in the
series. It grew out of a conference held at the Downstate Medical
Center on January 15, 16, and 17, 1976. It was Doctor Herbert Pardes,
former Chairman of the Department of Psychiatry, who took the initiative in opening new channels of communication between formal research
on the one hand and the demands and insight of clinical practice on
the other. He, together with a planning committee, formulated the
concept of an ongoing, clinically oriented, series of research findings. Dr. Robert Dickes, as current Chairman, has given continued
leadership and support to this venture. Dr. Dickes' initiative has
carried us beyond this first volume so that two other volumes are now
in the active planning stage.

We gratefully and affectionately acknowledge the contribution of
Caroline Apolito. She gave impetus to the venture from inception to
completion. She brought a personal touch that helped create a network of warm relationships with and among the contributors from many
parts of the country. She wielded an understanding and incisive edi-
torial pen. She provided the needed uplift and perseverance at many
points of crisis. Her dedication, spirit, insight, and intelligence
guided us throughout. For her, it was a labor of love and as such
made it so for all of those involved.

Norbert Freedman

Stanley Grand

January 1, 1977

CONTRIBUTORS

Jacob Arlow	Downstate Medical Center
Beatrice Beebe	Columbia University
Allen Dittmann	National Insitute of Mental Health
David Freedman	Baylor College of Medicine
Norbert Freedman	Downstate Medical Center
Louis Gottschalk	University of California at Irvine
Stanley Grand	Downstate Medical Center
Leonard Horowitz	Stanford University
Mardi Horowitz	University of California at San Francisco
Louise Kaplan	New York University
Peter Knapp	Boston University School of Medicine
Lester Luborsky	University of Pennsylvania School of Medicine
George Mahl	Yale University
Fred Pine	Albert Einstein College of Medicine
Benjamin Rubinstein	New York Psychoanalytic Institute
Louis Sander	Boston University School of Medicine
Sebastiano Santostefano	Harvard Medical School
Jean Schimek	New York University
Theodore Shapiro	New York University
Howard Shevrin	University of Michigan Medical Center
Lloyd Silverman	New York University
Donald Spence	Rutgers University School of Medicine
Irving Steingart	Downstate Medical Center
Daniel Stern	Columbia University
Regina L. Uliana	University of California at Irvine

CONTENTS

PROLOGUE: A GESTURE TOWARD A PSYCHOANALYTIC THEORY OF COMMUNICATION

Norbert Freedman and Stanley Grand

Twenty years ago, Rene Spitz (1957) published what we deem to be a monumental monograph--"No and Yes." We single out this work because Spitz may be regarded as the spiritual father of this volume. His was the first gesture in the direction of a psychoanalytic view of communication. Moreover, his work was buttressed by relatively hard data and was developmental in conception. Although we have a psychoanalytic theory of thinking, of drives, and of object relations, we do not possess a psychoanalytic theory of communication. This is remarkable in a discipline that rests heavily on the discourse between people. If this volume can make a fresh beginning in defining those principles which govern the symbolic commerce between people, our efforts will have been worthwhile.

How is this volume different from other volumes in the field of communication? This is a volume on communication which contains a dialogue in its own right--a dialogue between researcher and clinician. The researchers (all psychoanalytically trained) rest their conclusions on relatively hard data based upon sophisticated methods for the study of human interaction. These observations are then discussed by practicing psychoanalysts. It is hoped that this unique dialogue will contribute both to the general theory of communication and the psychoanalytic interpretation of discourse. There is a further difference between this volume and others in the field of communication. The volume not only provides a unique dialogue between researcher and clinician, it is also guided by a particular conception of communicative discourse. The conception we wish to highlight is one that regards discourse as a complex interweaving of manifest and latent structures--an integration of communicative and psychic structures. What do we mean by these two terms?

1

Communication refers to the interchange of messages between individuals. Communicative Structures refer to those manifest vehicles of
communication through which messages are transmitted. They are the
visible and audible manifestations of thought and language reflected
in the speech, gesture, paralinguistic and motoric arrangements of the
communicative act. Taken as a whole, they represent a complex organization of the transmission process which transcends the semantic and
syntactic elements of each of the components separately. Thus, Communicative Structure is the patterned display of the act of transmitting
a message to the listener.

In our era of mass media, communication and, by extension, communication research, has focused mainly upon the message and its manner
of transmission from source to destination. However, there is a danger in limiting the study of communication simply to the transmission
of information. Before a message can be shared, private images must
be retrieved, sorted, and selected. There is, after all, a communicator in communication--the organizer of the message. Consideration
of this aspect of the communicative act requires a conception of those
particular psychological organizations upon which manifest communicative structures rest. Such a view leads us directly to the second
term in our conception of communication, namely Psychic Structures.

Psychic structure, as defined in this volume, refers to those
enduring mental organizations of experience upon which manifest
communication rests. Historically, the definition of psychic structure has included a range of mental events as microscopic as the representation of sensations, images, and single words, to mental organizations as macroscopic as the major divisions of the mind given by
the terms id, ego, and superego. The definition, which we wish to advance here, does not exclude any of these, but rather, it seeks to
articulate more specifically those forms of mental organizations which
have a direct bearing upon the communicative act. As such, we shall
consider psychic structures to be those patternings and organizations
of experience, latent within the speaker and the listener, which constitute the necessary conditions for thought to be shared.

That there are mental organizations which are specific to the
communicative process is a fact widely accepted in cognitive as well
as psychoanalytic theory. What, then, is the specific contribution
which can be made by a psychoanalytic perspective? By virtue of its
role as a clinical discipline, psychoanalysis is privy to the private,
personal world of the communicator. Thus, it is in a unique position
with respect to its understanding of the subjective side of the communicative process. Moreover, the psychoanalytic theory, with its broad
psychobiological underpinnings and explicit recognition of drives, conflict, and object relationships, provides an important perspective on
the transition from private image to shared thought. Let us, then,
sketch out a set of postulates about particular psychic organizations
which we believe to be crucial to promoting this transition.

1. The Self in Communication

    Communication would not be possible without an awareness of self
as speaker, and other as listener. This postulate is basic, since the
temporary or chronic loss of the sense of self inevitably entails a
disruption in the communicative flow--a lacuna in the "basic dialogue"
between self and other. Anni Bergman (1971) has sensitively depicted
such lacuni in the communicative development of a symbiotic child. In
her essay "I and You," she describes how, in the absence of a self-
organization, the child avoids the use of personal pronouns, leaves
gaps in her utterances, never expresses a wish directly, and parrots
words or phrases heard. Indeed, the child exhibits a tendency to repeat words over and over until they become nonsense syllables.

    The continuing sensory and motor interchanges between infant and
caretaker, from the first days of life, set the stage for the development of the self and the capacity to transmit a message from the
"me" to "you." Logically, the self, as a psychic structure, is the
foundation for communication, but not its actualization. Without it,
true symbolic communication is not possible. With it, communication
is possible but not guaranteed. It is a precommunicative structure
developmentally, for discrimination even of the rudimentary "I" and
"non-I" precedes true symbolic representation. The development of
psychic organization--discrimination of the animate from the inanimate, the I from the non-I, the maternal object from the stranger--
corresponds step-by-step with the ability to establish semantic representations.

    The recognition of this developmental progression has led us to
take an ontogenetic approach in this volume, and we begin with a
series of infancy studies. We believe that the burgeoning field of
psychoanalytically oriented infancy research has much to contribute
to the foundation of communication theory.

2. Sensorimotor Organization in Communication

    Communicative structures are embedded in a set of bodily experi-
ences derived from muscle action and sensory innervation. According
to this postulate, the motor system provides the experiential base
for the capacity for symbolic representation. The transition from
action and sensorimotor experiencing to symbolizing is vividly illustrated by Spitz's depiction of the progression from the rooting response (a scanning reflex action), to headshaking, to the semantic
gesture "no." More generally, through bodily action, the experience
of physical space and form is transformed into cognitive space and
form.

    The sensory quality of bodily experience provides the foundation
for the representation of the drives and object relations. The stimulation of the oral zone, the touch of the body surface, sphincter

innervation, and genital arousal, all in the context of the basic dialogue between infant and mother, infuse the contents of communication
with a substrate of bodily representations. Sharpe (1940) has emphasized the way in which these original instinctual contributions return
during the associative process of psychoanalysis in the form of metaphor. Bodily determined metaphor is the core of communication in psychoanalysis, providing the connection between sensory experiences on
the one hand, and realistic representation on the other. It is the
stuff which gives vitality and drive to the communicative experience.

In the beginning, there are only sensorimotor experiences. This
is a view shared by psychoanalysis and contemporary cognitive theory
alike. While both theories recognize the common root, the two views
depart in terms of the continuing role of sensorimotor functions in
mature discourse. In contemporary cognitive theory, the sensorimotor
phase is but a passing episode. As complex symbolic processes emerge,
beginning with the second year of life, the motor and sensory systems
become progressively less relevant for verbal communication. But, in
the psychoanalytic view, these bodily innervations are the carriers
of the drives. They have a motivational function and exert an ongoing
influence on communicative structures during discourse.

There is, then, an issue of whether bodily experiences are epiphenomena or are continuing regulators of communication. Many papers
in this volume touch directly or indirectly upon this issue. If the
evidence points in the direction of a continuing regulatory and motivational role for sensorimotor experience, then objective psychoanalytically oriented research can make a unique impact upon the study of
communication.

3. The Organization of Consciousness in Communication

In any interpersonal dialogue, there occurs an intrapsychic dialogue as well. This is a dialogue between that which is in the center
and that which is in the periphery of awareness. According to this
postulate, communicative structure signifies an organization of consciousness in which there is an interchange between the intended message in the focus of awareness, and the matrix of unintended associated memories and images which form the background context of meanings.
The articulation of a message, then, reflects a particular organization of consciousness in which the central focus shades off into subtle
gradations of awareness, much like the "fringes" in William James'
(1950) "Stream of Consciousness"--the figure and ground of communication. The effects of the fringe upon the central focus of communication are often powerfully evident, as for example, in a case reported
by Rosen (1969) of a young woman who, during the course of a session,
unexplainably began to express obsessional fears about her treatment
and about the possibility that "the price of cure" in terms of "sac-
rifice of her self-determination" was too great. On leaving the office, she suddenly turned to the analyst and said: "I know that I

should have mentioned this; it has been on my mind all during the
session, but I will not be able to come tomorrow. I will explain next
time."

Whether such phenomena, visible in the peculiarities of communication, are interpreted in topographic (i.e., the unconscious pressing
toward consciousness) or structural terms, need not concern us here.
What is important is the recognition that a set of dynamic mental contents, operating outside of focal awareness, interacts with experiences in focal awareness. Clinically, psychoanalysis sets itself the
task of deciphering such latent meanings in the manifest communication. However, the structural separation of communication into conscious and nonconscious processes interacting with each other is, in
its own right, important for understanding communicative effectiveness. Thus, as Spitz (1966) has already noted, the structuralization
of mental contents and functions into sectors of development which become conscious or which remain unconscious, and the proportion of the
two to each other, have vitally important consequences for subsequent
development. We may conclude that the separation of conscious communication into figure, and nonconscious communication into ground is
the very arrangement which lends structure and effectiveness to the
communicative effort.

Experimental studies presented in this volume show how subliminally presented messages may register in the nervous system and may
affect the communicative process. But psychoanalytic research has
passed the stage of simply documenting the existence of an unconscious
process and saying, "Eureka, it is really there." Granting the existence of the intrusion into focal awareness of dissociative experiences, we need more information concerning how such experiences are
transformed if our knowledge about these phenomena is to progress beyond simple demonstration to a knowledge about unconscious regulation
and control. Here is an area for close integration between the data
of the psychoanalytic investigator and the data of general behavior
research.

4.   The Search for a Discovery of the Object in Communication

There is no communicative experience without mental representation, and there are no mental representations which do not entail object representations. In our fourth postulate, we affirm that all
private experiences are communicative experiences at their core, for
all inner experience yearns for an object that hears, listens, and
senses. In 1874, Brentano, presenting his empirical base for psychology, argued that we do not love or hate, but always love someone
or hate someone. While this view, which is commonplace today, came
to him as a major insight, he humbly credited the scholastics of the
middle ages, notably Acquinas, for this discovery. We can note this
communicative wish even in the most private of experiences, the dream.

Bergman (1971), quotes from Lessing: "Alba always tells me her dreams
in the morning. Alba sleeps for herself but Alba dreams for me."
Stone (1961) and others have shown how even those subtle, most private "noncommunicative" aspects of the interpersonal dialogue reflect
the wish to reach an inner object. It is this transferential wish in
the contemporary discourse which shapes and molds words, meanings, and
syntax.

Object relationship structures are at the core of the communicative effort. They define the direction of communication and the transition from private to public thought. As a minimum, these structures
entail an intention to reach an object, and it is this intentionality
which directs the transition from inner to outer speech. We recognize with Watzlawick (1967) that, logically, it is impossible not to
communicate, even in silence. All behavior in a dyadic content may
be said to have a regulatory and controlling function. Yet, the individual's decision to invoke a public and shared symbol, be it word
or gesture, is an act beyond the mere intention to reach the other.
It also signifies the hope of realizing the internal representation
in a contemporary context. Thus, object relationship structures entail not only a search for, but the discovery of objects as well.
Failure to establish object relations, in this broader communicative
sense, reflects a loss of contact with the other and a breakdown in
the experience of empathy. Object relationship structures, therefore, entail the wish to establish empathic contact with the other
and the hope that the internalized object can be realized in the
dialogue.

The significance of object relationship structures as central
motivational forces in communication is documented in many sections
of this volume. It enters into an individual's performance during
information processing, play behavior, conversational interchanges
and, of course, in psychotherapy and psychoanalysis. Phenomena described in this volume point to certain reciprocities between object
relations and communicative structures which raise issues regarding
the primary significance of transference in determining the course of
communication. These phenomena suggest that primary linguistic and
kinesic organizations have an independent developmental program quite
apart from an individual's object relations, and may impede or facilitate shared communication regardless of the quality of such relations.
It is in this area that psychoanalytically oriented research can begin
to tease apart the unique contributions of psychic structure and communicative structure to the process of communication.

5. The Integrative Functions in Communication

Communication always entails a dialectic, or what Spitz calls the
presence of antithetical tendencies. There is not only a "no," or a
"yes," but prior to that, a centrifugal and centrepetal tendency.
Psychoanalytic thinking is replete with polarities: drive and de-

fense, self and object representation, libido and aggression. The manifestations of these antithetical tendencies are vividly documented in even a cursory observation of recorded communicative behavior. In this volume, we shall see a whole series of such polarities: reaching and self-touching, separation and rapprochement, object-focused and body-focused gestures, and intimacy and distance. What is at issue here is how such polarities are integrated. A vivid example of such integration is Freud's (1919) linguistic analysis of the word "uncanny"--unheimlich. Unheimlich, as an expression of anxiety about strangeness, contains both the idea of secrecy (heimlich) and the wish for intimacy (heim), as if, in the very encounter of unfamiliar places, there occurs the secret wish to reestablish the intimacy of home. Words and gestures have a remarkable way of combining polarities into a single integrated unit. Thus, our final postulate holds that any communicative structure implies an integrative structure which achieves the coordination of polarities.

The integrated man has become the aristocrat of the psychological world. He is someone who is sought out and emulated, and his communication becomes a model for identification. The theoretical literature contains a number of concepts which are presumed to account for such an effective communicative achievement. Yet, these concepts are singularly devoid of operational definition. There is the concept of neutralization in which the drive determinants of behavior have lost their overriding impact; there is the concept of sublimation in which primitive identifications are now realized for the attainment of ethical or altruistic objectives; and, there is simply the notion of the synthetic ego functions, the ability of the ego to "synthesize" antithetical tendencies. Each of these concepts is invoked to describe the individual's integrative achievement. However, none of them depict the process by which such integration is accomplished.

The microscopic analysis of communication behavior may provide a more operational view of the integrative process. Papers in this volume are directed toward this objective. Work detailing the phasing in of rhythmic synchrony between caretaker and infant, or the rhythmic alternation of body movements phased in with syntactic structure, provide good examples of patterns which may be the building blocks of this process. Structuralization of these patterns can be observed at varying levels of communicative complexity. At the most complex level, the integrated communicative structure is one in which drive discharge and sensory feedback alternate with planning and anticipatory functions in particular sequential arrangements. Such arrangements are manifestations of a psychic organization which lends coherence to communication. The researcher's ability to detail sequential phenomena such as these provide a specificity to the integrative process which has only been broadly sketched out by clinical observations.

Here, then, are the themes of this volume. The organization of
the self provides the foundation for the communicative effort. The
organization of body experiences, involving motor action and sensory
innervation, creates the condition of vitality and drive. The organization of consciousness and the dialogue between focal and peripheral awareness lends structure to the communicative effort. Yet,
it is the continuing search for the discovery of an internalized object in contemporary discourse which lends direction to communication. Indeed, it is the object relationship structures which are
most centrally relevant in the shift from private image to communicated thought. Finally, there is an integrative organization which
coordinates the polarities operating within the individual's psychological makeup, and hence lends coherence to communication. These
psychic structures form the roots of symbolic thought manifest in
word, gesture, or sentence.

There has, in general, been much skepticism regarding the usefulness of a dialogue between researcher and clinician for the resolution of paradoxes created by psychoanalytic thinking. We clearly
disagree with such a view, and expect that the dialogue reported in
this volume should serve to mute much of this pessimism. But there
are other benefits to be derived from the dialogue presented here,
and we would like to outline these consequences as well. First, the
psychoanalytic researcher, by virtue of his specific orientation, can
point to phenomena which have generally been neglected by the nonanalytic observer. Thus, the studies presented here should enrich
the general understanding of the communicative process. Second, the
investigators' ability to bring sophisticated research methodology to
bear on clinical hypotheses should serve to both specify more clearly
and limit the overextension of such hypotheses so that theory and
practice may be placed on firmer footing. Finally, and most important of all, is the hope that the research findings reported in this
volume will serve to generate new directions and hypotheses for further clinical investigation.

Communicative structures and psychic structures are, of course,
two aspects of the same process. The exclusive focus upon one, the
scrutinizing of a minute communicative effort; or the other, the consideration of broadly conceived mental organizations, is likely to
mar the unity of its totality. This view was aptly stated by Brain
(1951) in the following passage: "If you look at a tapestry through
a magnifying glass, you will see the individual threads but not the
pattern: if you stand away from it you will see the pattern but not
the threads. My guess is that in the nervous system we are looking
at the threads while with the mind we perceive the patterns, and that
one day we may discover how the patterns are made out of the threads."

REFERENCES

Bergman, Anni. I and you: The separation-individuation process in the treatment of a symbiotic child. In John B. McDevitt & Calvin F. Settlage (Eds.), Separation-individuation essays in honor of Margaret S. Mahler. New York: International Universities Press, 1971.

Bergmann, M. S. The intrapsychic and communicative aspects of the dream: Their role in psycho-analysis and psychotherapy. The International Journal of Psycho-Analysis, 1966, Vol. 47, Parts 2-3: 356-363.

Brain, W. R. Mind, perception and science. Oxford: Blackwell Scientific Publications, 1951.

Brentano, F. Psychologie vom empirischen standpunkt, 1874.

Freud, S. (1919). The 'uncanny'. Part III. Relation of imagination to reality. Standard Edition, XVII. New York: International Universities Press, 1955.

James, W. (1890). The principles of psychology. Vol. 1. New York: Dover Publications, 1950.

Rosen, V. H. Sign phenomena and their relationship to unconscious meaning. International Journal of Psychoanalysis, 1969, 50:197-207.

Sharpe, E. F. Psycho-physical problems revealed in language: An examination of metaphor. International Journal of Psycho-Analysis, 1940, 21:201-213.

Spitz, R. A. No and yes. New York: International Universities Press, 1957.

Spitz, R. A. Metapsychology and direct infant observation. In R. M. Loewenstein, M. Schur, & A. Solnit (Eds.), Psychoanalysis: A general psychology. New York: International Universities Press, 1966.

Stone, L. The psychoanalytic situation: An examination of its development and essential nature. New York: International Universities Press, 1961.

Watzlawick, P., Beavin, J., & Jackson, D. Pragmatics of human communication. New York: Norton, 1967.

SECTION 1
EARLY OBJECT EXPERIENCES
IN THE DEVELOPMENT
OF COMMUNICATIVE STRUCTURES

INTRODUCTION

In beginning this volume with a set of papers which focus upon early object experiences in the development of communicative structures, we are attempting to highlight our view of an essential continuity between the earliest experiences of the infant vis-a-vis the caretaking environment and later communicative behavior--a "developmental line" of communication--to use Anna Freud's term. However, in focusing upon early, regulatory phenomena which occur during a phase of development which Hartmann and others have characterized as "undifferentiated," we are immediately confronted by a central paradox. Since communication is a process of information exchange, which in its essential nature implicates a matrix of conscious intentionality and all that this matrix implies for the complexity of psychic apparatus functioning, can one consider the regulatory phenomena of this early period really communicative?

Considering this paradox, the contributions to this first section are mainly concerned with what might be termed precommunicative behavior. The papers included here provide the reader with descriptions of the precursors to the development of psychological structure; a unique view of the interactive and regulatory processes operative in the early dialogue between mother and infant, and which, it might be added, may be re-evoked throughout life to sustain the possibilities for symbolic interchange. The contributions by Sander, Beebe and Stern, and David Freedman provide important perspectives on this early period.

Sander, taking an interactionist perspective on the bonding between infant and caretaker argues that the infant, far from being a static congeries of potential functions shaped by the reinforcements of a more or less adequate caretaker, is already at birth a highly complex actively self-regulating component of an equally complex and highly organized relational system. Sander develops a sophisticated systems model of schema formation and suggests that the organization of governed exchanges around attentional and intentional processes represent precommunicative regulatory structures present and observable early in life.

11

    Beebe and Stern focus upon the vicissitudes of an Engagement-
Disengagement process at the four month-old level and relate this
process to the structuralization of boundaries and defenses as well
as the emergence of object schemata. These authors, rather than
focusing on mutual regulation, address themselves to the opposite
side of the coin, i.e., the "stimulus barrier" to the interlocking
responsivity of infant to mother in this "split second world" of
interacting partners. This structuralization of boundaries is manifest in the detailed observations of the "chase and dodge" sequences
which contribute to the differentiation of self and object, and reflect the growing repertoire of behaviors which regulate the prevalence and duration of focused encounters. The exquisite responsiveness of the infant, through orientation and visual regard, highlights the infant's capacity to modulate or regulate the flow of incoming stimulation.

    Finally, David Freedman's paper is the first to explicitly ad-
dress itself to those psychic structures required for communication.
Through "experiments of nature" manifest among the congenitally
blind, deaf, and those subjected to extreme social isolation, Freedman proposes that stable self- and object-representations are prerequisite to intentionality in communication. By focusing upon
disturbances in the opportunity for empathic contact, Freedman highlights the importance of the infant-mother bonding to the development of such stable, integrated self- and object-representation
structures. As Pine suggests in his discussion of these papers,
this is the red thread which ties the early nonverbal behavior to
later structuralized communication.

    In all, the papers in this section provide a body of important
data supporting an essential psychobiological continuity in the line
of communicative development. Such a continuing line distinguishes
a psychoanalytic theory of communication from those views which postulate discontinuity between prelinguistic and linguistic stages of
communication. Further, the psychobiological line is also distinct
from views which recognize the continuity between prelinguistic and
linguistic phases, yet fail to take account of biological roots. In
this respect, the data reported in this first section are congruent
with recent developments in cognitive theory, which, under the impact
of Piaget have emphasized sensorimotor "intentions" as the foundation
for language and communication. Thus, these papers begin to chart
the origins of sensorimotor intentions in the human dialogue and
offer a view of an already highly differentiated beginning to the undifferentiated phase of development. Section 2 attempts to link
these early organizations of the basic dialogue between mother and
infant to the development of verbal dialogue in communication.

REGULATION OF EXCHANGE IN THE INFANT CARETAKER SYSTEM:

A VIEWPOINT ON THE ONTOGENY OF "STRUCTURES"

Louis W. Sander[1]

Boston University School of Medicine

Boston, Massachusetts 02118

PRECOMMUNICATIVE STRUCTURES--A SYSTEMS VIEWPOINT

In beginning a symposium with the title "Communicative Structures and Psychic Structures," there is a certain logic in starting
with the immediate postnatal period. This is a time quite before
the age at which one begins to think of communication as yet existing between the infant and the people around him, and certainly
before one thinks of the infant in terms of a psychic structure.
However, in taking an ontogenetic approach to the subject, we are
asking whether or not communicative processes may be determined in
some lawful way by the earliest features of interpersonal transactions or exchanges, the precommunicative structures, such as those
which characterize exchanges between neonate and caretaker. It is
this early period, in particular the first two weeks to two months
of life, which our group has investigated. We have been interested
in what can be said about these early events which might relate to
the notion of "structure" in the arrangement of those later behaviors
we label as communication. Even further, can anything sensible be
suggested that might possibly contribute bridging links between
early events and "psychic structures?" Whatever they might be, we
will probably have to be content with such bridges as ways of thinking about the problem rather than as concrete answers.

---

[1]Dr. Sander is supported by a research scientist award of the NIMH:
PHS #K05-MH-20505. Grant support has been provided by the Grant
Foundation "An Investigation of Change in Mother-Infant Interaction
over First Two Weeks of Life," USPHS Grant #HD01766 "Adaptation and
Perception in Early Infancy" and University Hospital general research
support funds.

Over the course of our work, we have developed a way of viewing
the organization of the interpersonal exchanges between infant and
caregiver which is based on the idea that these behaviors are first
and foremost in the service of regulation of behavior, and of functions of the interacting partners. In other words, the behavior of
each, which we can observe in their interaction, serves to regulate
both the behavior of the other and of their own complement of component functions. For some 200 years, the term regulation in biology
has had the meaning of "governed exchange." It is possible that the
nature of the exchanges and the means whereby "governing" is accomplished may provide the clues to a framework of persistent interactive configurations which is basic both to initial interpersonal
exchanges and to later communicational processes. Much depends on
what can be included within this concept of "regulation."

The psychoanalytic framework has been concerned from its beginning with the matter of regulation, as evidenced by the model proposed by Freud in the "Project For a Scientific Psychology" (Freud,
1954). This suggested, in the main, a model whereby excitation from
various sources arising both from within and from outside the individual might be regulated by processes essentially within the individual. This provides, for example, the general perspective in relation
to the organization of behavior as a configuration being generated
between drive and drive restraint, both influences operating from
within the individual. In the perspective which we shall be trying
to present, namely that of infant and caregiver as constituting an
interactive regulative system, regulation is referring to the regulation of the actual behavioral exchanges which describe the ongoing
interaction in the system, and which can be thought of as maintaining
the relative stability of both the individual and the system over
time. The interacting partners are both contributing behaviors which
regulate, and providing behaviors which are regulated. This is a
view traditionally more relevant to the description of the organism
in its environment of life support, with the "governing of exchange"
representing the operation of the life processes maintaining the
organism over time. The organization of the individual is part and
parcel of the organization of the system. The biologist does not
view the individual organism as a "monad," capable of independent
existence, but always as embedded in, and requiring intimate, complex,
and regulated exchange with the surround. The idea we will pursue
here is that the biological principles governing life support processes will suggest the lawful framework for a conceptualization of
"precommunicative structure." It is the systems approach which makes
this possible.

AN INTERACTIONAL INTERFACE BETWEEN INFANT AND CAREGIVER--ITS COM-
PLEXITY AND ORGANIZATION AT THE OUTSET

If we can go now to the empirical content of the transactions

and interactions between infant and caregiver, i.e., to the exchanges
between them, it is evident that current research is providing us
with a rapidly changing picture of the nature of the events which
make up this initial interaction. In the traditional view from
which organization of behavior has been discussed as the property
of the individual, the organization of behavior has been thought of
as developing. One began, in the discussion of its ontogeny, with
a somewhat vague "undifferentiated period" in the first weeks of life
from which the infant gradually developed an increasing organization
of interactions, through a process of secondary reinforcement, as
needs and discomforts were responded to by the caretaker (Brenner,
1955). Current research in early infancy is beginning to provide
provocative evidence that human existence normally begins in the
context of a highly organized relational system from the outset.
This relational system interfaces two live, actively self-regulating,
highly complex, living (and adapting) components--the infant and the
caregiver, each already running, so to speak. One does not activate
the other from a static position. At this point, we can pause to
consider briefly the nature of this interface and what we mean by
its organization and its complexity. We can then turn to a discussion of the possible implications which the actual characteristics
of these exchanges have for the symposium subject.

It is easy to envision an infant-environment regulative system
when one begins at the level of the foetus. Even here it used to be
imagined that the foetus was developing in response to its genomic
determinants in a kind of isolation provided by the optimally stable
surround of the womb, quite shielded from environmental intrusion.
However, the sensitivity of foetal development to variations in the
uterine environment is becoming more specifically appreciated (e.g.,
effects such as those of maternal age or uterine "depletion," etc.).
Changes are taking place in the traditional view of genomic "givens"
or "endowment" of the newborn as the even wider sensitivity of the
foetus to the larger environment of the mother is documented (e.g.,
effects of psychological and situational stress, nutrition, smoking,
alcohol, pharmacological influences, etc.). The newborn at birth
clearly is already a phenotype. There is evidence now that even the
sex of the infant may have an interactional determinant, namely, the
influence of the timing of insemination, whether prior to or following ovulation (Guerrero, 1974).

Interactional determinants of development are further illustrated by recent evidence of the decisive effects of interactions within
the first postnatal days, both on the mother and her subsequent maternal behavior (Klaus et al., 1972), and on the infant and certain
of its characteristics of regulation of state (Sander et al., 1972).
One of the implications here is for a change in our concept of "autonomous" ego functions and the "conflict-free" sphere, and perhaps for

a change in our concept of "apparatus," i.e., perception, motility,
etc. Do they mature as relatively static givens or structures which
later become available for the ego to "use" as operational tools at
a time when it can be said the ego begins? On the contrary, these
functions are involved at once in the regulation of events in the
system. The later strategies of their use may depend on the early
role they play in this regulation. For example, the infant in the
first two to three weeks of life can be observed to look at the
human face, become activated and excited, look away, quiet down--
then look back, become activated and excited again, look away, quiet
down. The regulation of excitation through visual input is carried
out by a variety of side glances and peripheral fixations, with visual focus on the adult's ear or chin. Some neonates have difficulty
looking away; others can be "captured" by a stimulus for more than 50
minutes at a stretch, and finally terminate the interaction by breaking into crying (Stechler & Latz, 1966). In other work, we have
found an effect of major differences in caretaker environment on the
development of looking behavior within the first two months of life
when the infant is presented with the stimulus of the human face. As
has been so beautifully demonstrated by Stern (1971), reciprocal gaze
regulation between infant and mother comes to have quite individually
different characteristics by three months of age in different infant
caretaker dyads.

The point that is being made is that from the very outset, the
interface of interpersonal exchange between the infant and caretaker
serves the function of regulation. Moreover, the interactional interface begins on the foundation of an organized behavioral complexity. Here, for example, can be mentioned the demonstration by Freedman (1971) of the preference of the newly-born infant for the normal
face configuration as contrasted with the "scrambled" face. There
are multiple modalities of exchange in this complexity as well as a
high degree of specific fittedness. For example, Freedman (1971) has
also demonstrated that upon the very first picking up of the newly-
born infant to a cradled position in the arms, the baby will turn
its head to the appropriate side, and orient its gaze directly to
the caretaker's face, i.e., this is a specificity of coordination
which does not have to be learned. Furthermore, Moore and Meltzoff
(1975) have presented a beautiful demonstration in the two-week-old
neonate of imitation of adult facial gestures, such as those of mouth
opening and tongue protrusion. This finding, related to simultaneity
of complex behavioral configurations in the partners, is exceedingly
difficult to explain using traditional models.

Condon (1974a) has made a most fundamental contribution to our
subject both in his demonstration of linguistic-kinesic synchrony in
the neonate as early as 12 hours of life, and in the insight of his
philosophy behind the research: namely, that we interact in terms
of already-organized configurations. To quote his expression, "we

participate in shared organization." He has also proposed a hierarchy of rhythmicities which constitute self and interactional synchrony (Condon, 1974), and has proposed its relationship to the organization of communication and language. By this method of frame-by-frame analysis of sound film taken of the awake-active neonate exposed to human speech, the frame-by-frame identification of change points in the infant's movements show them to be **exactly** synchronized with the frame of occurrence of onsets of words and of phonemic boundaries analyzed from the corresponding sound tract.[2] Bower (1972) has provided a different line of evidence for an already organized three-dimensional spatial-perceptual interface between the external object and the visual, postural, and motor organization of the infant.

TEMPORAL ORGANIZATION OF THE INFANT-CAREGIVER INTERFACE--A HIERARCHY OF RHYTHMS.

Our own picture of the infant-caretaker system and the complex interface of exchange between them, which must be "governed," or regulated, has been obtained from a somewhat different perspective, namely, that provided by an investigation of infant states along the sleep-awake continuum, and their relation, around-the-clock, to the occurrence and type of caregiving interventions distributed over the same span of time. One is struck by the range of endogenously generated rhythms which come to light as one becomes familiar with the picture of events occurring over the 24 hours of the day. Each of these domains of rhythmic functions, in some way, will interface with one or more of the caretaker's activities.

For the well-organized normal infant, the 24 hours, first of all, is constructed in terms of a basic circadian rhythmicity. This is illustrated in Figure I in which the duration of total sleep, total REM sleep, and total quiet sleep of a well-organized normal infant on day three of life are plotted in terms of their occurrence during each of the six or more interfeed intervals of the 24-hour day. Within the 24 hours, there is a further organization, the ultradian,[3] of both sleep and awake periods, which governs the duration and distribution of naps. Infants differ from each other in the

---

[2]This pioneering work has been carried further in an anthropological study by Byers in which speech interaction in various primitive cultures is similarly analyzed. Byers marshalls evidence to support the hypothesis that a basic 10 cps rhythm, roughly that of EEG alpha frequency, governs the precise timing in the interaction of the speech trains of the participants (Byers, 1975).

[3]Ultradian refers to periodicities of less than 24 hours but greater than one-half hour, and infradian refers to rhythms of less than one-half hour (Halberg, 1960).

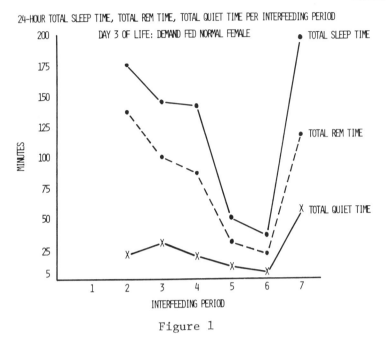

Figure 1

length of naps and of awake periods, the two lengths being significantly correlated within individuals in a sample of infants; those infants with long sleep periods will tend to have long awake periods. Infants also differ from each other in the degree of differentiation of nap lengths into a first and second longest nap per 24 hours (often occurring in sequence, although not always in the same order), and a number of briefer naps (Sander et al., 1975a). The pattern, number, length, and distribution of naps and awake periods is the site for the most obvious adaptive modifications necessary to synchronize infant sleep-wake behavior with environmental periodicities in a 24 hour framework. Temporal coordinations organizing the 24 hours can be thought of as providing a slow or low frequency background of state-change as context for the more rapidly changing events in the foreground of the interaction.

In addition to the 24 hour level there is a basic rhythmicity within the nap produced by REM/NREM cycles of approximately 50-55 minutes in length (Parmelee, 1974). By now these cycles have received a great deal of study, some of the most recent indicating that the length of REM/NREM cycle has a correlation with brain size, a basic time-space link in the biologic world (Zepelin & Rechtschaffen, 1974). The nap is organized in relation to the sequence of REM/NREM cycles within it in the demand-fed infant (in which the infant is not awakened to feed but allowed to awaken on the basis of endogenous influences). Figure II shows the distribution of REM/NREM

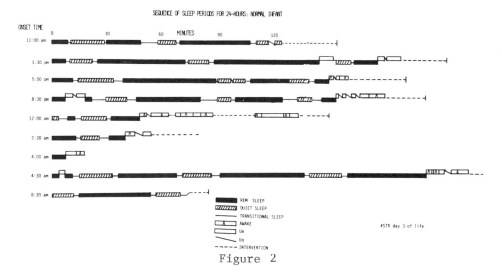

Figure 2

cycles within naps for the same infant which were plotted by interfeed intervals in Figure I.

Within the REM substage, frequency spectrum analysis brings to
light briefer cycles of motility peaks, ranging from 1-6 minutes,
more prominent at some times of day than others. In stable periods
of normal quiet sleep, cycles of fluctuating respiratory amplitude
can be seen approximating 8-10 sec in duration. This compares in
duration with the 9 sec cycle of rise and fall of affective intensity
in the mother-infant interaction which has been encountered by
Brazelton et al., (1975). Sucking bursts have a similar duration,
i.e., of 9-10 sec, with rhythms of sucks within the burst approximating 2 cps. (Wolff, 1968). Sucking behavior has been exhaustively
investigated in relation to individual differences, and as a sensitive
indicator of habituation and dishabituation by which a variety of perceptual discriminations have been discovered to be available to the
neonate (Lipsitt, 1964). Stern (1971) reports regulatory intervals
in gaze regulation between infant and mother as brief as 0.5 sec, and
as we have seen, Condon (1974a) and Byers (1975) have been studying
events in the dyadic exchange in the neighborhood of the 10 cps frequency of EEG alpha rhythm, a rate at which speech and motility have
been found to be synchronized within the speaker, and between the
speaker and the listener (self and interactional synchrony [Condon,
1974]).

The picture of this range of rhythmic events, several of which
may be synchronizing with caregiving activities at the same time but
in a different frequency range, gives a hint as to the multimodal,
complex, and yet highly specific interface between infant and care-

taker in which the regulation of exchange becomes established at the
outset of postnatal life. Each level may involve its own cybernetic
controls, the cycles of longer duration and slower frequency providing a context for a content of events with rhythms at the higher
frequencies. Endogenous generation of these rhythms within the infant, along with the features of phase-shifting, entrainment, etc.
which characterize biorhythmic processes, gives substance to the
concept of an active self-regulating determinant in the organization
of individual behavior. This self-regulation gains systems significance as it relates to synchrony or asynchrony with similar organization in the individual's surround, synchrony then providing the
basic structure for the organization of behavioral events in the
system. Halberg (1960) has pointed out that from the point of view
of biorhythmicity in the biologic system, phase-synchronization,
regulation, adaptation, and integration are all part and parcel of
the same phenomenon. Adaptive behavior is integrative in this sense.
This provides a general basis for viewing developmental process,
as well as life process, from the standpoint of synthesis and integration within a system, rather than from the standpoint of an
ontogeny of conflict and defense within an individual (Sander, 1975b).
In relation to the longitudinal perspective of the developmental
process, Waddington's notions of trajectory and homeorrhesis in
development fit more easily with the former than the latter viewpoint (Waddington, 1969).

TEMPORAL ORGANIZATION IN THE INFANT-CARETAKER SYSTEM: RESEARCH
FINDINGS

    The work which our group has been carrying out over the past
10 years began with a method for monitoring certain activities of
both infant and caretaker 24 hours a day using a bassinet monitor.[4]
This was combined with daily event-recorded feeding observations,
observed sleep and awake onsets, and event-recorded observations of
infant behavior when different face stimuli were presented in a

---

[4]Drs. Sander, Stechler, Julia, and Burns carried out the initial
major study, USPHS HD01766: "Adaptation and Perception in Early Infancy"; Dr. Sander, Dr. Chappell, and Ms. Snyder carried out the subsequent study funded by the Grant Foundation: "An Investigation of
Change in Infant and Caretaking Variables Over The First Two Weeks
of Life." The present collaboration is between Drs. Sander, Gould,
Teager, Lee, and Ms. Snyder in a project directed by Dr. Gould:
"The Study of Monozygous and Dizygous Twins to Ascertain in Risk
Factors of SIDS," USPHS Contract #N01-H3-3-2789. A second collaboration with this team and Dr. Rossett concerns a study of effects of
alcohol intake during pregnancy on neurophysiological competence of
offspring which is being funded by the National Council on Alcohol-
ism.

systematic way. The day-by-day course followed by three different
infant caretaking systems over the first two months of life in
regard to these sets of variables provided the major comparisons in
the analysis of the data. Nursery caretaking, individual around-the-
clock fostering, and natural mother caretaking were the three different dyadic systems with which we began the investigation. From the
data, a picture of postnatal temporal organization in the infant-
caretaker system began to take shape.

Birth can be viewed as a time of rupture in the framework for
temporal organization of a foetal-maternal regulatory system (Sander,
1976). New and prominent rhythms appear in the newborn at birth such
as those related to hunger and satiation, respiration, elimination.
At the same time, key entraining rhythms of the previous maternal
uterine environment are lost (such as basic circadian rhythmicity of
mother's motion and quiet, and of a variety of maternal blood
levels). Furthermore, after birth, the infant begins to be exposed
to striking fluctuations in the environment, such as those of light
and dark, of sound levels, etc. as well as to recurrent encounters
with specific cues such as mother's face or voice. The initial task
of caretaking in the neonate-caretaker system can be formulated as
that of the re-establishing of a new basis for temporal organization
in infant functions. For example, events in the infant, such as its
own sleeping and waking periods, must become phase-synchronized both
with its own new endogenous rhythms related to hunger or elimination,
and with recurrent exogenous events in the new environment such as
day and night, the day subsequently to become divided into sub-
periods of morning, afternoon, and evening.

Some of the findings encountered in the comparison of the three
different infant-caretaking systems can be summarized in relation to
this viewpoint. There are a great many bits and pieces of evidence
which we have put together in picturing the interaction of endogenous
infant and exogenous environmental determinants in the initial adaptation, and the way each contributes to the emergence of a relatively
stable framework of temporal organization characteristic for a particular infant-caretaker system. It is not possible, here, to do
more than list some of the main categories of our findings, with
reference to relevant publications where possible.

1. The first days after birth, regardless of caretaking environment, are characterized by a longer daily duration of awake and
active states than is found again until the end of the first month of
life (Sander et al., 1972). In these first days, there is a relative
disorganization, followed by a reorganization of sleep and awake
periods which includes not only the duration and occurrence of naps
and awake periods within the 24 hour framework, but appears to include
shifts in the finer structure of REM/NREM cycling and its characteristics. Relative disorganization of sleep and awake states is associated with increased crying of the infant, increased intervention

time, and multiple interventions which all diminish again as reorganization emerges. Over the first postnatal week, for the infant
roomed-in with its own mother on a demand feeding regimen, a coordination appears between infant state and caretaker activity such as a
relation of infant state to intervention time, or to mother's position of holding the infant, or to her vocalizing to the infant, etc.
(Sander et al., 1975).

2. There is an effect of caretaking environment on the rate of
emergence and extent of day-night differentiation of sleep and wake-
fulness in the infant over the first months of postnatal life (Sander
et al., 1972). There is a sex difference in this effect. In the
demand-feeding regimen provided by a single caretaker, rooming-in
around-the-clock from the first day, a basic day-night organization
of states appears between the fourth to sixth postnatal day (Sander &
Julia, 1966). Among other things, this involves the settling of more
than half of the longest sleep period (nap) per 24 hours in the night
12 hours. For this particular sample of nine infants, this was accomplished for all the infants by the 10th postnatal day. However,
it was only the natural mother, rooming-in with her baby around-the-
clock, whose records, by the seventh day, showed a beginning ordering
of the entire 24 hour span in regard to time of occurrence of naps
and awake periods (Sander et al., 1970). Within the definition of a
demand-feeding regimen, the natural mother was freer than the foster
mother to "shape" the time of occurrence of naps and awake periods
over the 24 hours. "Shaping," here, can be viewed as an intuitive
process carried out by the mother. It is aimed at phase-shifting of
ultradian rhythms (related to napping and awake spans) so they will
coincide with the most comfortable household schedule, e.g., keeping
the baby awake longer in the evening so it will sleep longer in the
early morning, attempting to feed it more so it will take longer to
become hungry, waking it up if it is napping too late in the afternoon and therefore will not be sleepy in the evening, etc.

3. By the end of the first week of life there is an individual
specificity in the interactions between an infant and the caretaker
who has been providing its sole care from birth. This specificity
can be thought of as a complex gestalt involving timing, sequence,
cue, etc., a complex in which the familiar sequence of caretaking activities over the awake span is carried out.

In a cross-fostering design involving two foster caretakers, evidence was obtained showing that by 10 days, the individually fostered
infant has formed a specific adaptation to the individual who is fostering it, so that a change of foster caretaker is associated with
significant changes in crying and feeding behavior. Further, in regard to specificity, a sample of natural mother-infant dyadic systems
shows greater idiosyncracy of regulatory interactions than does a
sample of infants, selected for normality, who are individually fostered by the same foster mother. Regulation, which is based upon in-

dividual differences characterizing the infant and the caretaker, becomes highly specific for the pair and leads to the unique and idiosyncratic characteristics of exchange in the natural mother system. Evidence of early specificity in perceptual processing was obtained by masking the natural mother's face on the seventh day of life over an entire awake period (the mother having roomed-in with her baby from the first day). A striking surprise reaction on the part of the infant occurs precisely at the time of initiation of feeding, and is followed by effects on infant state and feeding variables. These evidences of individual specificity of adaptations in infant-caretaker exchanges can be considered to illustrate an initial bonding. They point as well to the role of individual specificity in regulatory processes.

    4. Finally, there was a set of findings related to the course followed by infants over the first two months of life for whom specifically synchronized temporal organization was not established within the system within the first 10 days of life. These were infants who remained in the stressful, four-hourly scheduled, noncontingent, neonatal nursery caretaking with multiple caretakers for 10 days before beginning individual around-the-clock fostering. Effects were demonstrable in 1) the subsequent characteristics of sleep and awake state distributions in these infants; 2) their more frequent reaction to the visual stimulus, human face, by fussing and crying; 3) the course over the two months of the study of their looking behavior to visual stimuli; and 4) the greater week-to-week instability of the rank-order of infants within the sample in regard to a variety of variables (i.e., an instability of individual differences).

AN ILLUSTRATIVE MODEL FOR REGULATION OF EXCHANGE IN THE INFANT-CARE-TAKER SYSTEM

    An illustrative model can be drawn of the way the infant-caretaker exchange is regulated when the system reaches a level of relative adaptation, let us say, by the end of the third postnatal week. In the usual instance, by this time there is a basic structure to the 24 hour day, with a longest awake period occurring late in the day or early evening, and a number of earlier briefer awakenings; the majority of a longest sleep is occurring in the night 12 hours, with briefer naps during the day and perhaps some predictability as to their duration and occurrence in morning and afternoon. There is a broad background of temporal organization in the system which is becoming shared between caretaker and infant; the organization of caretaker expectancy is beginning to match the periodicity of recurrent states of the infant. Taking the complete awake period as the basic unit of observation, a characteristic course or sequence of events begins to jell, as illustrated in Figure III. By the third postnatal week in the adapted system, there is an order and sequence to the course of events. The time course of the awakening can be segmented into subunits of regulatory interactions, each with its own

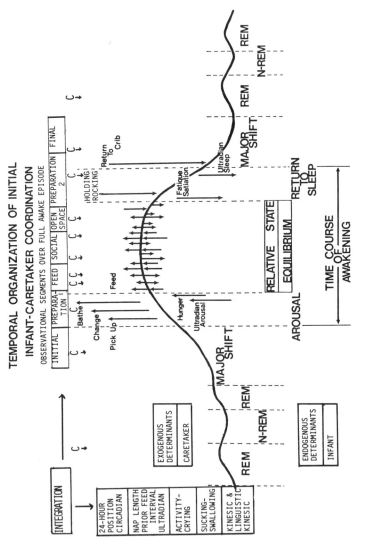

Figure 3

aims or goals and specific exchange patterns. In the diagram seven such segments are labelled: initial, preparation #1, feeding, social, open, preparation #2, final. Dyads can be compared in regard to these segments, their boundaries, content, duration, variability from observation to observation and from day to day.

The model proposed in Figure III illustrates several considerations regarding the structure of infant-environment exchanges which are given new perspective if approached in terms of regulation from a systems viewpoint: 1) the nature of adaptation or fitting together between infant and caretaker; 2) the role of integrative mechanisms; 3) the conditions for differentiation. These will be taken up briefly in this order.

1) The nature of the fitting together of infant and caretaker is illustrated in Figure III by the mutual interaction of endogenous (infant determined) and exogenous (caretaker determined) influences to achieve a relatively stable sequence, timing, and duration of exchanges. A capacity for mutual adjustment harmonizes the expectancies and interventions of the caretaker with the periodicities of infant states (also modifiable through mechanisms of phase-shifting and entrainment) to construct a time course whose determinants are shared between infant and caretaker. This provides a shared background of relatively slowly changing events related to state as a context for the foreground, or content, of their more rapidly changing direct interactions on the sensory-motor level. Ashby's (1952) model of the "ultrastable" system provides the basis for conceptualizing regulation in the adaptive system as a combination of these two levels of feedback relating biorhythms and cybernetic mechanisms (for discussion, see Sander et al., 1975).

A first criterion for match or mismatch in the regulatory exchanges is constituted by the direction and timing of infant state change. This is the infant's first level of initiative in the system and requires the caretaker to read "direction" of change. This can be viewed as an initial inference as to the infant's aim or intention, e.g., "I think the baby wants to go to sleep now." In Figure III, correspondence in "direction" or lack of it, is represented by the correspondence of direction of the arrows on the infant's and on the caretaker's side of the time line. The interaction, then, is itself a first order determinant of events over the awake period-- a sequence which constitutes a first syntax for the dyadic conversation. Chappell has developed a method of scoring appropriateness of caretaking interventions in terms of the time course of state change over the awakening (Chappell & Sander, 1976).

2) The role of integrative mechanisms. Integration and integrative functions can be seen to be built into biologic systems at many levels: in the design and construction of the nervous system itself (Sherrington, 1906; Lettvin et al., 1959); in the nature of bio-

rhythmicity and the features of phase-control and phase-synchrony
which are basic to functional coherence in the temporal organization
of the body's multiple physiological subsystems; in the evolved
fittedness between components making up the biological system which
sets the stage for them to be bonded in interactive regulation; in
the continuum of "state," which is itself a synthesis of different
physiologic components; in behaviors which themselves represent an
integration, harmonizing the polarity of complexity and unity. I am
referring here to attention, and the deployment of and focus of
attention. Adapted behavior, as represented in the concept of the
schema, represents integration as well, in which the final common
path of a goal-directed act implies the assimilation of a highly
complex context. Sign behavior and symbolic representation obviously belong among these integrative elements.

    In Figure III, integration is depicted on both the horizontal
and vertical axes. The horizontal axis concerns the integration of
the sequence of events up to any point in the awakening; the vertical
axis represents the integration of the array of rhythms, which also
must bear on the exchange at any point. At each point over the sequence of the awake period, the mother will be organizing her deci-
sion-making process and her actions in an integration of: 1) where
she is within the 24-hour framework of the day/night cycle; 2) how
long a nap the baby has had prior to its awakening; 3) where in the
familiar time course of this particular awakening she now is with the
baby; and 4) the "effectiveness" (fittedness) of her actions up to
this point (reciprocal or contingent sequences), and of her moment
to moment behaviors in the "present" moment; 5) what the remaining
sequence of events in the awake period is likely to consist of; and
6) how she would like the remainder of the awake period to go. At
each point in the figure, the infant, by the mechanism of state regulation, is also integrating or attempting to integrate the sequence
and the different time levels in the array of his endogenous rhythmicities which enter into the behavioral encounter with the caretaker.

    The "meaning" of the infant's behavior for the mother is the in-
tegration of the context-content relationship, i.e., "meaning" in
communication represents integration also. For example, it can be
readily seen that the meaning of the baby's cry for the caretaker
(in the adapted system) will in part be determined by where in the
order of events in Figure III (i.e., where in the context), the cry
event is occurring. Crying behavior at each of the sequence of
points illustrated by the letter "C" will have different implications
for its cause, aims, and appropriate intervention. As the initial
coordination or adaptation is being effected over the first 2-3 weeks
of life, there is opportunity for negotiation at each point in regard
to whose behavior initiates, and whose behavior is contingent. Since
contingent effects will depend on who initiates, it is clear that
"control" in the "conversation" is at issue from the very beginning.

With the perspective of regulation of the system at the interface between endogenously self-regulating partners, initiating and
responding become fused. This introduces integration as a feature of
regulatory mechanisms, one which sets the stage for the organization
of the system on the basis of psychic functions. In the "normal"
situation, with a healthy well-organized neonate and a sensitive and
able mother, phase synchronized in relation to the low frequency
background state context, there is a fine grained exchange or flow of
"control" in the foreground in which both participate reciprocally in
maintaining the stability of the interface. The intuitive mother's
actions, altering the flow, over time, in cybernetic regulations, can
be thought of as her "perceptions" of events in the relational system
--in respect of which the infant's actions represent both initiation
and response. Here, the openness to assimilation of complexity
(which can be thought of as accompanying simultaneity in the background context of state) sets the stage for the expression of systems unity in the aim of the volitional or intentional (accommoda-
tive) act. Perhaps the most specific behavior which represents this
unity of integrative process is that of attending (focusing attention) which, in the model being proposed, will also imply participation or reciprocal exchange, combining elements of both initiating
and responding. The reading by one participant of the direction of
the focus of attention of the other is one of the most elemental and
basic of perceptions which is made in the system by either mother or
infant, and which clearly soon enters powerfully into the list of behaviors which are regulated. On the basis of the reading of attentive focus, the aim of intention later will be inferred. Regulation
in the system at this elemental level thus becomes based on behavior
which is itself an integration, and as coordination on this level
between partners becomes established, it provides a next order of
complexity on which new exchanges can appear in the system.

3) The systems perspective of regulation sheds light on a third
set of considerations, namely those features which provide the conditions for differentiation. The concept of phase-synchrony, emerging
from biorhythm research, gives empirical substance to the notion of
equilibrium in the regulative system. In Figure III, the synchrony of
caretaker expectancy and infant state course over the awake span is
indicated as a relative equilibrium. At least by three weeks of life,
this makes possible a span of time in the sequence in which the caretaker and infant can experience a relative disengagement--the segment
designated as the "open space." The mother places the infant in the
reclining baby seat to "entertain" him/herself where mother can be
seen while she goes about her other duties.

Here, infant behavior is optimally disengaged from both endogenous and exogenous control for the exercise of an individually idiosyncratic and selective, volitional initiative. This is an equilibrium in which neither endogenous infant determinants preempt infant
behavior to return variables to their "regions of stability" (Ashby,

1952), nor does caretaker initiative capture infant response contingencies. The infant's own active selective exploration of himself, and the low intensity stimuli or discrepancies in the surround, provide differentiating self-regulatory feedbacks most specifically related to the goals of his action. In line with the re-afference theory of Von Holst (1950), initiation plays the central role in the regulation of behavior, providing the neurophysiological conditions which allow the unscrambling of "re-afference" from "ex-afference" by the persistent template of "efference copie" remaining from the initiation. This is a hypothesis which proposes a central mechanism which differentiates what happens to the organism from what he makes happen--an essential differentiation for control at the simplest level of motor behavior, e.g., the swimming of a fish in a current of water. As soon as goal direction enters the picture, the infant's initiation of voluntary action begins to determine the feedback control which is often referred to as the infant's active organization of his world, extending self-regulation through an increasing repertoire of behavioral (sensory-motor) schemata (Piaget, 1936). Mutual regulation of initiation constitutes the frontier of interpersonal encounter--in reciprocal exchange the initiative is traded back and forth. In the "open space" segment of the adapted system, the conditions are optimal for the infant to differentiate effects contingent to his/her own initiation. The experience of contingent effects has a profound impact on the alerting and focusing of infant attention. The conditions for the differentiation of self and other can be seen to reside in the condition of equilibrium in the system, and the relative disengagement of (or disjoin) of a self-regulatory core from preemption by either endogenous or exogenous determinants. At such equilibrium the richness of selectivity or option for the infant to initiate new activity or idiosyncratic goal organization would be maximal. This resembles Winnicott's conceptualization of the "intermediate area" quite precisely (Winnicott, 1958).

Discussion

Thus far, a viewpoint has been presented of the regulation of exchanges between neonate and caretaker based on empirical details which are becoming available of the characteristics of the interactional interface between them. Obviously, the picture is as yet quite incomplete but perhaps sufficient nevertheless to suggest connections to the ontogeny of "structures" underlying the organization of communicative processes and perhaps even of psychic organization.

Bassinet monitoring of infant state on the sleep-awake continuum has been drawn upon to illustrate steps in the organization of exchanges in the infant-caretaker system in a 24 hour a day framework. An illustrative model was suggested combining cybernetic and biorhythmic mechanisms of regulation by which stable interactional coordinations can be maintained as the adapted state is achieved in

the system. The model represents as well a prospective "open systems" view of developmental process which, from the biologic perspective, implies an acknowledgment of the essential integrative or
synthesizing nature of life process and of the various functions
sustaining the organization of the system. The interactions among
the various regulatory mechanisms which become established as stable
regulation becomes maintained in the infant-caretaker system, can be
thought of as constituting precommunicative structures. Some of
these have been illustrated already: 1) that a basis for intersub-
jectivity is provided by the temporal organization which is shared
in the adapted system by the interacting partners; 2) that a basis
for meaning exists in the background-foreground or context-content
relationship. Context is provided for the more direct exchanges between infant and caretaker by the lower frequency, more slowly
changing rhythms; 3) that a basis for inferring direction or aim
exists in the system in terms of the time course of infant state
change; 4) that inference as to intentionality, a basic requirement
for later communicative competence begins in the reading and control
of attentive focus in the context of the adapted system and the elab-
orations discussed in relation to 1), 2), and 3).

Can the natural longitudinal ontogeny through which the interactive regulative system, as we have modelled it, progresses over
the first three years of life suggest further conceptual links to the
ontogeny of psychic structure? This is a huge domain which, in no
sense, can be adequately dealt with within the scope of this paper.
It will be possible only to point to a few features of the model and
suggest that the ontogeny of self-regulation provides an entree to
the ontogeny of psychic structure. It suggests a continuum of regulatory function from a biological level of self-regulation to a psychological level of "the self" as an organizing self-regulating
structure within the personality (See Spitz, 1957).

From the level of the cell upward, self-regulation is a basic
property of living matter as is primary endogenous activity. In the
presence of the latter, the former provides the essential coherence
or unity of the organism for continued existence in its environment
of evolutionary adaptation. Self-regulatory mechanisms are organized,
therefore, in relation both to endogenous activity and to the surrounding life support system, whatever its level of relative complexity. In an effort to define and trace an ontogeny of self-regulation
in the human infant, we have focused especially on the sequence of
levels at which the infant can introduce new activities into the
interactional system, proposing that each new level perturbs the
regulatory system and demands a corresponding new adaptation or coordination between the infant and the caretaking environment in relation to the new level of activity (Sander, 1962). The process begins
at the outset of postnatal life with the level of activities serving
basic regulation, e.g., the time course of infant state change over
an awakening. The initiation of behavior, occurring always in the

presence of sensory input, gains a unique specificity relevant to
idiosyncracies of the individual as soon as goal direction begins to
guide action. The gradually advancing sophistication and intentionality of individually initiated goal-directed behavior in early development can be proposed to bear a direct relation to the ontogeny
of self-regulation. Effects, which are contingent to infant initiated action, play a central role in organizing the focus of infant
attention and in determining goal directedness. In an ontogeny of
self-regulation there must be a special place for the organization
of attention and awareness related to evaluation of the outcome of
self-initiated goal-oriented behavior. A sequence of adaptive
issues based on new activities, which the infant can initiate in the
system, provides an empirical framework within which an ontogeny of
self-awareness might be tentatively formulated.

Mutual coordination of attentive focus characterizes the adapted
system, and is evident in coordinated reciprocal games, gaze regulation, and smiling interaction. Such coordination provides the empirical base from which regulation can begin on the level of inference as to the inner organization of the partners. This would constitute an initial step in the building of "a semantic congruence
between the contents of two minds" (Marshall, 1971). Such inference
leads, then, to the emergence in the system of regulation on the
basis of inferences as to intention. Inference regarding the intentions of the partner plays a prominent role in the negotiation of
adaptive issues arising between infant and caretaker, especially
issues III, IV, and V which we have previously formulated (months
6-20 [Sander, 1962]). When the conditions are present for the carrying out of intentional goal-directed action involving internal representation (as achieved with the onset of object permanence in
Piaget's sense), a role for "inner awareness" in regulation related
to the outcome of the volitional action and its match or mismatch
with one's own intention can be proposed. An ontogeny of awareness
and an organization of self-awareness in relation to the generation
of schema underlying interpersonal regulations has been proposed by
Spitz (1957). In the sequence which Spitz describes, very much based
on regulation within the infant-caretaker system, in terms of the
severe restrictions to volition which peak around 15 months, especially in relation to socialization of body function, the stage is
set for the consolidation of the self, as a self-regulatory structure, in terms of an operational or adaptive organization of self-
awareness.

Of critical importance from the regulatory systems point of view
at this time is the validation, or invalidation by the caregiving
partner of the toddler's inner perceptions of his own initiations,
and intentions, his own motivational states, goal-realizations, etc.
As regulation at this level of inference becomes coordinated and
stabilized, the system achieves a new richness of equilibria and begins to support stabilities in interactive regulation which now per-

mit the consolidation of "partially-independent" internal self-regu-latory structures in personality organization related to the "self." Elsewhere, we have pointed out (Sander, 1975) that the role of in-tentional and directed aggression provides the basis for a process akin to "reversal" in the second 18 months of life by which the dis-embedding (or conservation) of "self-as-active-initiator" proceeds within the personality organization (Sander, 1975).

Obviously, if development over the life span can be viewed in terms of a regulatory systems model such as we have sketched, the experience at maturity represented by the expression "I am" must be viewed as culminating an evolutionary pyramid of integrative designs and functions which culminates as well the ontogeny of both "self" and the organization of self-awareness. A context of communicative structures is needed for the ontogenesis of such an expression, one which can be provided only by interpersonal exchanges at an appro-priate level of self-differentiation and organization. When the system provides exchanges which predictably validate or confirm such experience, a new basis is provided for further differentiation of aspects of psychic structure, especially those culminating the on-togeny of self-regulation.

REFERENCES

Ashby, R. Design for a brain. London: Chapman & Hall, 1952.

Bower, T. G. R. Object perception in infants. Perception, 1972, 1:15-30.

Brazelton, T. B., Tronick, E., Adamson, L., Als, H., & Wise, S. Early mother-infant relationship. In R. Porter & M. O'Connor (Eds.), The parent-infant relationship. CIBA Foundation Symposium #33 The Associated Scientific Publishers, Amsterdam, 1975.

Brenner, C. An elementary textbook of psychoanalysis. New York: International Universities Press, 1955.

Byers, P. Rhythms, information processing and human relations: Towards a typology of communication. In D. Klopper & P. Bateson (Eds.), Perspectives in ethology (Vol. 2). New York: Plenum Press, 1975.

Chappell, P. & Sander, L. The changing organization of caretaker-infant interaction during the first week of life. In M. Bullowa (Ed.), Before speech--the beginnings of human communication. Boston: Cambridge University Press, in press.

Condon, W. S. Communication and order: The microrhythm hierarchy of speaker behavior--play therapy in theory and practice. Presented at School Psychologists Convention. New York: March 15, 1973.

Condon, W. S. & Sander, L. W. Neonate movement is synchronized with adult speech: Interactional participation and language acquisition. Science, 1974, Vol. 183, 99-101.

Freedman, D. Behavioral assessment in infancy. In G. B. A. Stollinger & L. Bosch, Jr. (Eds.), Normal and abnormal development of brain and behavior. Leyden University Press, Boerhaave Series, 1971.

Freud, S. Project for a scientific psychology. In M. Bonaparti, A. Freud, & G. A. Kris (Eds.), The origins of psychoanalysis: Letters to Wilheim Fleiss 1887-1902. New York: Basic Books, 1954.

Guerrero, R. Association of the type and time of insemination with the menstrual cycle with the human sex ratio at birth. New England Journal of Medicine, 1974, 29:1056-1059.

Halberg, F. Temporal coordinations of physiologic functions. Symposia on Quantitative Biology, 1960, 25:289-310.

Klaus, M. H., Jerauld, R., & Kreger, N. C. Maternal attachment, importance of the first postpartum days. New England Journal of Medicine, 1972, 286:460-463.

Lettvin, J. Y., Maturance, H. R., McCulloch, W. S., & Pitts, W. H. What the frog's eye tells the frog's brain. Proceedings of Institute of Radio Engineers, 1959, Vol. 47, #11, pp.1940-1951.

Lipsitt, L. P. & Kaye, H. Conditioned sucking in the human newborn. Psychonomic Science, 1964, 1, 29-30.

Marshall, J. C. Can humans talk? In J. Morton (Ed.), Biological and sociological factors in psycholinguistics. London: Roger Press, 1971.

Moore, M. K. & Meltzoff, A. N. Neonate imitation: A test of existence and mechanism. Presented at Society for Research and Child Development Biennial Meeting, Denver, Colorado, April, 1975.

Parmelee, A. H. Ontogeny of sleep patterns and associated periodicities in infants. In F. Falkner, N. Kretchmer & E. Rossi (Eds.), Modern problems in paediatrics (Vol. 13). Basel: S. Karger, 1974.

Piaget, J. The origins of intelligence in children. (Trans. Margaret Cook). New York: International Universities Press, 1952. (Originally published, 1936.)

Sander, L. Issues in early mother-child interaction. Journal of the American Academy of Child Psychiatry, 1962, Vol. 1, #1, 141-166.

Sander, L., Chappell, P., & Snyder, P. An investigation of change in the infant-caretaker system over the first week of life. Presented at Society for Research and Child Development Biennial Meeting, Denver, Colorado: April, 1975.

Sander, L. W., Julia, H., Stechler, G., Burns, P., & Gould, J. Some determinants of temporal organization in the ecological niche of the newborn. Presented at the Biennial Conference of the International Society for the Study of Behavioral Development. Guilford, England: University of Surrey, July, 1975. (a)

Sander, L. W. Infant and caretaking environment: Investigation and conceptualization of adaptive behavior in a system of increasing complexity. In E. J. Anthony (Ed.), Explorations in child psychiatry. New York: Plenum Press, 1975. (b)

Sander, L. W. Primary prevention and some aspects of temporal organization in early infant-caretaker interaction. In E. Rexford, L. Sander, & T. Shapiro (Eds.), Infant psychiatry: A new synthesis. New Haven: Yale University Press, 1976.

Sander, L. W. & Julia, H. Continuous interactional monitoring in the neonate. Psychosomatic Medicine, 1966, 28:822-835.

Sander, L. W., Stechler, G., Burns, P., & Julia, H. Early mother-infant interaction and 24° patterns of activity and sleep. Journal of the American Academy of Child Psychiatry, 1970, Vol. 9, 1, 103-123.

Sander, L. W., Julia, H., Stechler, G., & Burns, P. Continuous 24 hour interactional monitoring in infants reared in two caretaking environments. Psychosomatic Medicine, 1972, 34, 270-282.

Sherrington, C. S. The integrative action of the nervous system. New Haven: Yale University Press, 1906.

Spitz, R. A. No and Yes--on the beginnings of human communication. New York: International Universities Press, 1957.

Stechler, G. & Latz, E. Some observations on attention and arousal in the human infant. Journal of the American Academy of Child Psychiatry, 1966, 5, 517-525.

Stechler, G. Infant looking and fussing in response to visual stimulation over the first two months of life in different infant-caretaking systems. Presented at Society for Research and Child Development Biennial Meeting, Philadelphia, Pa., April, 1973.

Stern, D. N. A micro-analysis of mother-infant interaction behavior
    regulating social contact between a mother and her 3 1/2 month old
    twins. Journal of the American Academy of Child Psychiatry, 1971,
    Vol. 10, #3, 501-517.

Von Holst, E. & Mittelstaedt, H. "Das Reafferenz Prinzip," de
    Naturwissenschaften, 1950, Vol. 37, 464-476.

Waddington, C. H. The theory of evolution today. In A. Koestler &
    J. R. Smythies (Eds.), The Alpbach Symposium 1968, Beyond Reduc-
    tionism. Boston: Beacon Press, 1968.

Winnicott, D. Transitional objects and transitional phenomena.
    Collected papers through pediatrics to psychoanalysis. New York:
    Basic Books, 1958.

Wolff, P. H. The causes, controls, and organization of behavior in
    the neonate. Psychological Issues, 1966, Vol. 5 #1, Monograph
    #17. New York: International Universities Press.

Zepelin, H. & Rechtschaffen, A. Mammalian sleep, longevity and
    energy metabolism. Brain, Behavior and Evolution, 1974, Vol. 10,
    425-470.

ENGAGEMENT-DISENGAGEMENT AND EARLY OBJECT EXPERIENCES[1]

Beatrice Beebe and Daniel N. Stern

Department of Psychiatry

Cornell University Medical Center-New York Hospital

New York, New York 10021

INTRODUCTION

The last decade's research has revolutionized our view of the capacities of the human infant in the early months, forcing a recognition of his considerable receptivity to environmental stimulation and his own capacity to seek stimulation and initiate social interactions. Particularly significant has been an appreciation of the central role of the infant's capacity for vis-a-vis orientation and sustained visual regard, which are considered to be among the most fundamental paradigms of communication, and central to the developing attachment between mother and infant (Walters & Parke, 1965; Robson, 1967).

Less, however, is known about the infant's capacity to modulate or regulate his social stimulation, particularly in situations of overstimulation. The management of incoming stimulation within a

---

[1] This work was supported by The Grant Foundation, the New York State Department of Mental Hygiene, the Jane Hilder Harris Foundation, and an NIMH Postdoctoral Research Fellowship.

The assistance of Stephen Bennett, M.D., Fred Pine, Ph.D., Joseph Jaffe, M.D., Samuel W. Anderson, Ph.D., Donald Hutchings, Ph.D. and Robert Prince, Ph.D. is gratefully acknowledged.

comfortable range has been seen as a central adaptive task of infancy
since Freud's Project for a Scientific Psychology (1897). He formulated the notion of a stimulus barrier which protected the neonate
from uncomfortable levels of stimulation by shutting off the perceptual function. With increasing appreciation of the infant's capacity
for an active role, more recent formulations have stressed the infant's own active contribution to the task of regulating the intake
of environmental stimulation (Spitz, 1965; Benjamin, 1965; Brody &
Axelrad, 1970). It is important to note that internal arousal is
so closely tied to external stimulation for the infant that behavioral
modes of modulating the latter always have implications for the former. That is, the infant's regulation of his environmental stimulation will also regulate his arousal. (The notion of internal arousal
or activation level is becoming more problematical, but some similar
notion is required.)

     If the infant's behavior in a social interaction is under con-
sideration, then the external stimuli are no more or less than another's behavior, and the infant thus becomes a partial creator and
modulator of his own interpersonal "object experiences." In this
paper, a spectrum of interpersonal object experiences along the dimension of engagement-disengagement will be examined. By "object
experiences," we mean the infant sensorimotor experience of modulating or regulating his own behavior in relation to the behavior of an
interpersonal object. The proposition will be made that the behaviors which constitute the gradations of this engagement-disengagement
spectrum are the actual experiential events from which inferences are
made about early coping and defensive operations, as well as about
the process of separation-individuation. Lastly, it will be proposed
that the behaviors constituting the gradations of the engagement-
disengagement spectrum, that is, this series of object experiences,
are the early building blocks for later internal representations.

METHOD

A. GENERAL ISSUES OF LEVELS OF ANALYSIS

     One source of difficulty in studying infancy is that the organi-
zation of the organism and nature of its transactions with the environment seem quite foreign in comparison with the adult, or even
the young child, where the child's capacity for locomotion, manipulation of objects, and primitive symbolic functioning offer a basis
from which to infer motivation and intrapsychic structure. We lack
appropriate analogous behavioral units in infancy.

     With this consideration in mind, we have used the method of
frame-by-frame film analysis in the hope that it may provide a route
to psychic functioning in infancy analogous to play, free association,
or the dream in the older child or adult. This method has the following advantages: (a) behavioral units appropriate to the capacity of

the infant organism, with demonstrable functional significance in
the interaction, can be identified; (b) the "stream" of events constituting the interaction can be followed moment-by-moment, in its
natural sequence; (c) the film can be viewed and re-viewed sufficiently slowly to identify the fleeting, "micromomentary" (Haggard
& Isaacs, 1966) events which have impressed us as having fundamental
significance in the interaction; (d) the analysis of events can be
sufficiently detailed to capture the subtlety and complexity of these
fleeting phenomena.

B.   ISSUES IN ASSESSING ENGAGEMENT-DISENGAGEMENT

     The central finding was that the three to four month infant has
a remarkable repertoire of maneuvers with which to modulate his object experiences. An effort has been made to categorize this repertoire so as to further differentiate qualities or modes of relatedness
to the interpersonal object in the free play situation at three to
four months. Any effort at categorization, however, confronts problems of nomenclature and operationalization. We propose to describe
this repertoire in terms of an engagement-disengagement spectrum
(Table 1). Although based on behavioral observations, the description of the spectrum and the ordering of its gradations is a heuristic
model.

     Whether engagement-disengagement is the best term for this ob-
vious and crucial dimension of human experience, remains an open
question. This term has been chosen due to its relative neutrality.
Although gradations in the spectrum will be made, it is important to
emphasize that this is not strictly a unidimensional, linear scale.
The gradations do not imply "magnitudes," but rather complex qualities or modes of object-relatedness. Each gradation in the spectrum
in itself encompasses a subtle range of object experiences (Table 2).
Nevertheless, some "directional" implication in this spectrum is retained, in the sense that it is anchored at one end by an intense,
affectively positive focal engagement (Figure 1),[2] and at the other
end by a complete cessation of the play encounter and a termination
of relatedness.

     To define and operationalize gradations of the engagement range,
it is necessary to take into account the simultaneous operation of
a number of different behavioral events. In real life, the process
of engagement, its quantity and quality, is a composite of a number of

---

[2]Figures 1, 2, and 3 are photo examples of film, with split-screen
from two cameras, one on infant and one on mother (or experimenter),
who are seated opposite each other in a vis-a-vis position. The
numbers at the top of the photos refer to frames occurring 24 per
second.

Table 1

Gradations of the Engagement-Disengagement Spectrum	Visual Attention			Orientation					Reactivity to Mother			Direction of Movement			Facial Expressions		
	Foveal Image	Peripheral	None	Center vis-a-vis	$5° - 30°$ para-central zone	$30° - 60°$ near peripheral zone	$60° - 90°$ far peripheral zone	$>90°$ out of vision	micro-momentary	Inhibited	Unrelated	Approach	Withdraw	None	Positive	Negative	Neutral
Facing & Looking	X			X					X			X			X	X	X
Side Looking	X				X				X			X	X		X	X	X
Visual Checking	X↕	X↕		X↕	X↕	X↕	X↕		X			X	X		X	X	X
Dodging		X		X	X	X	X		X				X			X	X
Inhibition of Responsivity		X	X	X	X	X	X			X				X			X
Fuss/cry											X	X	X			X	
Turn to Environment			X					X			X		X		X	X	X

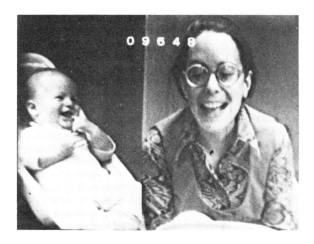

Figure 1. This is a photo example of film, with split-screen from
two cameras, one on infant and one on experimenter, who are seated
opposite each other in a vis-a-vis position.

criteria of relatedness. Accordingly, the range or spectrum of
gradations of engagement-disengagement takes into account the following criteria: (1) whether and how the mother is perceived visually; (2) the orientation and changes of orientation of the infant
relative to the mother; (3) whether the mother is reacted to; (4)
the direction of the infant's movement relative to the mother; and
(5) the nature of the infant's facial expressiveness or affect
generated.

C. CRITERIA OF THE SPECTRUM OF ENGAGEMENT-DISENGAGEMENT

1. Types of Visual Perception

        The four-month infant has two primary modes of visual
perception: (a) foveal, and (b) peripheral.

        (a) When the infant is looking directly at a "target
object," in this case the mother's face, the image is processed in
the foveal area of the retina. It is here that form or pattern recognition of the image occurs. With the use of foveal vision by four
months, the infant can distinguish different faces and can make primitive distinctions in the configurations or facial expressions of the
same face (Brown, 1975).

        (b) Peripheral vision processes the movement of ob-
jects falling on the retina outside the foveal area. In so doing,
it tracks the direction and speed of any moving object, and accordingly monitors the presence and movements of objects at which the

Table 2

Finer Gradations of The Engagement-Disengagement Spectrum

1. Facing and Looking

    a. sustained positive
    b. fluctuations positive,
       negative, neutral
    c. sustained mild negative
    d. intent watching

2. Side Looking

    a. positive
    b. negative
    c. neutral

3. Visual Checking

    a. horizontal (one-sided)
    b. side to side (checking
       on the run)

4. Dodging (not looking)

    a. head through center with-
       out look
    b. head away $5^{\circ} - 30^{\circ}$
    c. head away $30^{\circ} - 60^{\circ} +$
       body back/away
    d. refusing a reorientation
       by mother
    e. active pulling away
    f. head away $60^{\circ} - 90^{\circ}$

5. Inhibition of Responsivity

    a. stare-glaze
    b. limp head-hang at center
    c. limp head-hang at side
    d. head held 90°

6. Fuss/cry

7. Turn to Environment (Escape)

infant is not directly looking. By four months, this "peripheral visual monitoring" is estimated to be effective in the full 180° of the horizontal visual field (Tronik, 1975). The importance of the foveal mode in establishing primary attachment to the mother is well established (Rheingold, 1961; Walters & Parke, 1965; Bowlby, 1969; Stern, 1974). Much less emphasis has been placed on the significance of peripheral visual monitoring for understanding the range and nature of interactions that transpire outside of focal, foveal engagement.

    2.   Head Orientation in the Horizontal Plane

       The infant can navigate changes in head orientation of a full 180° by four months. Five distinctions can be made: direct "center vis-a-vis" opposite the mother; a "para-central zone" encompassing up to 30° on either side of the center, in which the infant can still look or make side glances; a "near peripheral zone" of 30 to 60 degrees; a "far peripheral zone" of 60 to 90 degrees; and a zone past 90° where peripheral processing is no longer possible (turn to environment). Although the horizontal plane has been

stressed, it is more accurate to think of movements in all three
spatial dimensions, such that movements in the horizontal plane
often involve movements in the vertical plane as well.

3.   Reactivity to the Mother

Reactivity to another human being is a crucial but broad
concept. For the purposes of this paper and the level of analysis
its methodology allows, a small but crucial sector of the entire
area of "reactivity" will be defined. This reactivity occurs at
the "micro" or split-second level, and has been termed "micromomentary" (Haggard & Isaacs, 1966). Both mother and infant live in a
"split-second world." From previous work, it is known that maternal
and infant acts, such as changes in facial expression, head movements,
discrete hand movements, etc., last the range of half a second (Beebe,
1973; Stern, 1975). From the case illustration to be described below,
the average duration of such maternal and infant behaviors were half a
second and one-third of a second, respectively.

Documenting reactivity requires defining the stimulus,
the response, and their relationship. The issue of deciding what
constitutes a stimulus, as against a response on either partner's
part, is particularly complicated. Some of the mother-infant or infant-mother sequences occur almost synchronously, others overlap (in
that one starts before the preceding behavior of the partner is completed), and in other cases, there is a short lapse between the end
of one partner's behavior and the onset of the other's "response."
Given this situation, the presence of "reactivity" rests on the demonstration of contingent or functional relations with specific temporal
criteria. The mean reaction times (from onset of one member's behavior to onset of partner's behavior) for contingent sets of maternal-infant and infant-maternal sequences were on the order of a third
of a second (.38 and .31 respectively). On the basis of the contingent analysis described below, and ongoing work in this laboratory,
we assume, for the purpose of this chapter, the existence of mutual
micromomentary reactivity between mother and infant. We do not mean
to imply that they are always reacting to each other in this fashion,
but rather that they are capable of it for stretches of time. Thus,
both can be remarkably sensitive to, and capable of rapidly readjust-
ing to the other's behavioral adjustments.

Three separate categories or forms of reactivity are differentiated:

(a) Split-second responsivity can occur for the infant during foveal or peripheral visual processing, and is termed
"micromomentary responsivity" (Haggard and Isaacs, 1966). These reciprocal responses between mother and infant occur so quickly that
one can usually not grasp them with the naked eye. Thus, many behaviors detected with the method of frame-by-frame analysis go

unnoticed in normal observation procedures. Their rapidity suggests that, at least for the mother, these events occur partially out of awareness or conscious control.

(b)   Another form of reactivity has been termed "inhibition of (micromomentary) responsivity." The term inhibition is used to describe the sudden cessation of reactivity, when the infant suddenly becomes motionless, either limp or with a frozen rigidity, particularly during a period of strenuous maternal stimulation (Figure 2). It is a sudden breaking of a previous micromomentary responsivity.

(c)   A third category has been termed (micromomentarily) "unrelated." In this case, functional analysis fails to show contingency within a time criterion of two seconds from the onset of the stimulus behavior.

(4)   Direction of Movement

Direction can be roughly categorized as approach, withdrawal, or neither. These directions apply to larger head and body movements in all three axes (vertical, horizontal, and saggital). A withdrawal, for example, may be an integrated head movement to the side and down, which can occur in any of the sectors of horizontal head orientation described previously. An approach may encompass not only a horizontal movement toward the mother, but also an up and forward movement in the vertical and saggital axes (Beebe, 1973).

(5)   Nature of Facial Expressiveness

Many fine nuances of subtle expressiveness exist from birth (Charlesworth, 1973; Beebe & Bennett, 1975). Nevertheless, we roughly categorize expressions as: positive (mouth openings and widenings, which, if foveal visual regard is sustained, can crescendo into full "gape smiles" (see Beebe, 1973); neutral, and negative (lipins, grimaces, frowns).

D.   GRADATIONS OF THE ENGAGEMENT-DISENGAGEMENT SPECTRUM

An overview of the criteria scored, which comprise the engagement-disengagement spectrum, are shown in Table 1. These criteria have been utilized to make rough gradations in the spectrum. Each of these rougher gradations has been given a common descriptive name that corresponds to normally observable interactive events. These are: "facing and looking," "side looking," "visual checking," "dodging," "inhibition of responsivity," "fuss/cry," and "turn to environment." The rough gradations of the engagement spectrum indicate the changing nature of the infant's behavior relative to the criteria defined above. It also shows what compromises the infant makes with respect to information intake, or what aspects of functioning "drop out" as the

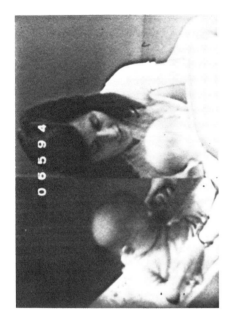

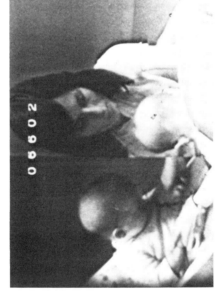

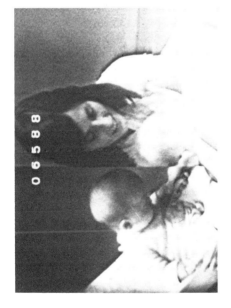

Figure 2: A,B,C. These are photo examples of film, with split-screen from two cameras, one on infant and one on mother, who are seated opposite each other in a vis-a-vis position. The numbers at the top of the photos refer to frames occurring 24 per second.

infant progresses through this spectrum from engagement to disengagement. Table 2 subdivides the spectrum into finer gradations which
detail the behaviors of the rougher categories.

1. "Facing and looking." As can be seen in Table 1, in facing
and looking, the infant processes the fullest range of information.
He perceives the form of the mother's face with foveal vision, and is
oriented vis-a-vis. He maintains potential micromomentary responsivity to changes in the mother's movements and expressions, through his
own expressions, and slight changes in head orientation. The full
range of the infant's rich array of facial expressions is available
here, and is most likely to appear during sustained visual engagement
(Figure 1).

2. "Side Looking." In contrast to facing and looking, side-
looking sacrifices center orientation, introducing a slight withdrawal
but maintaining foveal perception. Side-looking can have a dramatic
effect in modulating the nature of the infant expressiveness (and
maternal responsivity as well). Smiles, for example, may appear "coy,"
and neutral expressions appear "equivocal." Side-looking is an un-
stable posture, usually held only momentarily, and often leads to a
further orientation away and loss of visual engagement.

3. "Visual Checking." Proceeding to the next gradation of disengagement, "visual checking" is a term borrowed from Mahler (1963,
1968a, 1968b), and refers to a model of periodic brief visual engage-
ments, checking "in and out." The infant loses sustained foveal
visual engagement, and it is as if the infant is doing some "reconnoit-
ering" of the stimulation available. During orientation away, the infant retains the potential for remarkably tuned micromomentary responsivity through peripheral visual monitoring. Facial expressiveness in
this mode retains almost the full range (as the infant is looking, or
as he is leaving the facing and looking position), but the possibility for building a crescendo of intensity of expression, available in
the full engagement position, is lost during checking. A variant of
checking has been termed "checking on the run." The infant orients
and looks, but only for the briefest split second, and then looks
away again. The remaining grades will be defined and discussed more
fully below in the case illustration.

E. SUBJECTS

In this paper, one mother-infant pair will be used to illustrate
a selected portion of the engagement-disengagement spectrum. Similar
data has been collected for other pairs by our group. This particular mother volunteered from the local hospital community. The infant
was four months old, with a normal developmental course to date. This
particular stretch of film of this particular mother-infant pair was
chosen because it demonstrates especially well the mid-range of the
spectrum between the more obvious extremes of focal, foveal visual

attention, and complete disruption of the play encounter. The complex and subtle compromises between "engagement" and "disengagement" are seen in this sample in high relief.

F. PROCEDURE

Mother and infant were filmed seated opposite each other in approximately the same plane, with the latter in an infant seat. Two TV cameras were used, one on the mother's face and one on the infant's face. The resulting split-screen TV tape was kinescoped into 16mm film, with numbers printed on each frame (24 frames/sec). The kinescope was analyzed. For this particular pair, a 6-1/2 minute interaction was studied in detail, so that it is not possible to conclude anything about the characteristic patterns of the relationship. The sample comprised a "whole" uninterrupted sequence, from the time the camera was first turned on until the mother spontaneously stopped interacting with the infant.

CASE ILLUSTRATION

OVERVIEW

In this pair, the compelling clinical impression (which is statistically documented below in Table 3) was that a major portion of the interaction involved complex sequences of mother "chasing" and infant "dodging," and vice-versa, with each reacting to the other on an exquisitely tuned, micromomentary basis of latencies under half a second. To every maternal overture, the infant could duck, move back, turn away, pull away, or become limp and unresponsive. Through his virtuoso performance, this infant had near "veto power" over his mother's efforts to engage him posturally and visually.

Table 3 shows the contingent analyses which document quantitatively the manner in which each partner reacted to selected split-second movements of the other. The mother chased the infant by following his head and body movements with her own head and body, pulling his arm or hand, picking him up to readjust his orientation, even attempting to force the infant's head in her direction. In the course of the 6-1/2 minute interaction, a comparison of the first two and last two minutes revealed that the "chase and dodge" interaction increasingly resembled a "fight," with the mother making statistically significant increased use of pulling of the infant (see Table 4). The infant, for his part, began in the last two minutes to pull his hand right out of hers, with such force that he, several times, almost lost his balance. In addition, the infant, in the last two minutes, increasingly inhibited his responsivity (see Table 4). The mother routinely reacted to the infant's myriad avoidance maneuvers with fleeting but marked signs of negative affect: sobering, grimacing, biting her lip, jutting out her jaw, and occasionally thrusting the infant roughly away from her.

Table 3

Summary of Significant Interactions, by Chi-Square Test

"Stimulus"[*]		"Response"

1. Dodging:

    a) Mother loom   ---->   Infant (head back) head away
       (head-forward-and
       down-and-lean-in $x^2 = 17.7$, p $<$ .001 N = 249

    b) Infant dodge   ---->   Mother chase
       (head away   (pull, follow with head or
       head through)   body)

                                   $x^2 = 8.6$, p $<$ .01   N = 108

    c) Mother chase   ---->   Infant dodge
       (pull, follow,   (head away, head through
       tickle)   body back or side-away)

                                 $x^2 = 19.8$, p $<$ .001 N = 214

    d) and e) "refusing a reorientation"
       Mother pick up   ---->   Infant head center, eyes closed

                           $x^2 = 26.3$, p $<$ .001 N = 346

       and put on lap   ---->   Infant head away

                           $x^2 = 33.1$, p $<$ .001 N = 346

[*]Note:- A "response" is defined as occurring in the range of .25 seconds to .75 seconds after the "stimulus" onset.

    A comparison interaction with the experimenter immediately following the interaction with the mother, revealed that the infant's profound refusal to engage was due neither to fatigue nor incapacity, since the infant was able to maintain an oriented vis-a-vis, looking and maintaining a positively expressive encounter with the experimenter (see Figure 1). Nevertheless, in this age group, it is relatively common for an infant to be unresponsive to the mother while willing to engage a novel stranger. Although no definitive results are currently available, the strong clinical impression was that, in this particular case, the experimenter's rate of movement was

Table 4

Comparison First Two vs. Last Two Minutes

I. Increased Infant Inhibition of Responsivity in Last Two Minutes	$X^2 = 6.97$, p $<$ .01	N = 346
II. Increased Maternal Use of Pulling in Last Two Minutes	$X^2 = 8.66$, p $<$ .01	N = 346

considerably slower and calmer than that of the mother, and might also have contributed to the difference.

Dodging. Once the infant centered and looked, the mother's response was a "mock surprise" expression (mouth opening, eyebrows raised, partial loss of smile) concurrent with, or followed by, a quick head movement forward and down toward the infant. This movement has been termed maternal "looming." (See Figure 3.) The infant's predictable response to maternal looming was to turn his head away ($X^2 = 17.7$; p $<$.001). On the basis of Ling (1942) and Bower (1970, 1974), from the second week, infants respond to a looming or approaching inanimate object with obvious "defensive" behavior. These defensive reactions include attempts to increase the head distance from the approaching object, by moving the head back and away, eye widening, and negative facial expressions. This may be an example of a response which begins as reflexive, but later is pressed into social use to regulate the social interaction. Maternal looming was particularly disruptive of the infant's capacity to maintain a focused encounter in the center orientation. This "head away" reaction was immediate, beginning on the average 0.41 sec. after the onset of the mother's loom and 0.08 sec. prior to its termination. Thus the infant began his "head away" before the mother's action was even completed. It is striking that the very event which must be conceptualized as the sine qua non of an expressively positive, focused interaction, that is, getting the infant to orient to vis-a-vis and look, was in most instances cut off by the mother herself.

After the infant's head turn away (or other withdrawal response such as "head through," body-back or body-side-away), the mother routinely "chased" in some way, following with her head and/or body in the direction the infant had moved, pulling the infant's arm or body, or reorienting by picking up ($X^2 = 8.6$, p $<$ .01; Table 3).

These maternal chase behaviors generally were followed by another round of "dodge" behaviors by the infant: still further head movements away, including the remarkable one to a full 90° away on the

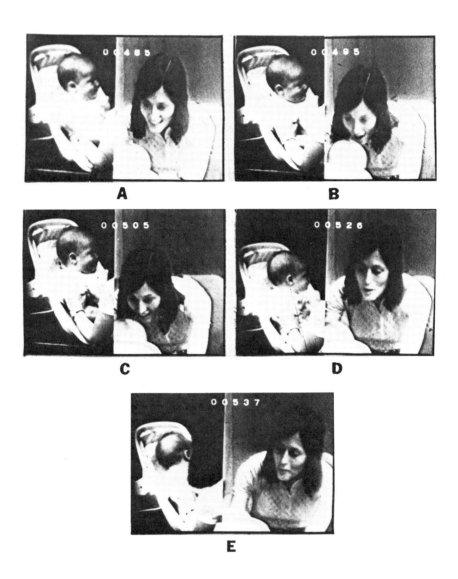

Figure 3: A,B,C,D,E. These are photo examples of film, with split-screen from two cameras, one on infant and one on mother, who are seated opposite each other in a vis-a-vis position. The numbers at the top of the photos refer to frames occurring 24 per second.

horizontal plane (Stern, 1971; see Figure 3, E); large head movements swinging a wide arc "through" the center vis-a-vis out to the other side, with eyes cast down or squeezed shut, possibly with a grimace or tight lip-in "line mouth"; or the infant might simply cease behaving. If the mother "chased" by pull or follow (with head or body), the infant dodged by head away, head through center, or body back or body side-away ($X^2 = 19.8$, p <.001). Average infant reaction time was 0.38 sec.

Such persistent dodging on the infant's part was generally followed by marked negative maternal affect, as evidenced by facial expressions (grimace, frown, bite-lip, sober; see Figure 3, D and E); occasional movements back and away from the infant. The mother often changed her mode of stimulation at this point (corroborating Stern, 1974).

An attempt to reorient the infant by picking him up was a frequent maternal intervention following a sequence of persistent infant withdrawal, and a statistical analysis was performed on the effectiveness of this maternal behavior in changing the tenor of the interaction. This particular interaction was chosen for analysis as an illustration of a maternal intervention that might be considered a potentially particularly effective way of re-engaging the infant. In fact, the opposite was true. Regularly ($X^2 = 26.3$, p < .001), as the mother picked the infant up, his head and body spontaneously recentered so as to line up the midline of his body with the mother; but this recentering was accompanied by eyes cast down or closed. As the mother put the infant down, usually on her lap, his head immediately turned away again ($X^2 = 33.1$, p < .001), so that by the time the mother had the infant repositioned on her lap, ready to begin anew, he had once again dodged her (see Table 3, D and E).

The infant's capacity to regulate incoming stimulation in the "chase and dodge" interaction thus involved acute vigilance, receptivity, and continued responsivity. Rather than "tuning out" stimulation, most salient in "chase and dodge," was the infant's exquisite sensitivity to the slightest maternal movements. Primarily through peripheral visual monitoring, the infant was capable of changing his orientation, posture, and gaze, from moment-to-moment, such as to maintain a certain postural and visual "distance" from the mother.

Inhibition of responsivity. Interspersed with persistent efforts to move his head away and pull his hand free, were stretches in which the infant seemed to lapse into "passive resistance," or perhaps more accurately, active nonresponsiveness, inhibiting his reactivity entirely. That is, no matter how vigorously the mother pulled, poked, or bounced, the infant would remain motionless, head hanging limp on the chest, head and eyes rigidly averted. Upon observing this behavior, the impression is of a profound refusal to engage (see Figure 2). Statistical evaluation confirmed the clinical impression that the infant made significantly greater use of inhibited responsivity in the

last two, as compared to the first two minutes of the interaction
(X^2 = 6.97, p <.01, see Table 4).

Turn to the environment. In the final interaction of the 6-1/2
minutes, the mother stopped behaving. After approximately 15 seconds,
the infant turned his head past the 90° position, swung his whole body
weight around in the direction opposite his mother, and turned his
eyes searchingly on the environment, losing any possibility of peri-
pherally monitoring the mother, and essentially "escaping" her presence, at least visually.

These significant interactions (summarized in Tables 3 and 4)
are a preliminary way of demonstrating how one particular mother-
infant pair negotiated this range of the spectrum.

DISCUSSION

The spectrum of engagement-disengagement has been the focus of
this paper for several reasons. Engagement and disengagement are
relatively neutral terms in the literature, and yet they capture
an important clinical sense of an interaction. The terms are sufficiently broad to encompass both a wide range of early object-
experiences and a number of theoretical perspectives from which to
view these experiences. The intent of this discussion is two-fold:
(a) to consider what relevance the spectrum may have for broader
theoretical issues of coping, defense, and separation-individuation;
and (b) to consider what implications the spectrum may have for precursors of internal representations of early object experiences.

The infant's capacity to engage and disengage his mother has
been formulated from several theoretical viewpoints. "Coping" can
be considered to be adaptive behavior which affects the environment
in the direction of the organism's own advantage, or freedom of movement while maintaining satisfactory attentional conditions for information processing and appropriate action. Every mother over- and
under-shoots the infant's optimum level of stimulation. From this
viewpoint, the spectrum specifies a set of normal adaptive or coping
maneuvers available to the infant to manage stimulation within a
comfortable range, and/or get his mother to alter her behavior (his
stimulation) if it is aversive.

One classical concept of infant "defensive behavior," in the
face of an over-stimulating environment, is to consider either withdrawal or decreased capacity for responsiveness as performing defensive functions (Greenacre, 1971). Optimal information processing and focal attention are progressively compromised as the spectrum
is traversed. Whether the infant is considered to be defending
against stimulation from within, or without, is an important distinction. It has been argued that only the former should properly be

considered defensive operations. However, because of the intimate
relation between external stimulation and internal arousal, the infant is in the position, via the described behaviors, to modulate
stimulation both within and without.

Regardless of the focus of interest, whether it is early coping
operations or proto-defensive maneuvers, the same spectrum of engagement-disengagement behaviors would apply.

It is impossible to consider early coping and defensive operations as distinct from issues of separation-individuation and early
boundary formation. As Lustman (1967) and Mahler (1967) argue,
boundary formation relevant to precursors of self-object differen-
tiations cannot be achieved without the development of defensive operations. The entire spectrum can be viewed as providing the infant
with a series of increasing visual-spatial boundaries in relation
to the mother.

In essence, whatever conceptual framework is used, it is again
this same spectrum of engagement-disengagement behaviors to which
one must refer. Indeed, the set of behaviors which constitute the
spectrum are the source for making inferences about these more highly
abstracted psychic constructs. Further, the spectrum operationalizes
these various theoretical perspectives.

If we consider each gradation along the engagement-disengagement
spectrum as a distinct object experience, consisting of its own per-
ceptual-cognitive-motor-affective components, then we can borrow
from Piaget's (1963) work to begin to suggest how these early object
experiences may later become psychic representations. According to
Piaget, the construction of the inanimate object-concept, or the internalization of mental representations, proceeds by way of the in-
teriorization of action schemes in relation to the object. A central
prerequisite, or precursor to the internalization of mental representations, is the inter-coordination of a number of schemes into a network (e.g., a rattle is to be looked at, to be grasped, to shake, or
to listen to). Only when the child's schemes are numerous, and internal structural links are established between them, does it become possible for him to differentiate himself and inanimate objects.

Although the "process" of the representation of the inanimate
object is well understood, less is known about the "product" of
this internalization in the specific realm of the internalization of
animate objects or persons. There is evidence to suggest that there
are two distinct subsets of the process of internalization, according to whether the object is animate or inanimate (Bell, 1970).

Regarding the problem of the internalization of the animate
object, the catalogue of the various action-schemes and their coordinations, which are specifically organized around mother, is

insufficiently comprehensive and detailed. The engagement-disengagement spectrum is an attempt to provide a description of infant behaviors relevant to such a catalogue.

It is, thus, necessary to expand our notions of the interpersonal
schemes available to the four month infant. Early interpersonal
schemes must include at least the content and mode of visual perception, the orientation in space relative to the animate object, the
affective tonality, the level of general activation, the direction of
movement with reference to the animate object, and the nature of the
temporal connectedness. These criteria of the engagement-disengagement spectrum provide formal categories of experience the infant is
developing with which to structure the interpersonal object. Moreover, the gradations of the spectrum describe different perceptual
and sensorimotor experiences or "modes of relatedness" relative to
the interpersonal object.

In Piaget's framework, it is the action schemes themselves, or
the infant modes of modulating his experience with the object, which
provide the infant with a "way of knowing" about the object, and
which is interiorized in the first mental representations. It is
proposed that the detailed knowledge of the infant action schemes
in relation to the mother, and their interactive regulation, provides not only a way of defining varying modes of "relatedness" in
the ongoing relationship, but also provides a way of assessing what
it is that is internalized in the construction of the animate "object-
relation." The hypothesis is that the dominant modes of the ongoing
relationship, based on detailed analysis of behavioral organization
and mutual regulation, will prevail in the internalized representation of the relationship. As Piaget has shown, the internalization
of the object does not proceed independently of the child's actions
with reference to the object. Hence what is initially internalized
is not an object per se, but an "object-relation": actions of self
with reference to actions of object.

The model of what is internalized, thus, includes mutually
regulated sequences of maternal-infant actions with a particular
temporal patterning. It is important to note that since the infant
is in a dyadic system in which the behaviors or action-schemes are
potentially so intimately temporally meshed with the mother's, one
aspect of what becomes internalized in the first object-relation is
a "time-frame of connectedness" or of mutual responsivity. What is
meant by time-frame of connectedness is the durations of behaviors,
the mutual sequential patterning of onset and termination of behaviors, their rate and rhythmicity.

Although the engagement-disengagement spectrum is presented
from the infant's point of view, the evidence presented in the case

illustration regarding the mutual influence in the "chase and dodge" interaction is a first step toward suggesting the kinds of inter- active regulations of the spectrum which might provide the "product" of emerging internalization, should this type of interaction charac- terize a particular pair.

Although the "chase and dodge" interaction in itself, or in this illustrative case, cannot be construed as pathological, if chase and dodge were heavily characteristic of the interaction, it might well have pathological implications. The fundamental nature of this mother's chase behavior was that it interfered with the infant's ca- pacity both to maintain focal attention and even to do visual "check- ing" of the mother's face. Particularly due to the infant's inabil- ity at this age to re-evoke the image of the absent object, pervasive "chase and dodge" might force the infant to make premature postural- visual separations without adequate means of remaining in (visual) contact. It is interesting to speculate as to whether the organiza- tion or behaviors seen here, that is "something chasing, out of the corner of the eye, but with no visual image," might be the basis for the earliest prerepresentational origins of the persecutory object. It is a mode of interaction in which the infant stays acutely tuned to the mother through peripheral visual monitoring, locked into the object relation temporally as he, at the same time, avoids her pos- turally and visually.

Normally, however, daily fluctuations in the mood or state of either partner, of situation etc., results in an expectably full use of the entire engagement-disengagement spectrum. Experience within all of the gradations of the full spectrum gives the infant a large range of different object experiences. We are suggesting that some composite of these object experiences are internalized to form the earliest representations of object-relations.

REFERENCES

Beebe, B. Ontogeny of positive affect in the third and fourth months of the life of one infant. Doctoral dissertation, Columbia Univer- sity, University Microfilms, 1973.

Beebe, B., & Bennett, S. Early facial expressions. Unpublished paper, New York State Psychiatric Institute, 1975.

Bell, S. M. The development of the concept of the object as related to infant-mother attachment. Child Development, 1970: 41, 291-311.

Benjamin, J. Further comments on some developmental aspects of anx- iety. In H. Goshell (Ed.), Counterpoint: Libidinal object and sub- ject. New York: International Universities Press, 1963.

Benjamin, J. Developmental biology and psychoanalysis. In N.
  Greenfield & W. Lewis (Eds.), Psychoanalysis and current biological
  thought. Madison: University of Wisconsin Press, 1963.

Bower, T., Broughton, J., & Moore, M. Infant responses to approaching objects. Perception and Psychophysics, 1970, 9.

Bower, T. Development in infancy. San Francisco: W. H. Freeman,
  1974.

Bowlby, J. Attachment and loss. Vol. 1. New York: Basic Books,
  1969.

Brody, S., & Axelrad, S. Anxiety and ego formation in infancy.
  New York: International Universities Press, 1970.

Brown, G. Y. Discrimination of normative facial expressions by 12-
  week-old infants. Biennial meeting of the Society for Research in
  Child Development, Denver, Colorado 1975.

Charlesworth, W. R., & Krewtzer, M. Facial expressions of infants
  and children. In Paul Ekman (Ed.), Darwin and facial expression.
  New York: Academic Press, 1973.

Freud, S. (1895). Project for a scientific psychology. Standard
  Edition, Vol. 1. London: Hogarth Press, 1966.

Greenacre. P. Toward an understanding of the physical nucleus of
  some defense reactions. Emotional growth, Vol. 1. New York:
  International Universities Press, 1971.

Haggard, E., & Isaacs, K. Micromomentary facial expressions as in-
  dicators of ego mechanisms in psychotherapy. In L. Gottshalk &
  A. Auerbach (Eds.), Methods of research in psychotherapy. New
  York: Appleton-Century-Crofts, 1966.

Ling, B. A genetic study of sustained visual fixation. Journal of
  Genetic Psychology, 1942, 61, 227-277.

Lustman, S. Psychic energy and mechanisms of defense. Psychoanalytic Study of the Child, Vol. XII. New York: International Universities Press, 1957.

Lustman, S. Scientific Proceedings, Panel Reports. Development
  and metapsychology of the defense organization of the ego. Journal
  of the American Psychoanalytic Association, 1967, 15, 130-149.

Mahler, M. Thoughts about development and individuation. Psychoanalytic Study of the Child, XVII. New York: International Universities Press, 1963.

Mahler, M. Scientific Proceedings, Panel Reports. Development and
metapsychology of the defense organization of the ego. Journal of
the American Psychoanalytic Association, 1967, 15, 130-149.

Mahler, M., & McDevitt, J. Observations on adaptation and defense
in statu nascendi. Psychoanalytic Quarterly, 1968, 37, 1-21. (a)

Mahler, M., & Furer, M. On human symbiosis and the vicissitudes of
individuation. New York: International Universities Press, 1968.
(b)

Piaget, J. The origins of intelligence in children. New York:
W. W. Norton, 1963.

Rheingold, H. The effect of environmental stimulation upon social
and exploratory behavior in the human infant. In B. Foss (Ed.),
Determinants of infant behavior, Vol. 1. London: Methuen, 1961.

Robson, K. The role of eye-to-eye contact in maternal-infant attachment. Journal of Child Psychology and Psychiatry, 1967, 8, 13-25.

Spitz, R. The first year of life. New York: International Universities Press, 1965.

Stern, D. A microanalysis of mother-infant interaction. Journal
of the American Academy of Child Psychiatry, 1971, 10(3), 501-517.

Stern, D. The structure of mother-infant play. In M. Lewis & L.
Rosenblum (Eds.), The effect of the infant on its caregiver.
New York: John Wiley, 1974.

Stern, D. Methodological issues in studying bidirectional influences
in mother-infant interaction. Biennial meeting of the Society for
Research in Child Development, Denver, Colorado, 1975.

Tronik, E. Personal communication, 1975.

Walters, R., & Parke, R. The role of distance receptors in the
development of social responsiveness. In L. Lipset & C. Spiker
(Eds.), Advances in child development and behavior, Vol. II. New
York: Academic Press, 1965.

THE INFLUENCES OF VARIOUS MODALITIES OF SENSORY DEPRIVATION ON THE

EVOLUTION OF PSYCHIC AND COMMUNICATIVE STRUCTURES

David A. Freedman

Baylor College of Medicine

Houston, Texas 77030

I

Because I take it to be implicit in the theme of the symposium, I will not dwell on the evidence that the ability to utilize the vocal/auditory system for the purpose of making speech sounds is neither a sufficient, nor even a necessary condition for the process of thinking. Suffice it to say that within the psychoanalytic tradition the necessity to differentiate between thinking and the communication of the products of thought was recognized very early by Freud. It will be recalled that in the course of developing the topographic model, Freud (1895, 1896) assigned the process of attaching word representations to thoughts to the preconscious. Thinking itself he conceived of as an unconscious neural process. In the intervening years, his conclusions have been affirmed by an abundance of empirical evidence. The phenomenon of echolalia in humans, as well as the extraordinary abilities of the mynah bird and parrot, provide proof positive that well articulated speech sounds can be produced by individuals who are entirely lacking in the ability to understand the message their words ostensibily convey. On the other hand, equally persuasive evidence is available from the study of the congenitally deaf (see below), and such comparative studies as those of the Gardeners (1969) to the effect that both the act of creative thinking and the ability to communicate the products of the thought process are entirely possible in the absence of a functioning vocal/ auditory system.

Such considerations to the contrary notwithstanding, there remains a considerable body of opinion which holds to the conception that the relation between thinking and speaking is epitomized by the double entendre "deaf and dumb." At least one psychoanalyst

(Edelheit, 1969) has proposed that the"... ego may, in fact, be regarded as a vocal/auditory organization -- a language determined
and language determining structure which functions as the characteristic human organ of adaptation." That this is not a unique
point of view was indicated by the proceedings of a recent American
Psychoanalytic Association panel devoted to the problem of the relation of language development to problem solving ability (Edelheit,
1972). The participants were sharply divided with respect to the
issue. Three, all of whom had direct experience with the congenitally deaf and other victims of congenital and perinatal sensory
deprivation, agreed that the ability to use oral language is only
secondarily related to the ability to think and solve problems. The
others, whose experience was apparently limited to the clinical
psychoanalytic situation, took a position closer to that indicated
by the preceding quotation.

That the divergence of opinion was directly related to the participants' prior experience seems to me fraught with significance
for our discussion. For it is the case both that the psychoanalytic
method is a talking procedure and that psychoanalytic theory, despite
the fact that it is rooted in the assumption that psychological development is an epigenetic process, has only in relatively recent
years considered the findings of the direct observation of the preverbal infant as a relevant source of data. Indeed, it is barely 25
years since Spitz (1950) felt it necessary to point out that infant
observation might provide information of relevance to the psychoanalytic theory of human mental development. Since then, an enormous body
of information has accumulated from this mode of research. It is, I
think, accurate to say that this literature is consistent in pointing
to the occurrence in the course of development of not one, but rather
of a series of parallel epigenetic processes. While these are necessarily more or less interrelated, it is also the case that they
proceed along separate and identifiable lines -- i.e., in the sense
postulated by Anna Freud (1965). Ultimately, of course, if one is
to explain the emergence of an integrated individual, one must also
assume a synthetic function, the operation of which yields the cohesive whole we designate as personality. While this is, of course,
relatively straightforward as it applies to the development of the
integrated individual, it is worth belaboring because I would like
to present evidence that the emergence of the vocal/auditory system
as an ego apparatus also involves both developmental processes --
i.e., is the result of the confluence of several independent lines
of development. Otherwise stated, the cohesive whole we take so
much for granted as our primary means of communication is a product
of the synthetic function.

II

A methodological digression. Because of the nature of much of
the data I have to present, it seems appropriate that I first clarify

the approach I have taken to the study of these problems. It is
apparent that the analytic situation has only limited value as a
medium from which to obtain early developmental data. Elkind (1970),
furthermore, has pointed out some of the difficulties inherent in
all human developmental research -- an area in which the very nature
of the subject matter drastically limits the ability of the investigator to use traditional experimental methods. Even if we leave
moral and ethical issues aside, the length of the human developmental
period as well as the complexity of the forces to which any given infant is subject, at any given time, makes the controlled experimental
situation into which only one variable is introduced, rarely applicable. As one alternative, Elkind suggests that the investigator may
resort to the identification of regularities as they occur in the uncontrolled situation. Such regularities, when they are clearly defined, can be regarded as reflecting the operation of some antecedent circumstance shared by the members of the population being
studied.

In view, however, of the vast congeries of common experiences
which all developing individuals share, it is often impossible to
determine precisely which elements of a complex recurring series
of phenomena are relevant to the emergence of a particular recurring
psychologic characteristic. Indeed, it is entirely possible for the
observer to be unaware of precisely those aspects of the infant's
ambience which may ultimately prove to be of critical importance.
Failure, for example, to take into account the probability that because of the infant's immature nervous system, as well as his lack of
experience, his perceptual as well as his cognitive processes are
radically different from those of the adult, has led more than one
observer of preverbal children to adultomorphize. The imputations
of the Kleinian school seem to me to represent only the most extreme
version of this. Less egregious examples can be found throughout
the psychoanalytic literature, beginning with the interpretation of
his grandson's behavior which played so large a role in Freud's (1920)
development of his theory of the repetition compulsion.

This is not, of course, to dismiss the use of direct infant observation, but to underscore that from a methodological standpoint
it -- like the controlled laboratory experiment -- has limitations.
Neither, for that matter, can the natural experiment which I have
espoused, and which I will now discuss, stand by itself. I offer it
for consideration together with some of my findings as an additional,
supplementary, approach to the study of early development. In a
sense, the converse of the conventional laboratory situation, one
which seeks to insert a single variable into an otherwise controlled
situation, in the natural experiment, one takes advantage of circumstances in which a single constant factor (or clearly definable group
of factors) can be isolated in an otherwise uncontrolled situation.
Working from this standpoint it is very difficult -- if at all possible -- to establish an unequivocal positive relation. On the other

hand, and herein it seems to me lies the value of the method, it is
eminently possible to establish a negative. That is, if one can
demonstrate that a given consequence follows in the absence of some
precondition which has been assumed to be critical, one has demonstrated that the presumed relation does not obtain. By way of illustration, I cite the progressive degradation of the situation of
the infant suckling at the breast from one to which our analytic
ancestors could impute all manner of psychological developmental
significance to a mere metaphor. It required the natural experiment of a generation of well functioning adults who had never experienced breast feeding to accomplish this transition, and to establish the fact that the specific experience of the mother's breast
was only an element -- and not a critical element -- in the complex
situation out of which the mother-infant bond emerges.

Because it has become so ubiquitous, however, the practice of
artificial feeding constitutes something of a special case among the
natural experiments. The situations which I will discuss are those
in which a relatively small cohort of developing individuals has
been exposed to circumstances which are highly atypical of generally
accepted normative experience. The victims of various forms of congenital and perinatal sensory deprivation have been my particular
interest. By no means, however, do they constitute the entire group.
One could also include here such varied populations as the youngsters
with skeletal deformities -- e.g., the victims of pre-natal exposure
to thalidomide and the offspring of parents who batter their children.
In each instance, it is possible to define some characteristics of the
involved population which are typical of every individual who has been
exposed to the given circumstance, and which do not occur in individuals who have not been exposed. Of these, it can be said that they
are the direct result of the given form of deprivation or distorted
experience. No congenitally blind person will ever see form or colors, and no congenitally deaf person will ever hear music. To borrow a term from the geneticists with respect to these functions, the
respective sensory deprivations are 100% penetrant.

Over and above those specific sequelae which are invariably
present, one can also detect some phenomena of which it can be said
that, while they are much more likely to be present in association
with the specific distorted experience, the association is not invariable. Again, to use the geneticist's idiom, for some qualities
the mode of deprivation has a limited penetrance. It was the observation of such very frequent but not invariable associations that led
to the possibility of viewing the various forms of sensory deprivation as media through which to investigate aspects of the developmental process. Just as the use of artificial feeding underscores
the importance of the anatomically non-oral aspects of the oral relation, so does the fact that there is variation in the psychological outcome associated with various modes of infantile sensory deprivation tend to throw into relief otherwise obscured aspects of the
mother-infant relation.

III

The possibility of viewing both the sensory deprivations and other forms of extraordinary infantile and early childhood experience from this standpoint occurred to me as the result of the observation, in collaboration with Mrs. Selma Fraiberg, of a psychotic, congenitally blind boy. Because this case has already been reported (Fraiberg and Freedman, 1964), I will limit myself to a very brief summary. The youngster, then aged 7, was referred to me for neurologic evaluation. The survivor of a pair of prematurely born twins, he was the victim of the pandemic of retrolental fibrous dysplasia which occurred during the period before the toxic effects of high oxygen tension were recognized. When, after examining the child, I turned to the literature, I found that the syndrome which he presented - ie., an autistic like state - had already been widely described in the congenitally blind. Indeed, something in excess of 25% of such individuals present a virtually identical clinical picture. I found the 25% figure particularly intriguing. At one and the same time, it both made the blindness seem very relevant to the occurrence of the psychosis, and precluded the possibility of ascribing the psychosis to the fact of the blindness alone. In keeping with what I have already outlined, it seemed necessary to view the blindness as analogous to a gene factor of limited penetrance, i.e., one which renders the individual vulnerable to other deleterious influences which in turn account, in this instance, for the autistic state.

Certainly in our original case and in many others we have seen since, it has not been difficult to identify additional potentially relevant influences. The disruption of the mother-infant bond which results from the absence of a visual response on the part of the child is considerable. Characteristically, mothers react to the fact of their infants' amaurosis as though it were a narcissistic blow. In addition, the babies' failure to follow visually or to show any form of visual response is interpreted as a rejection by many mothers. If a dialogue is to develop between such an infant and its mother, extraordinary compensatory measures are necessary. These prove to be beyond the capacities of many women who, in the average expectable situation, are perfectly adequate mothers. That appropriate interventions will, however, circumvent the barrier posed by blindness and allow the congenitally blind child to become aware of the mothering one as an object is indicated by the later work of Mrs. Fraiberg. She has recently described a series of nine consecutive cases in which, by facilitating the use of alternative modes of communication, she has prevented the development of an autistic state (Fraiberg 1974).

It will be apparent that in considering the issue of the development of the congenitally blind, I have drawn a distinction between the vocal/auditory system as a specific medium through which communication is carried on, and the process of communicating. I emphasize this theme both because it is a critical one for the symposium, and because

it is so clearly illustrated in the case of the autistic congenitally blind. When I first saw the youngster I have already mentioned,
he was incapable of communicating orally, or for that matter in any
other way. Four years later, when I last saw him and despite Mrs.
Fraiberg's best efforts, he was -- at 11 years of age --- still without
the ability to differentiate human objects or to communicate even his
basic wants. Today, chronologically an adult in his 20's, he continues to be autistic. At the same time, during my initial consultation,
his mother informed me that he sang very clearly, on pitch and -- when
singing -- was able to enunciate the words of the songs very clearly.
While I examined him, he repeated over and over again, "Peter not a
bad boy. Peter not a bad boy...." A year later, when he returned to
his New Orleans home from a stay in an institution in another city,
his mono-lingual English speaking parents complained to Mrs. Fraiberg
that he was talking gibberish. After she heard him, Mrs. Fraiberg
told me, "You know Dave, he isn't talking gibberish at all; he is
talking perfectly clear Yiddish. He is saying over and over again,
"der meshugene shlaft noch nit; der meshugene shlaft noch nit...."
("The crazy one isn't sleeping yet....")

     In this case, and it is by no means unique, the youngster's
well-developed vocal/auditory system could be characterized as functioning in a vacuum. The clinical evidence, which I will now present,
seems to me to support the conclusion that this, in turn, is the result of the patient never having differentiated self from object
and -- as a direct consequence of this failure -- never having differentiated the cognitive and affective structures which lead, under
average expectable circumstances, to the "need" to communicate. The
evidence I have to offer comes from both my own experience and the
literature. It embraces representatives of the following: (a) The
congenitally deaf, (b) The environmentally deprived, (c) An entirely
unique case -- a youngster being reared in a germ free environment
whom I have followed almost since his birth.

     In addition, I would like to say a few words concerning the vi-
cissitudes to which the average expectable child, who is being reared
in an average expectable environment, is exposed with respect to the
process of language development.

     The congenitally deaf. An abundance of data make it clear that
the inability to hear and speak does not per se interfere with the
ability to think. It is now 35 years since Eberhard (1940) wrote:
"The experiments show that the world of the young deaf child is already organized beyond the perceptual level and that this organization closely follows that of speaking people. They show clearly that
language is not essential for organized conceptual thought, at least
during its first stage...much of the first language development of
the young deaf child in school consists in the learning of words for
ideas that he already knows and uses in his everyday life, not as one
might believe a priori, in the development of conceptual thinking by

means of language symbols in a child whose world up to that point
has been a more or less unorganized one."

Her conclusions have been supported in the intervening years
by Furth (1966) who has shown that the congenitally deaf readily
learn to manipulate the symbols of symbolic logic, Vernon (1967)
who, on reviewing 31 independently conducted investigations, re-
confirmed the repeatedly discovered fact that the congenitally
deaf show no intellectual deficit if, in presenting their material,
the experimenters take adequate care to control for the lack of
speech and speech derived influences and by myself (1971). In an
earlier essay (Freedman, 1972), I added as a second condition, "if
the earlier development of the child has been compatible with the
establishment of adequate early object relations and their sequelae
in the form of internalized object representations and differentiated sense of self."

While my proviso is still valid, I have some question as to
the necessity of belaboring the point. For it is the case that the
probability that congenitally deaf children will differentiate self
and object and establish adequate object relations is approximately
the same as obtains for normally hearing youngsters. I make this
statement on the basis of my observation of five congenitally deaf
girls (Freedman, Cannaday & Robinson, 1971). The youngsters, who
were followed from age two and a half to age 5 years, were selected
because of the similarities of their cultural, economic, and medical
backgrounds. In areas that did not involve the use of language,
their performance on developmental tests was on a par with that of
their normally hearing age mates. Despite both the marked delay in
their beginning to use any oral language, and the gross deficiency
of their speech, they showed none of the already described characteristics of the congenitally blind. All had formed strong self-
identities as well as the capacity to enter into mutual interactions
and attachments to others. Lack of language aside, when compared
with normally hearing children they differed only in that they
tended to translate their wishes into action more readily than do
normally hearing youngsters, and were more likely to attempt to
solve problems without appealing for help. Because of these qualities, they tended to be regarded as brighter and more alert than
their normally hearing age mates. This impression, however, was not
borne out by developmental testing.

Despite the fact that their lack of hearing made them unable
to be aware of conventional oral expressions of prohibition, permission, praise, or blame, processes of internalization and identification did not appear to be adversely affected. All the subjects
were distinctly feminine in their interests and behavior, and they
had all developed well-defined internal regulators of behavior.

It is probably the case that the relative independence and somewhat frenetic activity manifested by these children are the earliest manifestations of factors that will eventuate in later typical characteristics of the deaf. Certainly their inability to appreciate the nuances of meaning conveyed by spoken language cannot help setting the deaf apart from the hearing, as the use of the vocal/auditory system becomes increasingly important in human activities. In contrast, however, to the situations of the environmentally deprived individual and of a very high percentage of the congenitally blind, by the time the use of speech and hearing become critical, the deaf individual characteristically will have experienced a considerable degree of psychic structuralization and differentiation of self and environment. His response to the isolation and frustration he must inevitably experience will be determined, at least in part, by the introjects he has already formed and, in his efforts both to account for and to compensate for his plight, he will be guided by established object-relations and expectations. One would, therefore, anticipate that his adaptive efforts will approximate those of the normally endowed individual.

A pervasive sense of loneliness is, for example, hardly to be recommended as a state of feeling. To be experienced, however, it does require as a precondition, some degree of differentiation of self and object and the establishment of internalized object representations. Rainer (1973) reports that such a feeling is quite characteristic of the congenitally deaf. The further observation (Altschuler and Rainer, 1958) that the admission rate among the congenitally deaf for schizophrenia is no greater than it is for the hearing is additional evidence in support of the proposition that psychic structures differentiate in this population along average expectable lines. Their problems in relating have to do with the lack of a medium through which to communicate, rather than a lack of differentiation and consequent lack of the feeling of a need to communicate.

The environmentally deprived. Whether one assigns priority to the scribe of the Egyptian Pharoah Ptelemachus or to Solimbene who performed the same function for the Holy Roman Emperor Frederic II, there is no doubt that the Environmental Deprivation syndrome has been recognized and reported since very ancient times. Because of the conditions under which the early investigators worked, it was however, impossible for them to make long term observations. Solimbene (See Provence and Lipton, 1962) notes that all of Frederic's experimental subjects -- those whom the nurses suckled but with whom they were not allowed to prattle -- died. A similarly high mortality rate continued to be prevalent into the early years of this century when, according to Spitz (1945), between 30 and 100% of foundlings in institutions in the United States and Germany died during their first year. By the end of the second year, the overall death rate was 75%. There was, in other words, no possibility of studying the emergence of either communicative or psychic structures. More recently, perhaps because of better hygienic and nutritional conditions, it has been possible for a very high percentage of found- lings to survive. The syndrome which they present has been described repeatedly (e.g., Goldfarb, 1943; Provence and Lipton loc. cit.).

Of its many components, two seem to be of particular relevance to this symposium. Referring to a group of 5-year-old children who were in institutions up to 18 to 24 months of age and then placed in families, Provence and Lipton described characteristic areas of dif- ficulty which appear to be the results of the earlier lack of experi- ence. The use of language for asking questions, expressing ideas and fantasies, and verbalizing feelings, for example, was not as well de- veloped as that of the family child at a comparable age.

They also note that it was rare to see a child who had lived as much as 18 months in an institution turn to an adult for help. How- ever, unlike the deaf child who, as I already have noted, tends to go about solving problems on his own, the deprived youngster quickly loses interest in whatever he is doing. Also unlike both the intact child reared under average expectable conditions and the congenitally deaf child, these children do not tend to see adults as potential sources of comfort, protection, or succor. The failure to utilize the parenting figure for such purposes remained significantly im- paired throughout Provence and Lipton's period of observation. At the same time, other evidences of the childrens' failure to establish adequate internalized representations of objects and to make attach- ments to objects are readily apparent. The vignettes which follow from one of my own studies are illustrative.

The subjects were six and four when they were discovered. Their psychotic mother, convinced that they were bewitched and defective, had kept them in isolation from birth. The details of their condi- tion when they came to attention are reported elsewhere (Freedman and Brown, 1968). For the purposes of this communication, I will describe some events which took place many months after they were placed in an excellent foster home.

The children smiled constantly and appeared, on superficial inspection, to be friendly and outgoing. Closer examination, however, made it apparent that their friendliness was more apparent than real. They made absolutely no distinction between those individuals with whom they had been in intimate daily contact (e.g., their case work- ers and foster parents) and total strangers. Five months after they were placed in foster care they were presented to a large conference. They showed no evidence of shyness or timidity when in the presence of an audience of over 100 people. They went as readily to the total strangers present as they did to their own parents.

Because of the persistence of their failure to become involved with other members of the family, the foster parents elected not to

adopt the children. When they ultimately were placed in adoption,
they left their home of 18 months without evidence of concern. At
no time did they refer to the foster parents or in any other way indicate a sense of loss. When the new parents decided -- in order to
make a clean break with the past -- to assign them new given names
they accepted the change without question. At ages eight and six,
when I last had the opportunity to see them, their speech continued
to be echolalic and they had not yet come to the use of the first
person pronoun. It would be difficult to say they were totally devoid of evidence of ongoing intrapsychic processes. Rather, it
seemed to me that there was minimal evidence of the coalescence of
isolated internalized fragments into cohesively operating structures.
They gave no evidence, for example, of the ability either to attach
meaning to the words they used or to conceive of language as a medium
of communication. Thus, on one occasion her adoptive mother asked
the nearly eight-year-old girl, "What do we say at the table?" The
child replied in a monotone, "Don't put your elbows on the table."
When the mother reiterated, "No, no, what do we say at the table?",
the youngster rattled off Grace in an equally mechanical and expres-
sionless manner.

Of the many related observations to be found in the literature,
those reported by Kingsley Davis (1940, 1946) and Marie K. Mason
(1942) seem to me to be particularly germane in that they again underscore the probability that nonlinguistic experience is critical if
the potentiality to develop linguistic ability is to be realized.

Davis studied a 6-year-old child who was found incarcerated in
a storage room. Apparently she had been confined to this room from
early infancy. There is documentary evidence that she had been an
entirely normal infant until she was between six and 10 months. At
that age, she was removed from foster care and returned to her mother
who kept her isolated up to the time of her discovery some five years
later. Although this child made some gains after she was found, e.g.,
she learned to walk and to feed herself, and she achieved some ability
to be neat, her development was extremely limited. I quote from a
note made some two years later, "Anna walks about aimlessly, making
periodic rhythmic motions of her hands, and at intervals, making gut-
teral and sucking noises. She regards her hands as if she had seen
them for the first time. It was impossible to hold her attention for
more than a few seconds at a time -- not because of distraction due
to external stimuli but because of her inability to concentrate. She
ignored the task in hand to gaze vacantly about the room. Speech is
entirely lacking...." (italics mine) Three years later, at the time
of her death at age nine, the child showed little change from this
picture.

In striking contrast to this youngster is the child reported by
Mason. Also a girl, she was born illegitimately to a totally aphasic
mother. Mother could neither read nor write, and communicated with
her family by gestures. From the time the pregnancy was discovered

she, and subsequently her child, was kept in a locked room behind
drawn shades. Six-and-a-half years later, carrying her child, the
mother made her escape, and the child came to the attention of public
authorities. Mason saw the child when she was admitted to a hospital
in Columbus, Ohio. The youngster had no language. She spent the
first two days in tears. Mason's overtures were greeted by a gesture
of repulsion from, to quote her, "the wan-looking child whose face
bore marks of grief and fear." Sensing that no direct approach was
possible, Mason attempted to involve her by playing dolls with another
little girl while ostensibly ignoring her. By this method, one which
would have been entirely inapplicable to such apathetic children as
Davis and I describe, she was able ultimately to engage the child's
interest and establish a mutual relation with her. Within a year-and-
a-half, she had acquired a vocabulary of between fifteen hundred and
two thousand words, could count to one hundred, identify coins, and
perform arithmetic computations to ten. Mason describes her at eight-
and-a-half as having an excellent sense of humor, being an inveterate
tease, and an imaginative, affectionate, and loving child. In less
than two years she made the transition from a world of silence and
isolation to an excellent adjustment in the average expectable social
world of childhood.

In comparing Mason's case to Davis' and my own, it seems evident
that the critical and distinctive difference in the former's life experience was the availability of a maternal figure to whom she could
make attachments. Both her ability to experience despair, and her
susceptibility to Mason's efforts to involve her, seem to me evidence
of her having already established intrapsychic representations. That
these, and the psychic structuralization they imply, were preverbal
is consistent with the already presented evidence to the effect that
the differentiation of psychic structures precedes the development
of communcative capacities -- constitutes in effect a necessary if
not a sufficient condition for their emergence.

The youngster I will now describe provides further evidence in
support of this thesis. He merits reporting because, in his case, it
was possible both to observe directly and, I believe, influence the
sequence of events by which linguistic abilities emerged.

Because of the possibility that he might be suffering from a
congenital immune deficiency syndrome, this otherwise healthy infant was delivered by Caesarean, and placed at once into a germ
free environment where he has remained throughout the intervening
four-and-a-half years. This has consisted of a series of progressively larger clear plastic air bubbles. More recently, he has also
had ready access to a play room constructed of plate glass panels.
Gloves, which are built into the sides of the isolators, provide
ready access to him. By means of these he can be picked up, handled,
and played with.

Certain consequences of the conditions of his existence merit mentioning. He has never felt another person's skin, smelt another person's body or breath, experienced the warmth of an embrace, or been able to mold himself to another person. Although, as noted, he can be picked up and handled within the confines of his plastic world, he has never been able to embrace another person or cling to someone in the manner Bowlby (1960) considers to represent a basic human need. Although he spends about half his time at home, the exigencies of his condition are such that he spends the remainder in the hospital. He has, therefore, not had the experience of either an exclusive or a single preeminent caretaker. He is, of course, subject to repeated painful assaults for the drawing of blood and the carrying out of other procedures. Needless to say, he receives much attention in the sense that celebrities receive attention. He has, for example, appeared on national television many times. Yet the conditions of his existence are such that he is all too easily left to his own devices. While he receives excellent hygienic care, the quality of the mothering experience available to him has been highly variable.

At the same time, he has never been encumbered by more than very light clothes or bedding. He has never experienced the transitory malaise of colds or other minor infections. At least before he achieved toddler status he had a much freer existence, and much more opportunity to exercise his muscles and explore his limited environment than does a child reared in more conventional circumstances. From the very beginning of his extrauterine existence he has also been exposed to a rich variety of visual and auditory stimuli. Against this background I would like to review some aspects of his developmental progress.

In some areas, e.g., motor development and locomotion, he has been consistently precocious. Although he is at this time also advanced beyond the norms for his age in his social and affective development as well as in the use of language, the course of the emergence of these capacities has not been smooth.

At six months, he made babbling noises in relation to his activities -- an age appropriate activity. He did not, however, direct his vocalizations even to familiar observers when they spoke to him. To do so would also have been age appropriate. Whether he was on his hands and knees, sitting, or standing, rhythmic rocking came to occupy increasing amounts of his waking time during the period up to his ninth month. Although he was responsive to the overtures of others, during this period he made no effort by sound or gesture to initiate an interaction with another person.

At eight months, our speech pathologist* estimated his language development to be at a four month level. At 12 months, if he babbled (a 6 month achievement), he did so only infrequently. He would also squeal occasionally as he went about his play activities. He did not, at 12 months, ever try to attract attention by shouting (an eight month achievement) or make the phrase-like babbles which Griffiths lists as a nine month achievement. Throughout this period, he manifested a wide range of affective behavior. He reacted with evidence of pleasure when he was held and tossed about, became visibly angry when he was frustrated, and protested appropriately when he was subjected to the various procedures carried out by the medical team. However, we were impressed that he rarely, if ever, initiated contact with others by either voice or gesture, and he engaged increasingly in repetitive rhythmical behavior. Although he played with the wide variety of toys available to him, he evinced no interest in involving others in his activities. Typically, his play activities were also accompanied by rocking.

His disregard of his environment, the delay in prelanguage development, and the persisting involvement in rhythmical self-stimulatory behavior led us to reasses the quality of the care this child was receiving. In considering our findings and what appears to have been the results of our interventions, it is important to keep in mind that his is an isolated case. Conceivably, much of what has been observed during the subsequent four years could have been the result of maturational processess alone.

At the outset we were impressed that despite, or perhaps because of, the highly varying environment in which he lived and the very large number of people to whom he was exposed, he had significantly less opportunity to establish affective ties with any one person or even with a small group of individuals than would be the case under more typical conditions of child rearing. When he was in the hospital, he was subjected to the routines of a busy service. Whether he was played with or not depended on the work load at any given time. There was little socializing in the course of such routine activities as cleaning and feeding. It is noteworthy, for example, that even at 24 months he did not regularly participate in the feeding of himself. The reason given both at home and at the hospital was that it would be too difficult to clean up after him. It seemed to us that the isolating effect of his environment as well as the often perfunctory manner in which caretaking activities were carried out might be relevant to the relative retardation of language and social development.

----

*Mrs. Karol Musher of the Division of Audiology and Speech Pathology, Department of Otolaryngology, Baylor College of Medicine, made this as well as later evaluations. She also directed the speech training program which was instituted.

On this basis, we instituted a campaign of intensified stimulation both in relation to caretaking activities and independently of
them. A systematic program of prespeech stimulation was instituted.
In order to increase, further, his awareness of coordinated sight
and sound, a television set was placed near his isolator. A specific caretaking person was assigned to him during his periods of hospitalization. When he was at home, too, systematic efforts were devoted to playing with him both during the discharge of caretaking
activities and independently of them. Whether because of these efforts or coincidentally, within a few weeks, there was a considerable
increase in the amount of his "prespeech vocalizing" in the form of
babbling, as well as evidence of greater word comprehension. For
many months, however, his speech development continued to lag. When
he was 13 months old, his receptive and expressive language as well
as his speech were judged to be at the six to eight month level.
Although three months later, when he was 16 months his oral receptive
language abilities were found to be at the 16 to 18 month level, his
speech continued to be at the 12 month level. By the time he was
two, however, he was functioning at or beyond age level in both the
receptive and expressive areas. His vocabulary did, of course, show
some idiosyncracies which reflected the special nature of his environment. At the present time, he continues to be a bright, highly verbal,
friendly, and affectionate little boy.

IV

Taken together, the data I have reviewed seems to me to converge
on the conclusion that the development of communicative structures
requires, as a prior condition, the presence of a psychic substruc-
ture. This, in turn, is not related to any specific mode of communicating, i.e., oral, manual, gestural. Rather, it is a level of mental
organization which must be present if communication is to occur. As
a psychoanalyst, I am inclined to characterize this state in terms of
the differentiation of self and object, and the presence of internalized and libidinally invested object representations. These I would
regard as the minimal conditions which must obtain before the motivation to communicate can emerge. While without them it is certainly
possible for an individual to make articulated speech sounds, these
would have to be autistic and echolalic; i.e., without communicative
significance. Given, on the other hand, the presence of an appropriate degree of differentiation of psychic structure, communicative
structures will develop whether or not the vocal/auditory connection
is available. Were I approaching this problem from the standpoint of
a Piagetian psychologist, I assume I would use a somewhat different
terminology and, perhaps, place more emphasis on cognitive as opposed
to affective considerations. In either case, it seems to me, I would
be postulating an epigenetic process -- one in which the emergence firs
of the motivation to communicate, and secondly of the preeminence of an
particular communicative modality is dependent on the convergence of

several lines of development. For each such line, one can identify maturational, in the sense of gene determined, anatomic changes and environmental influences, both of which eventuate in lasting changes in the emerging psyche. Given the complexities implicit in such interrelations as these, the psychic manifestations would necessarily reflect the idiosyncratic aspects of the developing individual's experience. From the standpoint of communication, they might well be manifested in the meaning the individual might find in a given message. The three clinical vignettes which follow are intended to indicate how the semantic significance of specific communications can vary as a function of the stage of the individual's cognitive and affective development.

Fraiberg (1951) has described some of the vicissitudes experienced by youngsters who are presented with information they are not yet prepared to assimilate. As one reads her material, it seems apparent that the difficulties have at least two sources. The child's need to retain theories consonant with his level of libidinal development is evident. Some distortions, however, are not readily explained on the basis of libidinal considerations alone. Her six-year-old patient Tony, for instance, was convinced that in order for his father to discharge sperm, it would be necessary for him to have his penis cut open. Tony explained that this was due to the fact that the sperm (which he always referred to in the singular) was "as big as a marble." He came to this conclusion, Mrs. Fraiberg ultimately discovered, because he knew about reproduction from a book which contained an enlarged drawing of a single spermatozoon. As drawn, it was as perceived by Tony "as big as a marble."

A three-year-old boy whom I have had the opportunity to observe responded to the announcement that his mother was going to get a new baby by pointing out that he was not broken and demanding to know why he was to be thrown away. This concern was traceable to the practice of discarding old and broken toys, as well as to a series of mongrel dogs his mother would bring home from the pound, find unmanageable, and then have "put to sleep."

Finally, M. Wulff (1951) described a significant cognitive dilemma in an 18-month-old girl with phobic and compulsive symptoms. When playing, the patient always tidied the room and cleaned the floor. As soon as she noticed a scrap of paper, a crumb, or a thread on the floor, she had to pick it up and throw it into the wastebasket. These neurotic manifestations had begun in association with toilet training, when her parents would exhort her "to be clean." When, on Wulff's advice, they relaxed all rules and demands concerning bowel training, the child's symptoms cleared up completely.

The implications of these anecdotes seem to me to go well beyond the obvious dilemma posed an immature child when he is confronted with information beyond his ability to comprehend. Given the still emerging

state of such a youngster's psyche, the significance he imputes to
such communications, as well as his efforts to adapt to them, must
inevitably also affect his still developing psychic organization.
To the best of my knowledge, this is a relatively little studied
aspect of the genesis of later psychopathology. It seems to me,
however, also to be one which holds considerable promise for future investigation.

REFERENCES

Altschuler, K. Z. & Rainer, J. D. Patterns and course of schizophrenia in the deaf. Journal of Nervous and Mental Disease,
1955, 127:77-83.

Bowlby, J. Grief and mourning in early childhood. Psychoanalytic
Study of the Child, 1960, 15:9-52.

Davis, K. Extreme isolation of a child. American Journal of Sociology, 1940, 45:554-565.

Davis, K. Final note on a case of extreme isolation. American
Journal of Sociology, 1946, 52:432-437.

Eberhardt, M. Studies in the psychology of the deaf. Genetic
Psychology Monographs, 1940, 52:4-55.

Edelheit, H. Speech and psychic structure. Journal of the American
Psychoanalytic Association, 1969, 17:342-381.

Edelheit, H. (Reporter) The relationship of language development
to problem solving ability. Journal of the American Psychoanalytic
Association, 1972, 20:145-155.

Elkind, D. Developmental and experimental approaches to child study.
In J. Hellmuth (Ed.), Cognitive Studies, Vol. 1. New York:
Bruner/Mazel, 1970.

Fraiberg, S. Enlightenment and confusion. Psychoanalytic Study of
the Child, 1951, 6:325-335.

Fraiberg, S. Blind infants and their mothers. An examination of
the sign systems. In M. Lewis & J. A. Rosenblum (Eds.), The effect of the infant on its caregiver. New York: Wiley, 1974.

Fraiberg, S. & Freedman, D. A. Studies in the ego development of
the congenitally blind child. Psychoanalytic Study of the Child,
1964, 21:327-357.

Freedman, D. A. Congenital and perinatal sensory deprivation: Some
studies in early development. American Journal of Psychiatry, 1971,
127:1539-1545

Freedman, D. A.   Relation of language development to problem solving ability. Bulletin Menninger Clinic, 1972, 36:583-595.

Freedman, D. A. & Brown, S. L.   On the role of coenesthetic stimulation in the evolution of psychic structure. Psychoanalytic
Quarterly, 1968, 37:418-438.

Freedman, D. A., Cannaday, C., & Robinson, J. S.   Speech and psychic
structure. Journal of the American Psychoanalytic Association,
1971, 9:298-317.

Freud, A.   Normality and pathology in childhood: Assessments of
development. New York: International Universities Press, 1965.

Freud, A.   (1895) Project for a scientific psychology. Standard
Edition: 1:295-387. London: Hogarth Press.

Freud, S.   (1896) Letters to Fliess: No. 52. Standard Edition:
1:233-239. London: Hogarth Press.

Freud, S.   (1920) Beyond the pleasure principle. Standard Edition:
15:7-64. London: Hogarth Press.

Furth, H. G.   Thinking without language. New York: Free Press, 1966.

Gardner, R. A. & Gardner, B. T.   Teaching sign language to a chim-
panzee. Science, 1969, 165:664-672.

Goldfarb, W.   The effects of early institutional care on adolescent
personality. Journal of Experimental Education, 1943, 12:106-129.

Mason, M. K.   Learning to speak after six and one half years of
silence. Journal of Speech Disorders, 1942, 7:77-83.

Provence, S. & Lipton, R. C.   Infants in institutions. New York:
International Universities Press, 1962.

Rainer, J. D.   Observations on affect induction and ego formation
in the deaf. Paper read at a panel on "Sensory deprivation: An
approach to the study of the induction of affects." Meeting of
the American Psychoanalytic Association, Dec. 1973.

Spitz, R.   Hospitalism: An inquiry into the genesis of psychiatric
conditions in early childhood. Psychoanalytic Study of the Child,
1945, 1:53-74.

Spitz, R.   Relevancy of direct infant observation. Psychoanalytic
Study of the Child, 1950, 5:66-73.

Vernon, McC. Relationship of language to the thinking process.
  AMA Archives of General Psychiatry, 1967, 16:325-333.

Wulff, M. The problem of neurotic manifestations in children of
  pre-oedipal age. Psychoanalytic Study of the Child, 1951, 6:169-
  179.

ISSUES POSED BY SECTION 1

Fred Pine

Albert Einstein College of Medicine

Bronx, New York 10461

I have been asked to give an integrative discussion of the
three papers on early object experiences in the development of communicative structures, and to give that discussion from a broadly
psychoanalytic point of view. In thinking about what an "integrative"
discussion requires, I come up with two possibilities: First, an interweaving of the three papers, discussing the parallels, consistencies, or inconsistencies among them; and second, the introduction of
some higher order concepts that subsume the issues raised in all
three papers. I shall pursue both approaches.

The three papers are all rich; however, I shall not go into any
of them in intricate detail but shall merely try to extract certain
recurrent themes. And they do seem to me to have considerable overlap. Given the assigned topic of this group of papers, it is not
surprising, or perhaps I should say it is a pleasant surprise, to
find that the unifying theme is indeed the position of communication
in relation to early object (that is, infant-caretaker) experiences.

How to explicate the relations among the three papers? Let me
try this: I shall start with the central idea of Dr. Freedman's paper, and then try to show the productive counterpoint to this idea
that is suggested in Dr. Sander's paper and in the papers by Drs.
Beebe and Stern. Dr. Freedman suggests that the differentiation of
psychic structures precedes the differentiation of communicative capacities. Self-other differentiation in particular, both makes possible and creates a need for communication between the members of
the differentiated pair. Let me refer to just one of his several
examples, the contrast between the children raised in relative social
isolation. Two siblings raised in isolation by a psychotic mother,
presumably (I believe it is implied) with severe distortion of self-
other differentiation, never developed functional speech, but remained

echolalic even after being found and placed with foster parents; a
contrasting child, raised in isolation with an aphasic nonspeaking
mother, presumably with an at least reasonable chance of normal development of self-other differentiation, did develop usable and even
reasonably rich speech after the end of the isolation.

But to show the links to the other two papers, I have to highlight two additional points in relation to Dr. Freedman's paper.
The first is that he is not only speaking of self-object differentiation, but also of a self-object tie; that is, he is speaking not
only of a cognitive achievement of awareness of separateness, but
also of that complex cognitive-affective-motivational achievement
that we refer to with the term object relationship--the tie to the
differentiated other. The second point that I would like to highlight is that he is focusing on the acquisition of language; that is,
"communication" in his paper refers principally, though by no means
entirely, to verbal communication. If, then, his paper argues for
the significance of the achievement of self-other differentiation and
of object relationship in the development of verbal communication,
that is, if he advances the idea that a tie to a differentiated other
is prerequisite to the development of language, then in contrast--and
here is one link among the papers--the papers by Sanders and by Beebe
and Stern show the impact of preverbal communication in bringing about
those very achievements of self-object relation and d..fferentiation.
Let me restate that: Freedman advances the idea that a tie to a differentiated other is prerequisite to the development of language (and
higher order communication in general); by contrast, though with no
contradiction, the other two papers show the impact of preverbal communication in bringing about that very object tie and the differentiation of self and other. Thus preverbal communication "instruments"
the relationship out of which language later grows.

What Dr. Sander indicates in his work is the fine attunement between infant and caretaker from the very outset of life. By seven
and 10 days, respectively, in the infant's response to the mother's
masked face or to a strange caretaker, we already can detect signs
of infant-mother bonding. Dr. Sander suggests that there is a prefittedness between infant and caretaker that, as I understand it,
must blend into a readiness for subtle mutual shaping--a process of
learning. While there is undoubtedly some general prefittedness (we
are all human beings with parallel biological makeup), and some even
more specific prefittedness (each mother and her infant share common
genes) in our own work (Mahler, Pine, and Bergman, 1975), we have
thought principally of the readiness to fit together--more the learning than the prefittedness. That is, we have suggested that the (meta-
phychological) adaptive point of view is already highly relevant in
day one, that the infant is born with a readiness for adaptation, for
shaping to the style of the mother via the nonverbal cues exchanged
between them. Whether the mother is equally ready for such shaping

depends more on the flexibility or rigidity of her character than on anything inherent in her age and stage. But, in any event, the point is, to return to the link to Dr. Freedman's paper, that this mutual preverbal cueing and its consequent shaping effects is the earliest glue of the object tie. That it already exists in the predifferentiated period, before "self" and "object," yet exists as differentiated entities for the infant, goes without saying. Indeed, that glue of the relationship, embodied in the intimate shaping to one another, is part of what makes the achievement of differentiation so difficult and what brings it about that differentiation is accompanied by inevitable feelings of loss.

Turning now to the paper by Drs. Beebe and Stern, we see additionally the other pole expressed via the preverbal communications network: namely, the differentiating function of the communication process. That is: Freedman says that verbal communication follows on the attainment of a tie to a differentiated other. And Sander adds that preverbal communications, through body contact and through daily rhythms, are the earliest carriers of and bring about that object tie. And now Beebe and Stern add further that those very preverbal (here largely visual) communication modes serve a boundary-creating function, that is, serve in the differentiation process.

The infant that Beebe and Stern describe at four months is not in passive communication with its surround. Even the more-or-less automatic intake function of the visual apparatus has already been harnessed. Even when seemingly in almost no visual contact with the mother, this infant is recording enough (a "sieve" mode of function of the visual apparatus, letting a bit of information through and sampling it)--to stay out of visual contact with her in diverse and subtly attuned ways. That the attunement here culminates in avoidance behavior should not blind us to the attunement. The authors view this behavior as related to separation-individuation--visual communication with the mother, through visual tracking and through gaze avoidance, serving a boundary-creating function. The infant can separate and come together with the mother--all visually.

Through observations of bodily relationships between mother and infant a bit later on, we have made parallel formulations (Mahler et al, 1975). Seeing the infant in the mother's arms in the second half of the first year, an infant no longer content to mold passively to the mother but instead straining its body away to look around the room, we have conjectured that the infant gets bodily information that includes "something that holds and restrains" and "something that pulls away." Since the correlation of these two with mother (the holder) and self (the strainer) is near perfect, this gives information that subserves self-other differentiation (or in Beebe's and Stern's terms, boundary formation). I would add that the visual tracking and gaze avoidance, or the "chase and dodge" of this mother-child pair, is one more source of information (like peekaboo games

and examination of the mother's face) out of which the infant gradually puts together the concepts "I" and "not I." But to expand on
that would take me afield into further work we have done on infant-
mother differentiation, so I shall let the matter rest here. Let me
just re-emphasize that differentiation is achieved through innumer-
able preverbal communication processes between mother and infant.

So that is the red thread of the three papers, and, it seems to
me, of one major side of infant development: namely, that preverbal
communication--we tended to speak of mutual cueing, of responsivity
to one another's cues--<u>cements</u> the object ties, <u>fosters</u> differentiation, and, when successful, permits <u>later</u> advances in function that
include, among other things, communication through language. Dr.
Freedman suggests, as I understand it, that the combination of differentiation (from the mother) and tie to her, creates the need, the motivation to communicate, a need that is met through language. In an
earlier paper (Pine and Furer, 1963), we advanced a related idea. We
suggested that there was a kind of trade-off of preverbal and verbal
communication--that is, that one of the things that eased for the infant the renunciation of direct bodily communication with the mother
was its replacement by vocal and then by verbal distal contact (which,
not so incidentally, also interferes less with the toddler's growing
need for motor autonomy). But I would like to use this question of
the "need" to communicate as a stepping stone to the other issue that
I would like to discuss that crosscuts the three papers.

That issue has to do with the whole question of consciousness and
of intentionality that lies unsettled as we discuss the growth of communication. When Furer and I wrote of the preverbal to verbal communi
cation "trade-off," we carefully avoided any imputation of intentional
ity or consciousness to the infant; we remained neutral (i.e., ignor-
ant) on the issue. These three papers are talking about very differen
kinds of communication processes, and it is worth at least highlightin
the differences and pointing up the unsettled questions. This time,
let me proceed chronologically through the three papers.

When Dr. Sander speaks of the regulation of exchange in the infant-caretaker system, he is speaking of relatively <u>automatic</u> processe
at least insofar as the infant is concerned. Presumably the earliest
these processes are genetically built in, and we would not feel easy
speaking of the infant's intention to adapt to the mother and to the
cycles of behavior that she induces. But by four months, in the Beebe
Stern infant, what we are seeing makes it look as though major <u>learnin</u>
has already taken place. Naturally the learning, like all learning, i
based on the built-in potentialities of the apparatus, but we see an
individually-tailored mother-infant interaction. We can speak of
learning. Can we yet speak of consciousness of (in this case) the to-
be-avoided mother? It is not clear just what we would mean by that.
Can we speak of the <u>intention</u> to avoid? We just don't know. This
gets us beyond observation to inference regarding intrapsychic phe-
nomena--and that becomes difficult.

These are uncertain questions in regard to the infant's active behavior, that is, his adaptive and avoidant behavior. They are equally uncertain questions vis-a-vis the infant's sending of non-verbal cues outward. Just when the early information that an infant emits merely by being, changes over into intended, let alone conscious, communication is a very large issue, and one that Dr. Sander alludes to. Even reference to the later "need" to communicate is more a metaphor than anything else. How and whether the child feels such a need, how it is represented at different (early) ages, is something we can at present only guess at. And further, there is no reason to believe that the development of intended communication is an all-or-none process or a once-and-for-all process. Quite the reverse; there is every reason to believe that automaticity, consciousness, and intentionality all rise and fall at different moments and vis-a-vis different specific communications throughout the life cycle.

So much, then, for a few of the interconnections among the three papers. Let me now turn to my other comments--the other aspect of the integrative task--comments based on ideas that subsume all three papers. For that, I would like to discuss the broad area of object relationship and the concept of the undifferentiated phase. I am now making a major shift in these discussion remarks, going outside of the three papers, but I shall re-tie my comments to them as I go along.

1. First to the question of object relationship. It is of interest to make ourselves aware of a shift that is taking place, one quite consistent with classical psychoanalytic theory, but still representing a major new interest. Suddenly, object relationship is everywhere. In earlier psychoanalytic theory, the object was important (indeed it was defined) in terms of its position as the end point in the search for gratification. Reading these three papers, we begin to get a sense that the object relationship is primary, and that the drives function to deepen and introduce conflict into that relationship. It is really a chicken and egg problem; and fortunately we need not make a choice between these two positions. In the never-ending cycle of development where events constantly turn inward on themselves, there is room for both, both the primacy of drive and of object relationship. Only our attempt to make conceptual abstractions from the developmental process leads to too sharp a demarcation.

It is not surprising that psychoanalysis first formulated a drive theory. This has to do with the observational perspective. Listening to the patient in psychoanalysis puts us compellingly into contact with the urges and their affective and ideational derivatives that Freud conceptualized in his astonishingly unifying drive theory. Baby watching, where the inside-the-head content is not available to us, but where the mother's ministrations are, makes the developmental role

of object relationship equally compelling. As such, these three papers reflect and are examples of one of the historical trends (i.e.,
infant observation) that probably contributed to an increasingly central concern with object relations (and to object representations as
well--which are partially derivatives of object relations and partially of drive processes).

There were other trends as well that contributed to the turn to
object relations. Child analysis, group therapy, therapeutic milieus
in hospitals, and our compelling everyday sense of the present and
historic impact of other persons in our lives--were all part of the
Zeitgeist out of which grew a more articulated object-oriented theory,
including both actual and internalized object relations, as represente
in the works of Winnicott, Mahler, and Kernberg among others. The delayed development of such a theory was probably overdetermined as well
and not determined simply by the listening-to-the-patient perspective
that I have already alluded to (see Pine, in press). Technical features of analysis, interacting with social valuation, probably also
had a role. Care to avoid opening up analysis to the criticism that
its cures were only "suggestion," probably contributed to a leaning
over backward to deny the real power of the analyst in the patient's
life; clinical experience with short-lived transference cures led to
skepticism about the power of relationships alone to bring about cure;
and most importantly, both the therapeutic opportunities and the per-
sonal-professional dangers that grow out of the phenomenon of transfer
ence led to efforts to keep the analyst-patient object realtionship
"pure."

Be that as it may, these three papers argue that the advance of
the communication process is not just an unfolding of basic biological givens; nor is it a product solely of detour behavior of drives
through the cognitive-motor apparatus that makes up language; but rather, that communication is part and parcel of the tie to important
objects--stimulated and shaped by, practiced in, and functional for
those relationships.

2. And finally, a comment on the concept of the undifferentiated
phase as infant research speaks to that issue. Dr. Sander suggests
that, in contrast to the idea that there is, in the beginning, a rather vague undifferentiated period out of which infant-mother relations only slowly become organized, there is instead a highly organized relational system from the outset. Indeed, the first two papers,
in particular, since they are about very early development, suggest
that a great deal is going on in that early period. Let me generalize
the issue:

In 1939, in Ego Psychology and the Problem of Adaptation, Hartmann wrote that "in some cases it will be advisable to assume that
both the instinctual drive processes and the ego mechanisms arise

from a common root prior to the differentiation of the ego and the id" (p. 102). That is a cautious statement about the origins of psychic life in the human infant. But it remains for us not to be stymied by the lack of differentiation in the undifferentiated phase concept itself. Hartmann wrote at what was an undifferentiated phase of our understanding of infancy. Infant research and conceptual clarification both allow for a more refined statement today.

What is undifferentiated and what differentiated in the so-called "undifferentiated phase?"--that is, in the earliest period of life. To answer, we can only make constructions from the non-verbal cues offered to us by infants. Let me again refer to Sander, who writes about the earliest days of life. He suggests that we can't think of apparatuses waiting to be "used" as "tools" of "the ego," but instead as serviceable from the start in the regulation of infant-object exchange. These tools can be thought of as differen-tiated; but differentiation, like intentionality, which I discussed a few moments ago, is not either-or, not once-and-for-all. It varies for specific aspects of the person and from moment to moment. That certain "tools" of ego function are already available at the start, does not settle the issue of differentiation across-the-board. What, then, can we say? Let me try to lay out a schematic framework, re-cognizing that it certainly needs elaboration and correction. Here I leave the domain of infant-caretaker communication for a moment in order to provide a broader grounding for a coming together of infant observation and psychoanalytic developmental theory more generally.

So, then, what is undifferentiated in the undifferentiated phase? Ego and id? Primary process and secondary process? Anxiety and pleasure? Self and other? Libido and aggression? Let us take a very brief look, noting where infant observation has helped clarify our thinking.

As for ego and id, we can say nothing about their differentia-tion at birth. These are theoretical abstractions and no more. But if we turn to the ego apparatuses (that is the inborn givens for per-ception, memory, learning, etc.) and the biological drives, it is clear that they are differentiated from the outset. Development sees their integration, not their differentiation--the apparatuses becoming functional for the expression, modulation, control, or gratification of drive, and the drives lending special cathexis to aspects of appa-ratus function (see Pine, 1970).

As for primary and secondary process, I think it is not pushing the point to say that infant observation has been suggestive regard-ing the differentiated presence of the roots of secondary process thinking in day one. I am referring to the focused tracking reported by Wolff (1959) and the perceptual preferences reported by Fantz (1961) and others--all in the first day of life. As displaceability is the

distinguishing feature of primary process, so fixity (here represented
by sustained perception-attention links) is the distinguishing feature
of the so-called "secondary" process. Some time ago Holt (1967) wrote
on the development of the primary process. Consistent with that, I
would suggest that the task of development is not the differentiation
of primary and secondary process, nor the differentiation of secondary
out of primary process, but the elaboration of each out of their simpl
origins.

As for anxiety and pleasure, we have to change our terms to less
specific affect words. There is no reason to believe that signal anxiety, as we know it later, exists at the start. Observation of infant
states shows at times gradual, at times more rapid, state and mood
variations. It is in the nature of affect, being quantitative, that
it can rise or diminish and that one affect can gradually turn to
another. While infant affects appear differentiable (to the observer)
at the extremes, and presumably are experienced differentially by the
infant, they blend at some midpoints. I believe their continuing
differentiation very early on is not at all clear. Interestingly,
affects are not all that reliably differentiated later in life either-
with pleasure changing to anxiety, with depression blending with anger
and the like.

As for self and other, after reading these three papers we should
tease apart two components: the concept of self and other, and the
relationship of self to other. Our own research on separation-individuation (Mahler et al.,1975) leads us to believe that the concepts of
self and other are undifferentiated at the start (not because we have
seen that, but because we believe we see evidence that differentiation
takes place later on). Dr. Sander's work suggests that the relationship of self to other (of infant to caretaker) is highly articulated
from the start, though it is not clear to me that that can be describe
adequately by either the term "differentiated" or "undifferentiated."

And, finally, libido and aggression: Here, as with ego and id,
we are dealing with theoretical abstractions. To the degree that we
observe infant states, we shall see (as with affect) both sharp dif-
ferentiations and transitional states between things that look like
forerunners of bodily pleasure and of anger. But the concepts themselves are far from precise, and are highly complex, and I can say no
more about them.

Let me draw to a close. Each of the papers in this section show
an aspect of the relation between the infant and the object in the
genesis of communication. I have tried to show a major link among
them regarding the role of preverbal communication in making for the
self object tie and differentiation out of which later more complex
affective and linguistic communication grows; and I have raised at
least one question that runs through them, having to do with the non-
observable phenomena of consciousness and intentionality in relation

to communication. All of the papers reflect a concern with (1) infant-caretaker relationships and with (2) a specification of critical psychological events of the earliest periods of life--concerns that I have discussed, respectively, from the points of view of the theory of object relationship and of the undifferentiated phase.

The papers are very full and I have barely touched upon the many issues that they raise, but it has been a pleasure to discuss them even in this brief way.

REFERENCES

Fantz, R. L. The origin of form perception. Scientific American, 1961, 66-72.

Holt, R. R. The development of the primary process: A structural view. Psychological Issues, 1967, Nos. 18, 19, 345-383.

Mahler, M. S., Pine, F., & Bergman, A. The psychological birth of the human infant. New York: Basic Books, 1975.

Pine, F. On the structuralization of drive-defense relationships. Psychoanalytic Quarterly, 1970, 39, 17-37.

Pine, F. On therapeutic change: Perspectives from a parent-child model. Psychoanalysis & Contemporary Science, 5. New York: International Universities Press, in press.

Pine, F. & Furer, M. Studies of the separation-individuation phase: A methodological overview. Psychoanalytic Study of the Child, 18. New York: International Universities Press, 1963, 325-342.

Wolff, P. H. Observations on newborn infants. Psychosomatic Medicine, 1959, 21, 110-118.

SECTION 2
THE TRANSITION FROM
BASIC DIALOGUE TO
VERBAL DIALOGUE

INTRODUCTION

        The papers in this section span a period of ten years of de-
velopment beyond the first year of life. It is during this span
of time that we witness a rapid growth in the individual's ability
to communicate: a growth entailing the transition from early interactive and regulatory processes characteristic of the infant-
mother bond of the first year, to the emergence of communicative
organization--a change from basic dialogue to symbolic verbal dialogue. While much of this growth can be attributed to the development of cognitive competence per se, such competence does not insure
the integrity of the structure of communication in human interaction.
While there is a plethora of literature describing the growth of
cognitive competence from the toddler stage through latency and
early adolescence, there is little data of recorded communication
samples tracing the evolution of communicative ability. Three such
studies are included in this section.

        These papers highlight the fact that at each stage of develop-
ment we can observe a recapitulation of the kinds of regulatory
processes prominent in the origins of the basic dialogue. The patterns of regulation, elaborated operationally by the interactive
and boundary creating processes reported in Section I, aim at the
establishment of the basic psychic organizations upon which communication rests. Thus, they aim at the elaboration of more or less
internalized object representations, at the progressive differen-
tiations of self and nonself, and finally, at establishing intentional structures.

        The basic patterns for these regulations of the infant-mother
dialogue had been laid down by Spitz' "No and Yes" some years ago.
Kaplan, building on Spitz' ideas, focuses upon the more or less derailed maternal dialogue. Her account and definition of this dialogue highlights, once again, the central position of the early
self-object organization for the development of communicative structures. The basic dialogue is defined by the consummation of reciprocal action cycles between mother and infant. The derailed dialogue
entails the interruption of such action cycles. Kaplan is able to
demonstrate, in her analysis of the behavior of preschool children,
how completed or incompleted cycles affect the child's later ability

to initiate social contacts, engage in shared play, and to manifest empathy.

Dittmann, observing children almost 10 years older than those observed by Kaplan, describes a regulatory structure which he terms "the listener response." It is manifest by the listener's rapid verbal or nonverbal response to the speaker, phased in with the phonemic rhythm of the speaker's communication. Such listener responses show a remarkable upsurge during early adolescence, and seem to be indicative not only of increased comprehension in receiving or interpreting messages, but denote a capacity to empathize with the experience of the other. Thus, while the form of the interactive process changes, the basic structure remains amazingly constant across the age spectrum.

Norbert Freedman's paper highlights the fact that the communicative regulations which sustain the delivery and reception of verbal symbols, need not be interpersonal, but can be intra-individual as well. The proposal is advanced that the kinesic behavior which accompanies any interchange is the visible manifestation of structures which sustain and regulate communication. Such an interpretation of kinesics, as a form of auto-regulation which gates optimal stimulus input, is developed within a two factor theory of communication, involving the use of the motor system in both the establishment of shared representation, as well as emphasizing the use of the body for self-monitoring and the reduction of interference cues.

Freedman presents data showing that the motoric monitoring systems reflect a continuous line of development observable at all age levels. This view of kinesic behavior has important implications for the understanding of the pathology of communication (cf. Grand's paper, Section 3) and for communication during psychoanalysis (cf. Mahl's paper, Section 5).

The view of the regulatory role of motoric behavior in communication assumes that sensorimotor operations through increasing schematization and internalization, function as sustaining structures throughout life. Schimek, in his discussion, highlights this view and suggests parallels to areas beyond that of kinesics. The view of a hierarchic integration of earlier modes as supports for higher levels of functioning provides, in Schimek's view, a promising alternative to traditional psychoanalytic concepts of the way the past influences adaptive functioning. Such a view seems particularly fruitful for the understanding of the development of the capacity to communicate.

THE BASIC DIALOGUE AND THE CAPACITY FOR EMPATHY

Louise J. Kaplan

New York University

New York, New York 10003

In reviewing recent experimental studies of altruism in young children, including their own work, Yarrow et al. noted the hazards of interpreting findings which depend on relating experimentally contrived adult nurturance to experimentally elicited child-behaviors such as sharing, concern for others, and understanding of others (Yarrow, Scott, & Waxler, 1973). Results of experimental study of these variables have been inconsistent. "Nurturance is reported as having facilitating effects, no effects and depressor effects on learning" (p. 257).

Yarrow comments on this state of affairs:

"When one refers to nurturance in a child's socialization, it is to affectional and rewarding interactions through time. Processes such as the child's identification with the parent, or the parent's becoming a generalized reinforcer for the child, have meaning only in terms of a history of experiences between parent and child...When nurturance is brought into the laboratory what are its dimensions? Usually, it is a microexperience of 5 to 20 minutes of friendly interaction with an unfamiliar adult just preceding the primary experimental manipulation" (p. 258).

Yarrow goes on to recommend that future research focus on the origins of empathic and sympathetic behaviors in the context of the original mother-child relationship. One approach he says, "... might be the investigation of the earliest processes of differentiation of self from other. Somewhere in this domain one must look for the beginnings of empathic and sympathetic responding and the conditions that support or constrain this development." He adds, "Perhaps there is need to concern ourselves with not only the beginnings of

altruism, but also with how altruistic motives are lost or bred out
of the individual" (p. 263).

This paper is a demonstration of one way that Yarrow's recommendations might be implemented. At the New York University Mother-
Infant Research Nursery, we are conducting a study of the separation-
individuation process in young children. Our study affords an excellent opportunity to observe how the processes of self-other differentiation relate to the development of empathy. Descriptions of the
fate of empathy precursors in three female children who attended
the nursery will follow a statement of the relevant theoretical issues. The descriptions will illuminate the relationship between
issues of early self-other differentiation and the origins of empathy.

Margaret S. Mahler's separation-individuation subphase hypothesis acts as the primary guide for organizing the behaviors observed in the infants and mothers at the nursery. The children usually enter the nursery at around six months, somewhat after the end
of the symbiotic stage and at the height of the differentiation subphase of separation-individuation. Soon afterward, the children are
already demonstrating behaviors of early practicing where maturing
locomotor abilities stimulate further differentiation from the mother.
The mastery of upright locomotion at around 13 months ushers in the
phase of practicing proper, and for a time the child's joy in functioning supercedes his interest in the mother. If the mother is
available for occasional "emotional refueling," most young toddlers
are satisfied. However, each elated step away from mother increases
a toddler's self-awareness. By 16 to 18 months, this increasing
self-awareness makes the toddler feel alone and vulnerable, and he
once again renews his interest in the mother. This renewed interest
is characterized by demanding coercive attitudes, aggression, and
no-saying. The rapprochement crisis is then said to begin, and it
usually overlaps for a time with behaviors typical of practicing
(Mahler, Pine, & Bergman, 1975).

The data of this paper concentrate on the transition period
between practicing and rapprochement. Nevertheless, we continue
to see children in the nursery until they are about 26 months of
age. We, therefore, have the opportunity to observe some of the
initial resolutions of rapprochement.

It has become evident from the nursery observations that each
phase makes its distinctive contribution not only to the child's
growing differentiation between self and other, but also to cognitive and affective variables that could be thought of as precursors
of empathy.

As the study progressed, it became useful to conceptualize the subphase of separation-individuation as phases in the basic dialogue* between mother and child. The nature of the dialogue changes with each move toward differentiation and separation. Some mother-child couples are better attuned in some phases than in others. Some mothers, for example, provide just the right kind of emotional availability during practicing. They encourage independence while remaining as a secure home base to which the child may return for occasional "emotional refueling." During rapprochement these same mothers may not understand the child's sudden aggression and no-saying. The self-assertiveness, which is typical of the child's role in the rapprochement dialogue, may become muted.

The various phases of the basic dialogue make differing demands on a mother's capacity for empathy at the same time that they make distinctive contributions to the child's later ability to empathize with others.

Before extracting examples of empathy precursors from the observational data, it was necessary, first, to come to some initial formulations about the specific affective and cognitive features that might be associated with instances of empathy in later life. One does not expect to find true empathic responses in infants and toddlers. The strategy would have to be to look for the earliest expressions of the components that are associated with empathy in older children.

One set of findings that was particularly useful in generating these initial formulations came from Rosalind Gould's (1972) observational study of fantasy expression in nursery school children. She described two behavior constellations in these children. The first constellation illustrated what she called, "identification with the protector-provider." Children, whose fantasy play was said to be representative of this first constellation, demonstrated the following characteristics: a sense of entitlement, pride in themselves and in their achievements, flexibility of defense, a capacity for problem-solving and the invention of compromise solutions, a willingness to ask for help, and a harmonious balance between fantasy play and other learning activities. In addition, Gould emphasized that these children were trusting with others, and demonstrated empathy or understanding and consideration for the motives and needs of other children.

On the other hand, children whose fantasy play was indicative of "identification with the aggressor" also demonstrated the following: a demanding coercive inappropriate sense of entitlement, rigidity of defense, global forms of condemnation of self and others, too

---

*The term "basic dialogue" is from Rene Spitz's paper "Life and the Dialogue." In H. S. Gaskill, ed. Counterpoint: Libidinal Object and Subject, it refers to the nonverbal action exchanges between the human baby and its mother.

much or too little fantasy play, anticipation of blame, and an inability to work out compromise solutions. This second group of
children did not demonstrate understanding in their behavior with
other children. Furthermore, they displayed anger frequently, and
when they were hurt, they were unable to ask for help or seek protection or comforting. In other words, they did not expect empathy
or understanding from others.

Some of Witkin's (1974) findings in his investigation of psychological differentiation in 10-year-old boys were also valuable.
Empathy, "... or sensitivity to the moods, needs and characteristics
of others, which genuine empathy implies, and interest in interpersonal relations as well as freedom to engage in them, characteristically were found not among the limitedly differentiated children, but
among the highly differentiated boys whom we have called 'emotionally
soft' " (p. 266). In contrast to the emotionally hard, highly differentiated boys, who demonstrated emotional remoteness and aloofness
and manipulative behavior with others, these emotionally soft, highly
differentiated boys gave direction to their lives, "in their long-
range pursuit of meaningful interests and friendships and their ability to persist in the face of difficulties, to set and maintain their
own high standards of achievement, and to take on and carry through
responsibilities appropriate to their age" (p. 261).

In his overview on parent-child relationships that relate to
psychological differentiation, Witkin states that the structuring
of experience that leads to differentiation begins in infancy. Some
mothers, he points out, respond to a baby with sensitivity to each
need rather than indiscriminately or according to their own needs.
Other mothers have global methods of response to the child. Witkin
notes, specifically, those mothers who indiscriminately respond with
floods of stimuli to drown the child's discontent. Because of their
own needs these mothers seem to interpret the child's discontent as
reflecting a need for outside excitation. These children are handicapped in their growing awareness and in their capacities to interpret specific needs. Witkin sums up, "The ways in which a mother
contributes to an articulated mode of experiencing through her per-
ceptiveness and sensitivity in handling a child merits further study"
(p. 360).

As we have indicated, Spitz's concept of the basic dialogue was
a vital focus for understanding the development of empathy. In his
(1964) paper, he emphasized not only the important role of maternal
empathy, but also those features of the basic dialogue which could
either stimulate or interfere with a child's acquisition of the emotional and cognitive characteristics that comprise empathic responding.

In this paper, Spitz highlights the developmental consequences
of the interruption of action-cycles in infancy. It was his conten-

tion that the behavior patterns in the early mother-infant dialogue
consist of action-cycles with anticipatory, appetitive, and consummatory phases. When an action-cycle is interrupted before consummation, the child experiences unpleasure or anxiety. After a critical quantity of anxiety accumulates, discharge through ordinary
channels is no longer sufficient. The child becomes preoccupied
with need compensations in order to complete or finish the interrupted dialogue. Spitz likens these compensatory activities to Freud's
idea of the dream as a safety valve which protects the psychic organization from the dangerous consequences of unfinished action-cycles.
He also cites the experimental research on dream deprivation and the
Zeigernik effect where in both instances the failure to complete
leaves a residue and an urge to repeat. In instances of the interruption of action-cycles in the mother-infant dialogue, we would
expect that the need to compensate and the urge to repeat would take
precedence over, and interfere with, later age-appropriate consummatory activities leading inevitably to further interruptions of current action cycles. In more extreme cases, one would expect that
even compensatory activities, such as compensatory play, would become disorganized and nonconsummatory. Spitz put it this way:

"There comes a point at which the compensation of the accumulated undischarged appetitive readiness cannot be carried through
without seriously interfering with the normal functioning of the
organism. A conflict arises now between the need to compensate
and the requirements of normal everyday functioning. At this point
a vicious circle begins, for the need to compensate conflicts with
the consummation of normal function creating an increasing quantity
of unfinished action-cycles. These now will cumulate in their turn
and lead to the disorganization and disruption of the compensatory
attempts. The culmination of this process is what I call derailment
of dialogue" (p. 761).

Thus, with consistent and repeated interruptions of the action
cycle at the appetitive phase--before consummation--we can expect
damage to the capacity to master and understand the environment and
a breakdown in the ability to utilize future opportunities for communication and dialogue.

With more or less empathic mothering, a total derailment of
dialogue is not to be expected. Action-cycles would be disrupted
only over specific issues and the child's compensatory acts would
be manifest in specific areas only, leaving room for age-appropriate
mastery and consummatory behaviors with regard to current action-
cycles. Furthermore, each phase of basic dialogue requires empathic
understanding of different kinds of action-cycles. The appetites
and anticipations of practicing differ from those of rapprochement.
Interruption of an action-cycle may be characteristic of a child's
practicing period, but later rapprochement resolutions may then go
on to compensate.

In these preliminary formulations on the nature of empathy, the distinction between empathy and sympathy became another central issue. The nursery observations informed us that sympathetic reactions were not at all unusual in the toddlers. They often responded to another child's distress or pleasure by becoming distressed or pleased themselves. It was patently clear that any faithful rendition of empathy precursors would have to include a dimension or two that went beyond sympathy or the intuitive sharing of another's feelings, motives, and needs. Indeed, the confusion between sympathy and empathy often obscures the meaning of true empathy. Sympathy is commonly thought to be a component of empathy, but we frequently forget that sometimes sympathy can interfere with empathy. Paul (1970) argues forcefully for maintaining sharp distinctions between the two terms.

"Empathy is different from sympathy; the two processes are, in fact mutually exclusive. In sympathy, the subject is principally absorbed in his own feelings as they are projected into the object and has little concern for the reality and validity of the objects special experience. Sympathy bypasses real understanding of the other person and that other is denied his own sense of being. Empathy on the other hand, presupposes the existence of the object as a separate individual entitled to his own feelings, ideas and emotional history" (p. 340).

Empathy, then, would have components that evidence real understanding. Gould's finding that empathy tended to be associated with confidence in problem-solving, Witkin's description of the empathic boys highlighted their abilities to persist in the face of difficulty and to pursue long-range goals, and Spitz's emphasis that derailment of dialogue interferes with effective mastery and understanding of the environment, all point to the importance of problem-solving behavior as a central component of empathy.

In addition to her citation of confidence in problem-solving, Gould alerts us to behaviors that might indicate internalization of protective mothering, delight in the self, sustained make-believe play, a capacity to initiate dialogue with others, and ability to ask for help from other-than-mother persons. Instances of displacement of anger, too much or too little fantasy play, anticipation of blame, and the inability to ask for help protection or comforting should be noted as indications that weigh against the development of empathy.

Witkin's research leads to the expectation that an early component of empathy might be found in a toddler's "interest in interpersonal relations and the freedom to engage in them." In addition, observations of a global style of maternal responsiveness to infant need and a tendency to interpret a child's inner needs as reflecting a need for outside excitation would be seen as interfering with the capacity for empathy.

Spitz's observations on derailment of dialogue further enlarges the perspective of empathy precursors. It becomes important to define the specific issues over which the mother-infant dialogue derails, and to look for the child's compensatory efforts around these issues. Do these efforts become manifest in play or in dialogues with other-than-mother persons? In cases of more than mild or temporary derailment of dialogue, does a child become unable to compensate either in play or in alternative dialogues?

CASE STUDIES

The major portion of the case study section of this paper is devoted to the development of three children from the practicing period through the early rapprochement period which overlaps with practicing. A brief postscript describing the changes that took place later in rapprochement will conclude the case study section.

HOPE

Until the height of the rapprochement crisis, Hope had the benefit of prolonged empathic mothering. From the beginning, Hope's mother was specifically attuned to Hope's needs. She responded appropriately to Hope's anticipatory signals as well as to her appetitive child-initiated gestures. Our one concern during the earliest months of the project was that Mrs. H might be too altruistic--that is, too self-sacrificing in her efforts to assure that Hope's needs were instantly met. Mrs H often seemed scattered in her thinking, and she neglected her own appearance. Yet, when it came to Hope's needs or Hope's appearance, Mrs. H was efficient and nurturant. We sometimes thought that the close attunement between mother and child might delay differentiation, and that self-awareness would come late to Hope. However, we were reassured when Mrs. H returned to school part-time just after Hope's first birthday. And, from the time we knew her at eight months until her 18th month, Hope was a charming, thoroughly responsive child. At 12 months, there were already clear signs of emerging self-awareness.

During her practicing period, Hope was the freest in exploring her environment. The mother was carefully attuned to Hope's need to return to home base for emotional refueling. When Hope's exploratory forays began to run down or when Hope began to look fatigued, Mrs. H did not wait for Hope to become distressed or overly-tired before offering comfort. She recognized Hope's refueling gestures and beginning approach to her immediately, holding out her arms and saying, "You need a little snuggle." Hope would have her snuggle, and within a few minutes was full of her usual bouncy energy.

In fact, at 16 months, even though Hope could have been said to be in the rapprochement sub-phase both chronologically and in terms of her self-awareness and cognitive capacities, her mood was still the elated mood of the practicing toddler, and her approaches to her mother were for emotional refueling.

When her mother was out of the room, Hope was able to use others for "refueling." In addition, she was trusting in her approach to other adults. Her approaches were thoughtful and not indiscriminate or demanding. In her manner of approach, she appeared to take into account something of the perspective of the other. For example, in her approaches to the observers, Hope began by touching their pencils. She smiled and then held onto the pencils as though writing. Soon she began a babbling adult-like talk with the observers and really wrote in their notebooks. She was able to accept the fact that she had her own notebook and pencil to "write" with. She moved off to her own table and wrote, like an observer, in her notebook. It was not an unusual scene to find Hope sitting at her own table seriously writing away and occasionally glancing up to babble to the observers.

Hope's approaches to the other children were usually spontaneous, direct, and playful. Yet, there were times when she had to be resourceful in her approach. One morning, Hope was sitting quietly in the toy high chair munching on the cookies she was taking from a small bag which she held tightly in her left hand. Suddenly, she found herself without the bag of cookies, as Fay, the nursery cooky-snatcher had deftly relieved Hope of the bag. Fay had then run quickly to the other end of the room and was hurriedly devouring Hope's cookies. Hope sat open-mouthed with surprise staring at Fay. She thought for a minute, lowered herself from the chair, and without hesitation began to very slowly approach Fay holding out her hand and saying firmly, "please...please" with each step she took.

What was significant was that Hope's mother never asks Hope to say "please" or "thank you." However, Fay's mother was continually reminding Fay to say "please." Fay rarely complied with her mother's demand. The dialogue between Fay and her mother consisted of frequent daily reminders from mother of pleases and thank yous which were ignored by Fay. It seemed to us that Hope had thought through what had seemed to be a reasonable way of approaching Fay. She was, of course, too immature to comprehend the subtleties in the dialogue between Fay and her mother. It must be reported that Hope's well-orchestrated "please...please" was no more effective in getting Fay to share the cookies than were Fay's mother's efforts to get her to share and be polite.

Hope was more successful with Ivan. Ivan had returned to the nursery after a prolonged absence. For two weeks he rejected all the advances of the other children, and sat near his mother's feet or shadowed her around the nursery. Ivan loved to play ball with his mother and, whenever he could, he coerced her into a ball game. When Mrs. I ignored Ivan's ball game entreaties, he would collect all the ball-shaped objects in the room and lay them at her feet. One morning

as Ivan entered the nursery, Hope interrupted a game she had been
playing and searched the room for a ball. She ran gleefully up to
Ivan with a ball in her hand. She said, "Hi!" and tossed the
ball to Ivan, accurately landing it in his hands. Ivan was soon
thoroughly involved in the ball game with Hope, and for a few minutes
was able to have quite a good time without his mother.

At nine months, Hope had already demonstrated strong sympathetic responses to other children's distress. Characteristically, she
did not turn away from these distress scenes though they apparently
touched off distress in herself. Hope would stare intently, her
eyes welling up with tears if another child fell, hurt themselves
or cried. At that time, she was overwhelmed with her emotions. She
would end up crying herself and crawling quickly to her mother for
comfort. In the same way, when another child was notably happy,
Hope's face would radiate joy.

Hope was just 16 months, when we observed a make-believe play
sequence which symbolically reversed the painful result of another
child's accident. It may also have been a compensation for Hope's
own distress at witnessing the accident. In this instance the border
between sympathy and empathy is blurred. It would be hard to prove
whether Hope was primarily interested in alleviating her own distress.
Nevertheless, her behavior did demonstrate internalization of protective mothering and a capacity for coping with distress by invent-
ing a symbolic resolution:

Hope is playing with the small brown bear. She is standing up, holding him in her arms and cuddling him. She is very absorbed in this
activity. Kris gives a little gasp. He is standing upright on the
slide facing the observers, when he falls over backwards, face up,
flat on his back. Hope looks quickly in his direction just as he was
falling off the slide. She watches as he begins to scream pathetic-
ally. Kris' mother comes over and picks him up, rocking him gently,
and caressing his head. Hope has witnessed the whole event, and
stands now, riveted with attention at Kris and his mother, next to
the slide, clutching her teddy bear. She remains fixed in this position for approximately one minute. Slowly and thoughtfully she
carries her bear over to the slide, and then climbs onto the slide
with him. At the part of the slide that Kris fell off, Hope pauses
and positions the bear exactly at the edge in a precarious position,
as if considering whether or not the bear will fall as Kris did, or
whether she will save him from that fate. After about thirty seconds
of this, she apparently decides against the disaster. She sits down
in a position to slide down, with the bear held carefully between her
legs. She follows the bear slowly down the slide, holding his shoulders with her arms, and the rest of him between her legs. When they
reach the bottom, she gently bounces the bear up and down, and then
mimics the same action with her own body. She heaves a big sigh,
picks the bear up, turns him around, and smiling broadly, gives him

a huge hug. She carries him off to continue her play. (Total of four minutes).

The first recorded instances of make-believe play appear in Hope's records. At 16 months, her mother reported a number of repetitive play sequences at home.

Hope had been having a sleeping problem for several months, and the bedtime ritual had elaborated itself into three hours of anguish for the parents. At one point, Hope's parents attempted to resolve the situation once-and-for-all by comforting Hope and then closing the door, saying "good-night," and letting her cry. For some time after that, Hope was found throwing her dolls angrily into her crib and yelling at them, "No! No!" Hope would then pick the dolls up one by one and hug them.

During practicing and early rapprochement, toddlers play "chase me" games with their parents and confidently expect the parent to run after them and catch them. Hope, when her mother began to leave for school at night, elaborated the chase me body-action game into a make-believe game. Hope would pack her toy suitcase with her toys and blankets. She stopped at the door and said, "Good-bye," as she proceeded to disappear into the next room for several minutes, all the while babbling to herself. She soon returned on her own, and there was no invitation to "chase me." Hope then unpacked her belongings and settled down. The game was repeated several times each night just preceding Mrs. H's departure for school with her briefcase full of books.

From 12 to 19 months, Hope was the child who demonstrated more mirror reactions than the others. Her positive delight in her mirror image was always apparent. She would find at least one opportunity each day to parade herself before the mirror and smile happily at herself.

In conclusion, I should like to call attention to Hope's confidence in her problem-solving capacities. She was able to tolerate the heightening of arousal level that accompanies cognitive dissonance. She expected that her cognitive appetites would be consummated.

When Hope was 17 months old, Guy, a child who had moved out-of-town several months previously, came to revisit the nursery with his parents. All the children stopped their activities momentarily. They were apparently interested in the "new" child. After a second or so of puzzled staring, gaze aversion was the reaction of all but Hope. Hope continued to stare at Guy. Her body movements became increasingly excited--her state of arousal was high. She approached excitedly waving her arms, staring, and babbling at Guy. Her mother picked her up to say, "hello" to Guy who was in his father's arms. Hope continued to stare, and to move her body in an excited way.

Suddenly, she reached over to me with her body, almost leaping out of her mother's arms and into mine. I held Hope, and allowed her body movements to guide me into the reception room. She knew exactly where she was going, and knew that I was the one to take her there. I was led to the wall where I had hung the photographs of the babies from the previous year. I imagine that I had been selected to carry Hope to the photograph because Hope had watched me hanging the photograph the week before. Hope searched about the montage of pictures. She pointed as she found Guy's face, and then she shrieked, "Baby! Baby!" Her fists were shaking up and down with excitement. She had a giant smile on her face. Hope gestured for me to put her down, and she ran back to the nursery pointing to the real Guy, announcing to one and all, "Baby! Baby!"

I hypothesized that Hope's inventive sustained make-believe play, her delight in herself, her confidence in problem-solving, and the sensitivity of her approaches to others were derivatives of a basic dialogue relatively free of interrupted action-cycles. Such qualities of mind were likely to be found in older children who were described as empathic.

FAY

For the first ten months of her stay at the nursery, Fay played quietly at her mother's feet, watching the other children soberly. Mother and child played together in a subdued manner. They were never exuberant or high-keyed. During her first year, Fay was very much like her mother. Mrs. F was a somewhat self-effacing person who kept a low profile in the group. Fay also kept a low profile. They were a well-attuned mother-child couple with one exception. Mrs. F had an intense need for propriety. She was concerned that she do the right and polite thing at all times. She expected the same of her young daughter. At the least indication that Fay might appear to be a greedy or selfish child, Mrs. F would fail to respond appropriately to her. Even at our first interview when Fay was barely five-months-old, Mrs. F admonished her for sucking on the corner of my couch. "Now Fay," she shook her finger, "people don't bite couches." Oral greed became the issue most likely to interrupt the generally smooth relationship between Fay and her mother. Mrs. F would forbid the eating of cookies, sucking on a bottle, and thumb-sucking except at prescribed times and in prescribed places. Mrs. F would take Fay off into a corner of the reception room and hide Fay's face when she discovered her sucking on her thumb. Subsequently, we observed Fay's preoccupation with searching on the carpet for the cooky droppings of the other children--these were the only occasions when she would leave her mother's side. She became a food searcher, and notorious cooky and bottle snatcher.

Just after her first birthday, and shortly after she had begun to venture away from her mother to engage in independent play, we

noted that Fay's preoccupations with food and bottles interfered
with her capacity to enjoy early practicing play. Her preoccupations led to numerous disruptions in sustained play activity. Fay's
absorption in an activity could always be interrupted by the high
arousal value of food.

When Fay returned to the nursery the next Fall, her mother's
schedule of propriety included the following items: Fay will no
longer be demanding of my attention; Fay will learn to do things on
her own; she will play fairly with the other children and share her
toys; most importantly, she will no longer need her bottle--except
when dressed and ready to go home. Fay was then 17 months old. Just
about the only mother-child interaction that Mrs. F permitted, and
indeed insisted on, was the naming of objects, the naming and classification of colors, and the saying of "please" and "thank you." At
first, Fay was steadfast in her refusal to name correctly. Some
months later she was using naming as a way of insuring positive
mother responsiveness.

Within a few weeks after her return to the nursery, the big
rocking-horse had become Fay's favorite toy. It became a kind of
home base that compensated for Mrs. F's unwillingness to continue
to serve as a home base for exploration. When Fay entered the room
in the morning, she would stand holding onto the horse's neck or his
reins, soberly and quietly watching the other children play. Her
behavior was much the same as the way she had watched at her mother's
side the year before. Fay was extremely possessive about the horse,
and no other child could ride on it without Fay breaking down into
howls of protest. Fay claimed the horse in a greedy manner, and she
would ride on it incessantly. We felt that her extreme attachment
to the horse was also compensatory for the sensuous body-closeness
and intimacy which had been minimal in the mother-infant dialogue.
Fay's sensuous delight and her greedy territoriality with the horse
was a source of consternation and embarrassment for Mrs. F. "If I
take her off she will howl and make a nuisance of herself for the
rest of the morning. If I leave her on, she will become known as
Greedy Rocking-Horse Fay." After several weeks, Fay could tolerate
sharing the horse, but she would stop her play and watch apprehen-
sively when another child was rocking on the horse.

During her first weeks of return to the nursery, Fay was unable
to get on the horse by herself, so the problem of greediness was temporarily avoided. The following incident describes Fay's first interaction with her mother over the rocking-horse.

Fay is trying to mount the rocking-horse. Her mother remains at the
couch wanting Fay to try for herself. Fay watches her mother helplessly and makes several sounds of entreaty. Her mother says in a
quiet, persistent way, "Oh, Fay, you want to get on the horse?" Fay
tried to climb, slipping and sliding, onto the horse, but is still

unable to reach the saddle seat. She stops with a loud sigh and
rests against the horse mouthing the edge of the saddle and absently
stroking the horse's neck. She watches the noisy antics of Kris
and Hope listlessly, continuing to mouth the saddle....She tries
again, and vocalizes again, but is barely audible above the squealing
of the other children. Fay looks sadly and uncomprehendingly at
everyone's amusement, and again babbles her dilemma. She continues
to hold onto the horse, first the saddle then the rein, and tries
to mount again. No success. As she slides to the floor, one of
her feet lands on a piece of zweiback. Fay suddenly runs to her
mother and says in an asking tone, "cookie?" Her mother says, "Yes,
good," and rewards Fay's verbalization with a kiss. (Total of five
minutes.)

By the next week, Fay had learned how to climb onto the rocking
horse by herself. In addition, she discovered where to find her home-
going bottle, and also how to embarrass her mother into letting her
have the bottle when she wanted it. From then on, each morning Fay
would rock back and forth excitedly on the horse with her bottle
hanging triumphantly from her mouth. She would stop her rocking only
momentarily to get a few sucks from her bottle. Although Mrs. F was
embarrassed by her "Greedy Rocking-Horse Fay," she was no match for
Fay's persistence and determination.

Fay's mirror reactions were fleeting, and her reactions were
hard to read. There were three instances recorded of a decidedly
pleasurable reaction. At 18 months, Fay's play was largely of the
vigorous-large-motor-play type. She was much more outgoing, and
she sometimes played with the other children and mothers. In addition, she had acquired a streak of playful mischief. She retained
her quiet, sweet disposition, but was becoming decidedly unlike her
mother in her boisterous liveliness.

Fay demonstrated few examples of symbolic make-believe play.
The few instances of this type of play were not sustained. Fay
used a stick to pretend to comb her hair, for example. Nevertheless,
she did develop an interest in one doll. With this doll, Fay would
play games that her mother had played with her, but which the mother
characteristically had interrupted before Fay was satisfied. One
morning, while playing with the doll in this manner, Fay caught her
mother's eye. She looked mischievously at her mother, and carried
her doll over to the rocking horse. She placed the doll on the rocking horse and began to rock the doll back and forth, all the while
looking at her mother with a big smile on her face.

Fay was most watchful of the other mother-child interactions.
She soon learned that she could initiate dialogues with other mothers, and invite them to play with her in ways that her mother had
refused. Each mother was selected carefully for her particular game
style; Ivan's mother for ball playing, Jane's mother for gymnastics

and tickling games, circle games and dancing with Hope's mother.
On the morning when her father brought her to the nursery, she approached all the mothers for one thing or another, referring to them
as "Mommy."

When Kris fell off the slide, Fay looked distressed and worried.
Her brow puckered as she watched Kris' mother comforting him. But
Fay then averted her glance, dropped the toy she had been playing
with, put her thumb in her mouth, and became low-keyed for several
minutes. Similarly, when Guy came to visit, Fay stared intently for
a second or two but then averted her glance almost immediately. Fay
was good at solving problems that involved her personal needs. For
the most part, however, she seemed unable to tolerate the arousal
and tension that other problems demanded.

Fay was able to make effective compensations for the few issues
of interrupted action-cycles, both in her play and in her capacity
to initiate dialogue with others. She also showed signs of sympathy
for other children. There was evidence in Fay's behavior of being
able to hold onto a basic feeling of protective caring mothering.
She had enough sense of self-worth and self-esteem to persist and
to cope with some of her problems.

At 20 months, Fay displayed a combination of regressive compensatory activity such as her continued oral greed and her sensuous
delight on the rocking-horse, progressive compensatory activity which
allowed her to seek help and interactions with other-than-mother
figures, and also age-appropriate play activity and a number of well-
consummated dialogues with her mother.

JANE

As in the two previous cases, Jane and her mother were also
much alike in temperament. Both were intense, slender, small-boned,
and very pretty. Mrs. J engaged in continuous aimless movement.
Jane's movements lacked continuity and flow. They were both hyper-
alert and neither warmed up easily. Mrs. J was a very devoted mother.
She was possessive and overly-involved with Jane, but certainly not
a depriving, rejecting or ungiving mother.

During counseling sessions with Mrs. J, which became necessary
after a deterioration in the already symptomatic relationship with
Jane, Mrs. J remarked that Jane had always startled easily, and that
she seemed to be aware of the difference between mother and other
as early as four months of age. I gathered that Jane had been a
hard to console infant from birth and that her sleep-wake cycles
tended to shift rapidly from light sleep to high arousal without
intervening states. The similarity in temperament between Mrs. J
and Jane helped Mrs. J feel close to her baby. Yet, the probably
innate high arousal of both child and mother was certainly a major
factor in the disruption of their basic dialogue.

Mrs. J's inability to be stationary prevented the possibility of her acting as a secure home base from which Jane might safely explore the world around her. Mrs. J was constantly interacting with Jane and pushing her to achieve. She indiscriminantly stimulated Jane with age-inappropriate activities and play. Mrs. J was the type of mother, referred to by Witkin earlier in this paper, who regularly responds with floods of stimuli in order to drown the child's distress. The mother interprets the child's distress as a response to lack of outer stimulation. When Jane was distressed, Mrs. J was unable to comfort her. Her solution was to tickle Jane, to throw her in the air, or to try to get her to laugh. Mrs. J was unable to locate the source of Jane's discomfort. She often felt that it was her failure to provide stimulation that led to Jane's distress. Before she came to know and trust the nursery staff, Mrs. J would often blame Jane's distress on inadequacies of the equipment in the nursery. Mrs. J's high-pitched attempts to comfort and distract Jane would inevitably lead Jane to a peak of undischargeable excitement. Similarly, Mrs. J would abruptly leave the room just after several minutes of intense interaction with Jane. Jane would suddenly find herself alone, highly aroused, and surrounded by strangers.

During her first year at the nursery, when her mother left her alone in the room or even ignored her briefly, Jane would throw her bottle away and scream accusingly at the other children as though they had robbed her of her bottle--an action she had learned would bring prompt maternal attention. Head-banging was another characeristic solution to finding her way out of a stressful situation-- the most stressful being separation from the mother. Jane was almost 16 months old before she walked alone, although she had the maturational capacity long before then. For several months she walked holding on to her mother's hands, even though in all other respects she was the most agile and motorically competent child in the nursery. Jane was unable to request help from her mother except in self-destructive modes. Like her mother, Jane was unable to locate the source of her distress. It was as though she did not expect to be taken care of unless she was desparate.

When Jane was 18-22 months old, much of the activity of Jane and her mother consisted of a desperate over-aroused attempt to establish a dialogue with each other. At home, Jane was "impossible," "becoming a little monster," and "treating her father like a stranger." The predictable end to a morning in the nursery was a cumulation of tension overload that became a violent temper tantrum. There were few recorded instances of Jane playing with the other children or with the toys in the nursery. Her only momentary happiness came in those few occasions when she and mother found a satisfactory play interlude together. These, however, also left Jane unsatisfied. The timing and synchronization of play movements were never quite right. Jane was insatiable in her need to possess her mother totally. She

was thwarted in her attempts to achieve some kind of consummatory
dialogue with her mother, but she was unable to do anything else but
persist in these attempts.

Jane's stranger anxiety was intense. She was totally unable
to approach others and explore the possibility of an alternative dialogue. She was on the alert, and wary of any approach to initiate
dialogue with her. If approaches were made to her in any manner
but cautiously, indirectly, and avoiding eye contact, Jane would
run screaming to her mother. If other children approached her, Jane
would hit them or scream at them. The arousal of stimuli "other-
than-mother" was too much for Jane to tolerate.

Jane did not engage in symbolic make-believe play. When she
began playing with a doll, she did not know what to do with it, and
she would often end by throwing it on the floor angrily. Jane pur-
posefully avoided the mirror, and by inference her own mirror image.
Until her 22nd month, the only recorded event of a mirror reaction
was the following:

Jane runs over to the mirror. She seems very directed. She gets
to the mirror and looks at herself. She hits the mirror with her
right hand. Her mouth is part open in what appears to be a neutral
expression. She stops and looks at herself again. Now she begins
to turn away. She hits the mirror one more time. Then she turns
away, but still moves her right arm with the same hitting motion.
In doing so, she hits the wall near the mirror. She now turns 180°
and looks at the observers. Her expression is now a frown. She
moves to the table and sits down. (Total of two minutes.)

When she was being dressed on nursery mornings, Jane would
happily repeat over and over again, "School...school." Yet, for
three months, Jane would enter the nursery ready for battle, her
face screwed-up in a furiously angry expression. Jane's smiles
were rare and her typical facial expression was a pout or a sullen
frown. Some smiles appeared when she saw another child in distress.
Her most frequent reaction to witnessing another child's distress
was to hit the child or to hit her own mother. In situations involving her own distress, she would also often hit another child or
hit her mother or both.

The mother-child relationship during these months was characterized by ambitendency which Mahler (1975) says, "...soon develops
into ambivalence and is often intense...in these situations the
toddler wants to be with and at the same time separate from the mother.
Temper tantrums, whining, sad moods and intense separation reactions
are at their height in these children" (p. 292). When Mrs. J did
pick Jane up to comfort her, Jane would alternately cling and push
her mother away in prototypical rapprochement style. Although, to
some extent, Jane's behavior represented the typical rapprochement

toddler's dilemma, it is not typical for the crisis to be so intense, prolonged, and unrelieved.

In certain surprising ways, Jane was an acquiescent, compliant child. She did want desperately to please her mother. She complied with many of the mother's teaching instructions and took to the initiation of toilet training with astonishing equanimity. Moreover, at 20 months, she was the only child who did not protest when put in a horizontal position for diapering. Jane was demanding and aggressive, but she did not lay claim to own her own body. Her heightened self-other awareness did not link up with feelings of a justifiable right to be and act for oneself.

Jane learned what her mother expected her to. Nevertheless, her own problem-solving and exploratory behaviors were severely curtailed by her hyper-aroused state and her apprehension that her appetites would lead, not to consummation, but to a further accumulation of tension and arousal.

POSTSCRIPT

HOPE

Sometime during her 20th month, we observed a subtle alteration in Hope's behavior. The changes corresponded in time to Mrs. H's report that Hope was becoming temperamental and willful at home. In the nursery, Hope displayed very little willfulness or self-assertiveness. She was mildly coercive in demanding that her mother sit near her while she had juice, and she began to say "no" frequently, but certainly less often than other children. Mrs. H's response to the incessant "No" saying of the toddler group was to play a game with the children at the close of the morning session. "Alright," she would call out in mock cheer leader tone, "let's have it for Yes."

During this period, Hope's general mood became low-keyed and somber. On occasion she would become hysterically high-keyed and run around the room screaming at the top of her lungs. We saw little of the even-paced elated buoyancy of the earlier days at the nursery.

When Hope was 23 months old, Mrs. H declared triumphantly that Hope had gotten over her "bratty period." "She obeys very nicely now, and she can really listen to reason."

In the meantime, we noted that Hope had become increasingly helpless. Whereas previously she was delighted to show off her accomplishments, now she engaged our attention by asking for help with everything--even puzzles she had successfully put together several months previously.

Hope's charming style of initiating an interaction by imitating the other person now became her sole form of approach. She often seemed unable to approach another child before imitating them.

In the event of altercation about possessions or territorial rights, Hope could not hold her own. She was beginning to strike the observers as "incompetent" and "unresourceful." Her mother was little help in stimulating Hope's problem-solving abilities. Mrs. H would sigh, "Hope can't get on the horse. You know, I can't figure out how to do it myself. I couldn't even begin to explain it to her." When it came time to commence with toilet training at 24 months Mrs. H expressed her total bewilderment about just how to go about the process. She decided to take Hope to Jane's house in the afternoons so that Hope could imitate Jane's successful behavior.

Hope's approaches to her mother did not include the typical rapprochement desire to share achievement with the mother. Hope's feeble attempts to arouse her mother's interest in new accomplishments were usually ignored. Hope's approaches up to the 26th month were still of the emotional refueling type. She would periodically climb on her mother's lap for a snuggle and a bottle of milk—an approach her mother continued to encourage.

Hope retained her joyous reaction to her mirror image and her interest in other people. She was animated and happy whenever she was with another person, but subdued when left to her own devices. The symbolic play that had flourished so extravagantly at the beginning of rapprochement disappeared altogether both in the nursery and at home.

The precursors of empathy that were apparent at around 18 months had all but vanished. Hope and her mother had their most attuned dialogue during the first year and one half. Mrs. H was not as able to respond to the rapprochement toddlers need for self-assertion and independent achievement. The rapprochement dialogue had been silenced almost as soon as it had begun.

FAY

Fay and her mother went on battling over Fay's greediness. Every so often, Fay would comply with her mother's wishes that she share her toys, and not eat too much, and not complain too much about not having a bottle. Yet, the next day we would observe a prolonged bout of constant thumb-sucking, overeating, persistent furious claims that the rocking horse and the stove were, "mine," and angry hurling of the training cup that was meant to substitute for her bottle.

Fay, however, had been successfully toilet trained by 22 months. Her delight in being able to please her mother around this issue was

apparent to all. Fay became our most competent trash collector and
table wiper. At home, and at school, she engaged in sustained make-
believe play sequences. She was a friendly child who willingly accepted the overtures of others. Fay was adept at defending her
rights with the other children. And, she knew how to work out a
good trade when she wanted something that somebody else had. Her
pride in independent achievement did not preclude her being able to
ask for help when she needed it.

Fay was skillful, and she happily referred her accomplishments
to Mrs. F for approval. Although Mrs. F did not like "bragging,"
she was obviously pleased with Fay. Mrs. F still overly emphasized
proper learning, but she was also competent at teaching Fay what Fay
wanted to know. Her efforts to make Fay into an independent, resourceful child were now taking root. What had seemed a somewhat
harsh ignoring of Fay's desires for help and body contact in the
first year, began to look more appropriate to Fay's development.
Occasionally, Fay's appetite for body contact and oral gratification
continued to interrupt her otherwise well-developing skills and com-
petencies. For the most part, though, she seemed pleased with herself, and she thoroughly enjoyed her relationships with other people.

JANE

At 26 months, we noted some easing of the strained relationship between Jane and her mother. Mrs. J had learned to relax a
bit, and she permitted herself to sit quietly in one place while
Jane played. Jane often interrupted her play to approach her mother
for the "refueling" she had missed during her earlier months at the
nursery. Jane would lean her back against her mother's knees and
suck contentedly on her bottle while Mrs. J gently stroked her hair.

Jane was now able to make friendly overtures toward the other
children and selected members of the nursery staff. A few instances
of symbolic play were observed. Jane would wash a doll's face or
put it to bed. However, the play sequences were brief, and Jane appeared to be tense. Jane still never smiled at herself in the mirror.
She continued to greet her mirror image with a pout or a frown. Weeks
would pass without a temper tantrum. Nevertheless, when Jane was
tired, the suspicious, wary, and quickly-distressed Jane, would return with full force. Even on her best days, Jane was wary and tense.
She continued to misinterpret friendly approach as an attack.

At home, Jane had begun to be affectionate and playful with her
father, and she was able to feel comfortable in her mother's absence.
Jane finally made claim to her body by insisting on doing everything
herself in her own way. Nobody, including her mother, could help her
with anything, and no one could share an activity with Jane. When she
had difficulty, if anyone intervened to help her, Jane would cry bitter
tears and sometimes have a temper tantrum.

SUMMARY

We have approached the study of empathy in young children by
describing the unfolding of empathy precursors within the domain of
the basic dialogue during the first two years of life--the period
of self-other differentiation.

Each phase of the basic dialogue between mother and infant
makes its specific contributions to the earliest expressions of the
cognitive and affective components of empathy. It would be premature to predict whether Fay or Hope will be the more empathic child
later on. But, an important lesson can be gleaned from the case of
Hope. If we were to have based predictions solely on her development up to 18 months, the conclusion would likely have been that Hope
would be unusually empathic. The subphase theory of separation-
individuation cautions that the whole story is not told until all
phases make their contribution. And even then, the later contribution of Oedipal relationships often reorganizes and redistributes
the developments of the preoedipal period.

As for Jane, it could be stated with some degree of confidence
that the continuing stranger anxiety, the prolonged lack of trust
in others, the need to blame for inner tension, the low self-esteem,
and a style of competence based on total self-sufficiency all speak
for an enduring character structure that would preclude the capacity
for empathy.

Ultimately, however, this was not intended as a predictive
study. The study set out to generate hypotheses about the precursors of the later components of empathy. The primary aims of the
study were to discover, illuminate, and describe some of the details
suggested by Yarrow's recommendation that the sources of empathy
might best be investigated by observing the earliest processes of
self-other differentiation.

Using the model of Spitz's theory of derailment of dialogue
and Mahler's formulations of separation-individuation, this study
suggests some of the conditions which may lead to a diminution of
the empathic capacity. Throughout, the emphasis has been on the
intimate connections between empathy and the capacity to tolerate
appetitive arousal in other cognitive and affective realms. Empathy
has been described as a problem-solving activity that depends on
separation between self and other, and trust in the self and in
others. On the other hand, a diminished capacity for empathy would
be likely to appear within the context of heightened stranger anxiety, low self-regard, and intolerance of appetitive arousal with repetitive efforts to discharge the residues of the unconsummated interrupted action-cycles of the basic dialogue.

REFERENCES

Gould, R. Child studies through fantasy. New York: Quadrangle
  Books, 1972.

Mahler, M. S., Pine, F., & Bergman, A. The psychological birth of
  the human infant. New York: Basic Books, 1975.

Paul, N. Parental empathy. In E. James Anthony & Therese Benedek
  (Eds.), Parenthood. Boston: Little, Brown, 1970.

Spitz, R. The derailment of dialogue: Stimulus overload, action
  cycles, and the completion gradient. Journal of the American
  Psychoanalytic Association, 1964, 12:752-755.

Witkin, H. A., Dyk, R. B., Faterson, H. F., Goodenough, D. R., &
  Karp, S. A. Psychological differentiation. New York: Wiley, 1962.

Yarrow, M., Scott, P., & Waxler, Z. Learning concern for others.
  Developmental Psychology, 1973, Vol. 8, No. 2, pp. 240-263.

HANDS, WORDS, AND MIND: ON THE STRUCTURALIZATION OF BODY MOVEMENTS

DURING DISCOURSE AND THE CAPACITY FOR VERBAL REPRESENTATION[1]

Norbert Freedman

Downstate Medical Center

Brooklyn, New York 11203

INTRODUCTION

Harold Bloom (1973), in his quest to depict the relationship of one poet to another, put forth a forceful idea--the anxiety of influence. The poet, in his effort to preserve the integrity of his creative thought, must continually ward off the intrusion of his predecessors. He turns his energies upon himself to retain this autonomy, and often achieves it at terrible cost. The verbal dialogue in human discourse is far from a poetic dialogue, but, it too, is governed by the anxiety of influence.

The articulation of experiences in a communicative setting is an awesome task, the understanding of which challenges our imagination. Communication requires the transformation of image and experience into symbolic form. Such a transformation entails both a state of being in touch with the sensory quality of experiencing and the disciplined shaping of the experience into shared symbolic form. Communication, as an act of sharing, implies communion. At the same time, communication calls for selection and disembedding, for there are numerous influences from without and interferences from within that must be excluded. Those experiences to be shared must first be ordered and brought into focus. The first task is that of representing; the second is that of focusing. Representing and focusing, of course, alternate in any communicative interchange.

[1] This research was supported in part by Grant No. MH-14383 awarded by the National Institute of Mental Health, United States Public Health Service.

Representing is an activity akin to what Werner and Kaplan (1963) refer to as symbol formation as applied to external speech. It must be distinguished from representation--it is the <u>activity</u> which casts the representation into public view, and this activity, of necessity, involves the experience of a motor act. Representing fundamentally involves connecting image to symbol, and always entails some intervening activity which sustains the connection. It also involves an intention to share the image and, hence, entails an object relationship. Focusing, on the other hand, does not imply that an image has already been selected for representation, for before a thought can be shared, it must first be retrieved, ordered, and sorted. There must occur a reduction of multiple alternatives. One of the most challenging aspects of communicative speech, as George Klein has noted (1965), is to exclude that which is not to be stated. Such selection or exclusion of alternatives requires the implementation of support activities, and particularly the affirmation of self and nonself. Where representing signifies "yes" and sharing, focusing implies "no" and disembedding--a momentary separation from the listener to gather and coordinate one's thoughts. Both representing and focusing are physically visible in any interpersonal transaction.

Any sample of a communicative interchange between two people (as seen for example on video tape), allows us to witness a dance, a dance in which torso, hands, and head move in rhythmic accompaniment to speech--a dance where, during pausing, there occurs a retrenchment and a focus upon the self. Such a dance can be viewed as the nonverbal signal system of a particular culture, much as it may be recorded by an ethnologist observing a tribal ritual. It can be regarded as an act of influencing behavior, a nonverbal description of the act of persuading and yielding and, indeed, this is the tack taken predominantly in social psychology today. It can also be regarded as the vestiges of a primitive past carried into the contemporary situation. In contrast, we have by now amassed some convincing observations which attest to the central role of movement behavior in the processing of information. Body movements have been linked to measures of cognitive style or linguistic competence, quite apart from the speaker's cultural background or the power relationship in communicative discourse (Freedman et al.,1972; Freedman & Steingart, 1975). Even blind individuals, who have not learned the significance of gestures as signs or signals, move their hands, head, or feet while they speak (Blass et al.,1974). From an information processing viewpoint, motions of the body during discourse are a requirement which sustain the processes of representing and focusing.

How then do we understand the impact of bodily activity upon cognitive processing? In general, we hold that bodily action evokes a <u>kinesic experience</u> which serves to confirm existing schemata, and may even help to "bind" image to word. We use, here, the term "experiencing" as a construct, as used by Escalona (1963) in describing the

infant's experiencing of the maternal object. It does not imply
that action causes thought to occur, but rather that it is felt by
the speaker to be an integral part of his communicative structure.
That physical activity serves as a nutriment, as a building block
for schema formation in infancy, has been widely accepted (Held &
Hein, 1963; Klein, 1965; Piaget, 1952; Rapaport, 1951). That activity continues to exert a sustaining influence in the encoding and
organization of thought throughout life has been much less documented.
It is contended here that body acts, as kinesic experience, provide
the kind of support which is essential for the secondary process.
While bodily activity has been linked to various aspects of cognitive
processing, what has not yet been shown is that such activity may refer to relatively independent subsystems having a bearing on the
processes of representing and focusing.

This paper, then, will present data pertaining to the role of
body movement, as kinesic experiencing, contributing to a more or
less effective verbal representation during discourse. The work to
be covered will review a series of studies carried out by my colleagues Felix Barroso, Wilma Bucci, Stanley Grand, and myself, at
the Clinical Behavior Research Unit at Downstate. We shall succes-
sively examine three major issues, each of which has a central bearing on the identification of those psychic structures which make communication possible.

The first issue is concerned with the identification and definition of two discrete structures which sustain the communicative process. There is an enactive kinesic system organized toward the representing of thought, and a supportive kinesic system organized toward
the attaining of focal attention. The enactive system is exemplified
by Freud's comment that "If her lips are silent, she chatters with
her fingertips"; or by the notion of depictive gestures, as used by
Werner and Kaplan (1963). The supportive kinesic system is akin to
what both Spitz (1945) and D. Freedman (Chapter 3) have described under the heading of coenesthetic organization; it has the properties
of diffuseness rather than localization. It lacks variations in intensity, and appears to make the person refractory to further sensory
stimulation. The supportive system emphasizes the importance of various forms of stimulation (auditory, visual, or motor) in disembedding
the self from the field. Effective communication requires an adequate
balance between enactive and supportive experiences. Grand, in a
paper to be presented later, will show how the imbalance of enactive
and coenesthetic experiences becomes the hallmark of the pathology of
communication. In the first section of this paper, we shall present
experimental observations which define the functions of kinesic representing and focusing.

The second issue is concerned with the evolution of representing
and focusing behavior. Both enactive and supportive systems have

their roots in earliest developmental stages. We already noted that
most cognitive and psychoanalytic theorists agree upon the central
role of body action in the early formation of psychic structures.
Piaget's sensorimotor period (1952), Freud's trial action (1957),
Bruner's enactive representation (1967), all attest to the physical
beginnings of thought. But as complex symbolic operations take over,
mention of bodily activity fades away, and it is viewed either as regressive manifestations or as epiphenomena of little functional consequence. Indeed, it is often asserted that the inhibition of motor
activity is central to the development of the secondary process. The
argument, here, is in the opposite direction. It may be wiser to
speak of an evolution rather than a decline or inhibition of motor
action. What is called for is a set of developmental norms to define levels of representing and focusing activity which are optimal
for verbal representation. Toward this end, in the second part of
this paper, we shall present findings from a developmental study
tracing changes in representing and focusing in successive age groups

   Thirdly, there is the issue of the integration of representing
and focusing structures. Adequate verbal representation requires,
in part, a balance between enactive and supportive systems; it also
calls for the deployment of such motor activity at optimal developmental levels. Moreover, such communicative structures, to be effective, must be ordered according to a planful and purposive sequence
We shall develop the specific hypothesis that the more effective verba
representation occurs when focusing precedes representing behavior.
This issue will lead us to shift from experimental and developmental
observations to the kinesic-linguistic study of clinical interviews.
We shall consider body movements and language context as they appear
in an associative monologue--a situation akin to the analytic setting

   In our observations evaluating these three issues, we have
largely relied upon movements of the hands. Hand movements have a
critical developmental root. Stone (1961) has noted that in phylo-
geny, the availability of a highly versatile pair of hands together
with the development of speech are the most important foundations for
human capabilities. Wolff (1952) considered the hands the fundamenta
vehicle for the study of the structure of thought. The majority of
Piaget's examples of schema formation during the sensorimotor period
refer to motions of the hands. Hand movements are not the only physical manifestations of cognitive processing in communication. There
are postural shifts, facial display, head nods, or foot movements.
The hands are the most frequent, regularly occurring, quantifiable,
and psychologically revealing bits of overt behavior available for
objective study. In our focus on hand activity, we regard these
movements as markers, as signposts of certain cognitive operations
which must be coordinated with other bodily adaptations (foot movements, eye gaze, etc.) for a fuller understanding of the processes
involved.

THE BASIC COMMUNICATIVE STRUCTURES: REPRESENTING AND FOCUSING

The bodily manifestations of representing are none other than
common communicative gestures, or as we have called them, object-
focused movements. The object-focused movement is a motion of the
hand accompanying speech, phased in with rhythmic or content aspects
of the verbal utterance, usually directed away from the body. The
bodily manifestations of focusing are provided by various forms of
self-stimulation--body-focused activity. Object- and body-focused
movements can be elicited experimentally by a specified set of psychological conditions, and these conditions even reveal their psychological function. Let us consider a 10-year-old as he is first asked to
define a word such as "vase" or "hammer." This task induces object-
focused movements depicting the shape of the object or the action
which illustrates its use. Then let us consider the same child solving a version of the Luchin's can problem. "Suppose I want to have
three pints of water, and suppose I have a can which I can fill with
one pint of water and a can which I can fill with two pints of water.
How can I get exactly three pints of water?" The action of pouring
the two cans into one is played out with the hands, while the child is
giving the verbal response to the solution. Then let us consider
the same child, again, when we ask him to perform the interference
task of the Stroop Color-Word test where the child is presented with
the word RED printed in the color blue, and is then asked to name
the color of the ink, disregarding the word. This task evokes continuous self-touching, mostly of the finger/hand variety. The object-focused movements for the first two tasks, and the body touching for the third task, seem almost obligatory, and the statistical
differentiation between tasks was massive. Observations such as
these led to some formulations concerning the role of object-focused
movements as a manifestation of representing activity, and body-focused movements as focusing activity.

When an individual punctuates, qualifies, depicts, or concretizes
his message, he creates, by means of a condensed motion (which not only
expresses or communicates his image, but which also buttresses in
feedback fashion), the image he seeks to represent. Object-focused
movements, when they occur, have all the constituents of representing:
a private image (a hammer), an arbitrary symbol (the spoken word), and
an action directed toward the object of presence. When there is
some strain between image and symbol, the action arises which creates
a kinesic experience at the very point at which the arbitrary symbol
must be articulated. Through depicting the size, shape, motion, or
relationship of the private schemata, the existence of the object is
confirmed--hence, object-focused movements. This motor act not only
buttresses the image, but acts to cement its connection to the symbol,
and it is this connecting process which seems to be the central psychological function of this activity. Through confirmation of image,
and through the work of connecting the image to the word, object-focused activity ensures the continuity of representing.

Just as object-focused movements arise when there is some strain between image and symbol, body-focused activity appears when an individual experiences an interference with his focus of attention (the word RED printed in the color blue). A disturbance in the pattern of stimulus input (inducing a confusion in ordering or selecting) calls forth the compensatory tactile stimulation of the body's surface. When a person is confronted with ambiguous cues, interfering cues, or conflicting cues during communication, the speaker is likely to turn to soothing, grooming, rubbing, or scratching. We suspect that these forms of tactile stimulation not only regulate sensory input, but have the role of confirming the boundaries of the self at the very time when the sharing of thoughts is also required. Just as object-focused movements are a confirmation of the existence of an object, so are body-focused movements a confirmation of the existence of the self during communication.

Experimental observations of representing and focusing behavior. The kinesic experiences, which appear to confirm the existence of inner representations, can be observed in experimentally created conditions. Barroso et al. (a, in preparation) was able to induce object-focused movements through presentation of the can problems described earlier. He noted that the child's actions depicted the action scheme, and also frequently preceded verbalization onset. Here, then, we are dealing not only with a confirmation of the image, but with a kind of cognitive rehearsal.

While the kinesic experience may buttress the clarity of the image, the foregoing study has not shown that such increased clarity will also buttress the linguistic representation and, hence, sustain fluency. This word-cementing function of object-focused movements has been shown in a most recent study by Bucci et al. (in preparation) Bucci compared the video-recorded communicative behavior of two groups of college students whom she termed "symbolizers" and "nonsymbolizers" Symbolizing was defined by the ease with which a subject was able to name a color in response to seeing a color blot. This, indeed, is the definition of representing. In examining the kinesic behavior of the subjects, she found that the object-focused movement rate among symbolizers was about four times the rate of that for nonsymbolizers. More significantly, verbal competence, verbal fluency, or speech rate was identical among the two groups. But the range of association, as reflected by the specificity of images depicted, was infinitely richer in the symbolizing group. It is as if the beat-like accompaniment of motor acts kept the symbolizers in touch with the sensory "stuff" of their mode of representation. Miller's (1963) experiment comes to mind in which he asked subjects to accompany words with action or inaction, and found that the bodily activity seemed to facilitate the meaning as well as the retention of word symbols.

The object-focused movements in Bucci's study included not only depictive representational acts, as in Barroso's study, but speech primacy movements which emphasize or qualify, but do not describe. Clearly, there is a range of object-focused movements, and their developmental significance will be considered in the next section. In spite of this range, all object-focused movements contribute to the connection between image and word. We may put forth a model in which the movement acts like a representative to congress. When there is difficulty in the constituency (the thing being represented), he or she hurries home to buttress the troubles which have arisen; and, when the needs of the district have been clarified, he takes the shuttle back to congress to write the bill. In similar fashion, object-focused movements may be deployed in different directions. At one point they are evoked to buttress the image, and at another point to buttress the word. Yet, their common beat-like accompaniment to speech appears to be instrumental in increasing the range of ideational flow. This cementing function becomes most evident in the clinical situation where one can observe patients with a difficulty in representing. Both chronic schizophrenic patients or geriatric patients reveal a depletion of object-focused activity. They still retain the memory of the verbal chain, but their ability to connect their utterances to experience has been shattered.

This interpretation of object-focused movements as cementing is at variance with current interpretations of kinesics. Are not object-focused movements a manifestation of a particular culture? To be sure, the size or shape of gestures differ between Sicilian or Anglo-Saxon. But some beat-like accompaniment of speech by the hands can even be observed during communication among persons in a London pub. Movements occur at a point at which an image must be symbolized, usually at the onset of a phonemic clause, and this may be presumed to be true regardless of the speaker's cultural background. Further, are not object-focused movements the manifestations of a nonverbal attempt to influence the transaction? They may be signs of affiliative needs (Rosenfeld, 1966), or persuasiveness (Mehrabian, 1969), yet the very impact of persuasiveness may be derived not from the extention of the arms, but from the fact that the listener senses that the speaker, via enactment, is in touch with his representational world. This is probably the source of the success of actor and orator alike. Mahl's experiment (1968), in which he observed the speaker who neither saw his listener not felt he was being seen, is most pertinent. Object-focused movements persisted under these conditions even when there was no listener to be influenced.

The appearance of object-focused movements in communicative speech depends on the presence of an image which must be represented. If such an image is not in focus, there can be no representation. Klein (1965), in particular, has noted that in communication, the individual must surround himself with support conditions which regulate environmental interference and sustain an optimal focal attention. Such a process becomes manifest by the patterns of body-focused activity.

For some time, we have been struggling to find an adequate formulation concerning the psychological functions served by self-stimulation during discourse. In an earlier study, in a simulated clinical interview situation (Freedman et al., 1972), subjects were exposed to two experimental conditions: confrontation with a cold, and confrontation with a warm interviewer. Not very surprising, the cold condition elicited much more body touching. Upon re-examining the situation, it became evident that what we call coldness was an interference situation. The subject was asked to tell what was on her mind, while the "doctor" exhibited disinterest. Verbal encoding had to continue while feelings of distraction or even anger were experienced.

The warm-cold situation induced self-touching through ambiguous cues. Yet, the central condition giving rise to self-stimulation in a communicative setting is the task of staying on the beam, while at the same time warding off intrusive cues. This condition is most clearly created by the color-word interference situation. In the study by Barroso et al. (in preparation), he was able to show that the naming of colors elicited some degree of self-stimulation, but a significant increase in this behavior could be observed when the interference condition was introduced; that is, when the individual had to continue focusing on the color of the ink while warding off the impact of the word. Moreover, those subjects in the Stroop situation who had more pervasive self-stimulation, also made fewer errors. Hence, the patterns of self-stimulation were not only related to interference, but also to performance.

The interpretation for this behavior is that the self-stimulation provides feedback action regulating the arousal created by the interference condition (Grand et al., 1975; Venables, 1963). If this is so, we must be able to distinguish between arousal and the regulation of arousal. Spitz (1957), in his neonatal observations, has similarly noted, in the rooting response, a pattern which starts with the arousal of tension and its discharge, followed by its reduction through tactile stimulation (mouth against breast). Turning back to adult behavior, criteria can be found which differentiate excitement-expressive from excitement-regulative behavior. In general, it would seem that motor discharge alone, i.e., kicking, bouncing, tapping, perform a primary discharge function; while activity setting off a double feedback, involving tactile as well as motor innervation, plays more of a regulatory role. Such activity not only regulates stimulus input, but leads to a confirmatory experience of body boundaries.

If self-stimulation is created by an interference in the focus of attention, then we may suspect a corresponding interference in the formal organization of thought. Interference cues may disturb processes of retrieval, selection, or ordering. It is in this sense tha we would expect a relationship between body-focused activity and the organizational aspects of language. We, in fact, found in a recent factor-analytic study (Freedman & Steingart, 1975), that the level and pervasiveness of body touching could be linked to various aspects of formal linguistic construction, i.e., whether language was frag- mented, Narrative, Complex, or Conditional. The more circumscribed the self-stimulation, the more complex the language construction; the more pervasive the self-stimulation, the more simple the language form. Object-focused movements, on the other hand, were not related to these formal aspects of language, but they were shown, in another study (Freedman et al., 1973), to be linked to the thematic or mean- ing aspects of messages, as this was evident in an individual's abil- ity to express aggressive feelings. It would seem, then, that we can find in the two kinesic structures, a link to two aspects of language encoding, with object-focused movements having a bearing on semantic encoding, and body-focused movements having a bearing on syn- tactic skills.

We are cognizant that self-stimulation in communication has been interpreted in terms of its social significance, as withdrawal or isolation; in terms of its clinical significance, as signs of depression; in terms of its psychoanalytic meaning, as manifesta- tions of narcissism. These views fail to emphasize the functional significance of self-touching as a means of regulating sensory input, and for establishing a condition in which information processing may occur (i.e., the retrieving, ordering, and selecting of thoughts to be encoded) under stress. It is a bit of self-imposed sensory iso- lation.

THE ROOTS OF REPRESENTING AND FOCUSING IN INFANCY

The antecedents of the two communicative structures can be found in the earliest months of life. The entire sensorimotor period can probably be divided into a phase (first 6 months), during which body- focused movements predominate, and a period (second 6 months), dur- ing which the rudiments of object-focused movements predominate. During the period of the circulatory reaction, we can speak of a predominantly sensory phase, for in body touching there is a double feedback involving both tactile and motor stimulation, whereas in the period where prehension is dominant, the feedback derives pri- marily from motor innervation.

The activity during the first four months of life reveal the close coordination between hand movements and the development of at- tention. Body touching ranges from diffuse, to a stuckness upon the mouth, to a relinquishing of the mouth at three to four months when the hands meet at the midline. (Note that this progression appears to be recapitulated in our developmental observations.) This is a period during which the child struggles with the attainment of focal attention. Attention, according to Bruner (1969) who inspired the title of this paper, moves from a period of distractibility, to

stuckness (when hands are focused upon the mouth), then to a state
of anticipatory tracking when the hands meet at the midline. It is
a shift from reacting to what is encountered, to finding what is intended.

Psychoanalytic formulations concerning this progression of self-
touching, together with the attainment of focal attention, emphasizes
that this is also a period of the confirmation of the sense of self
(Adelson & Fraiberg, 1971). When at three months the hands meet at
the midline, there occurs a convergence of visual, tactile, and sensory experience. The hand that moves is also felt, and is seen, and
this convergence, as Hoffer (1949) has noted, constitutes the emergence of the sense of self--"His fingers finger his fingers. Thus
he himself touches and is being touched simultaneously. This double
touch is a lesson in self-discovery" (p. 52).

The transition from hand-to-mouth, to hand-to-hand activity,
constitutes a bridge to the further exploration of objects. Once
visually guided behavior is established, the stage is set for the
step-by-step development of prehension (White, 1964). Yet, it
is not until about twelve months, that bodily motions are used as
authentic symbolic activity. Thus we see in the progression of
kinesic and cognitive development, the rudiments of our two communicative structures. Not only do body-focused movements precede the
development of object-focused movements, but the development of focal
attention is clearly a precondition to the development of representing; and, perhaps, the development of the sense of self precedes the
development of object representation. Throughout this period, the
actions of the body constitute the building blocks from which attention and representational schemas develop. Whether, and in what way,
these kinesic experiences continue to hold sway in communication after
complex symbolic processes have been developed, is an issue which we
shall consider next.

II   ON THE EVOLUTION OF REPRESENTING AND FOCUSING BEHAVIOR

The foregoing depiction of object-focused movements as representing behavior and body-focused movements as attention sustaining behavior, have provided a frame of reference portraying the role of
kinesics in effective verbal communication. Yet, how do these functions evolve? We have noted that the basic mechanisms are already
in existence within the first year of life. It should be possible to
describe a step-by-step evolution of representing and focusing activity during communication, just as it is possible to depict the lines
in the development of anxiety (from diffuse to signal) in the capacity to separate or in identity formation.

In conceptualizing the structuralization of object-focused activity, we have borrowed George Klein's (1965) notion that for effective communication, discharge must not be indiscriminate. Muscle

action must be directed toward reality, and it must be closely linked
to the signalling system. In the case of representing behavior, we
can assume that the more the motion of the hand is contiguous to the
utterance, the more likely does the action provide the necessary
link between image and word. The model is similar to that used in
the study of the development of visually guided behavior (White,
1964), where the ultimate developmental attainment is one in which
the action is right on target. In the case of object-focused movements, the target is the word. With this target in mind, we can then
visualize evolutionary stages.

The structuralization of self-stimulation, as it evolves with
age, is guided throughout by the aims of self-confirmation and the
regulation of attention. It is proposed that structuralization must
progressively assume the pattern of figure and ground, with object-
focused movements the figure, and body-focused movements the ground.
In adult communication, the main traffic between people occurs at
the midline at the level of the head, and rests on eye-to-eye contact. In adults, then, we would look for representing activity
which is allowed to function relatively immune from self-stimulation.
In general, the more circumscribed (in terms of the body area stimulated) and the more patterned the activity, the more likely is self-
stimulation so orchestrated that it sustains attention and facilitates verbal representation.

A method for studying the developmental progression of object-
and body-focused movements during encoding. We have developed a research methodology which, in a unique way, addresses itself to the
questions just raised. Normal male school children, 12 in each age
group 4, 6, 8, 10, 12, and 14, were exposed to simple information
processing tasks which could be performed by all children, and also
hold the interest of such a wide age span. Their performances were
video taped. One of the tasks was vocabulary definition. Children
were asked, "What is a hair brush? A hammer? What does the word
fear or ugly mean?" The motor behavior elicited in response to each
of these questions provided us with a rather precise and objective
index of the amount of object-focused and body-focused movements
that emerged along with the verbal response. The method is unique
in that it offers a circumscribed verbal encoding unit with definable onset and termination. It becomes possible to assess the incidence of motions--their onset prior to verbalization (focusing
time), and during verbalization (representing time). Such data
yield two basic bits of information: a developmental curve showing
the mean incidence of type of movement at a given age level; and,
secondly, an event sequence tracing the occurrence of the movements
in the verbalization span within an age level. The protocols of
all 72 children were scored, and means were obtained for each age
group. Mean definition scores clearly progress across the entire
age span, and the level of definition is higher for the first 10 of

the list of 20 words (action and form concepts), compared to the
second 10 words (abstract words). Summarizing the age trends, it
can be said that at the age of four, definitions are at the preopera-
tional level, at eight and 10 years of age definitions are at the
level of concrete operations, and among 12 and 14-year-olds, word
definition approximates the level of formal operations. For details
of the procedure, see Van Meel et al., manuscript in preparation.

DEVELOPMENTAL OBSERVATIONS

If we now consider the evolution of object- and body-focused
movements during vocabulary definition, we can immediately dismiss
one hypothesis--this we shall call the inhibition of motor activity
notion. Such a view would appear to be suggested by Werner and Wapner's (1949) sensoritonic hypothesis which posits a reciprocal relationship between action and ideation. It also has its origin in
Freud's Interpretation of Dreams and in his paper on the Two Principles: namely, that there is one system concerned with the discharge
of tension which is directed toward the free discharge of the quantity
of excitation, and another system which succeeds in inhibiting this
discharge, raising the level of cognitive performance. We hasten to
add that to equate the appearance of object- and body-focused movements with manifestations of motor discharge, is a superficial application of these theories; nonetheless, the opposition of motor behavior versus thought organization persists in current clinical thinking
Everyday observations tell us that there is a good deal of motor behavior in communicative speech, yet is this behavior a vestige of an
early past, or is it instrumental in ongoing processing of thought?
If it is possible to observe a motor function which increases with
age and complexity of thought, then it is likely that such movements
are not just residuals of the past, but serve an intrinsic encoding
function.

In the case of object-focused movements, we observed a straight
linear increase from four - 16 years of age. In the case of body-
focused movements, we observed an increase up to 10 years of age;
then it declined. Yet there was still a good deal of self-touching
activity at 14 years of age. Since each age level revealed a systematic increase in complexity of thought, surely such increasingly
effective verbal representations cannot be accounted for by inhibition of manifest motor action.

THE STRUCTURALIZATION OF OBJECT-FOCUSED MOVEMENTS

The structuralization of object-focused movements can be defined
by the increased movement-word linkage. One approach to demonstrate
this linkage of object-focused activity is through the classification
of gestures. In our original classification, we distinguished a hierarchy of object-focused movements ranging from those which are primarily representational in nature, to those which are speech primacy in

nature (Freedman, 1971). Representational movements are gestures which depict the content of a message, the action, or form of what is being represented. They are a sort of parallel enactment of the "story," as if words were not enough. Speech primacy motions, on the other hand, carry no message content, but are rhythmic accompaniments of speech, usually occurring at the onset of a clause. With successive age levels and encoding competence, the rate of representational movements declines, but the rate of speech primacy movements increases (Figure 1). Figures depicting the linear relationship described in this section and other statistical analyses can be found in the study by Van Meel et al. (in preparation).

A more precise account of the changing structure of object-focused activity during verbalization can be gleaned if we examine the occurrence of a single kind of movement, a representational act, as it surrounds a verbal utterance, and then trace the ensuing structure across age groups. While representational movements decline with age, they do occur in all age groups. We selected four words: small, square, knife, and hammer, and sought to locate the occurrence of the movement in the response sequence before, during, or after. Three distinct stages could be noted. At the four-year-old level, we could note both substitution and rehearsal: representational movements occurred prior to response onset, and were followed by some rudimentary efforts at verbalization. At the 10-year-old level, we observed a structure of supplementation and redundancy: movements started at the onset of speech, and lasted throughout the utterance. It was as if the child surrounded himself with a visual, perceptual, imagistic aspect of his message. Finally, at the 14-year-old level, we observed subordination: we already know that at this age level, word definition is accompanied by succinct speech primacy gestures;[2] yet representational actions do occur. However, they never precede the word, nor do they last throughout the verbal response, but they are limited to the elucidation of a single word. To use a poetic phrase, the act now pays homage to the word.

---

[2]The function of speech primacy acts, at this most advanced stage of representing, has been a matter of theoretical concern to us. One possibility advanced in an earlier paper is that they are condensed internalizations of earlier forms of enactment in which only the beat quality is visible and in which the enacted image has now been internalized and incorporated into the verbal channel. If the internalization hypothesis is correct, then there would be more enactment themes in the fabric of language. We are currently examining the content of language during speech primacy activity. Another intriguing hypothesis holds that speech primacy motions constitute a new emergent function necessary for linguistic encoding.

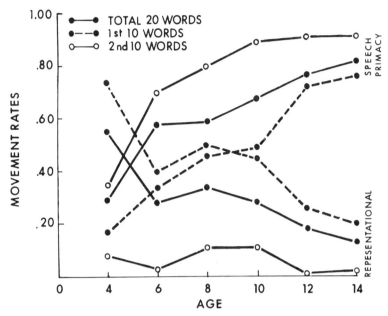

Figure 1 Mean representational and speech primacy rates for successive age groups: first ten, second ten and all twenty words.

Object-focused activity, then, evolves ever so closely to sustain linguistic representation, but undergoes three definite stages:
a stage of substitution and rehearsal, a stage of supplementation and
redundancy, and a stage of subordination. Each of these stages corresponds to an appropriate level in the development of thought. Each
of these stages, too, depicts a particular coding pattern characteristic of the communication of adults who differ in psychopathology
and personality organization. For example, supplementation is most
characteristic of the field-dependent individual who seems to use
gestures both as a means of appeal to the listener and as a means of
providing himself with visual feedback. Subordination, in contrast,

may be a characteristic of the field-independent person. This pattern appears to be a form of communicative autonomy, for in such a kinesic structure, body movements are used to sustain the word as the primary medium of exchange.

THE STRUCTURALIZATION OF BODY-FOCUSED MOVEMENTS

In our scoring of body-focused movements, we have distinguished three classes: bilateral and continuous motions covering various areas of the body; bilateral finger/hand motions, repetitive acts of fingers upon fingers or upon hand, usually at the midline; and lateral body-focused activity, involving a circumscribed body area such as the leg or arm. These three categories conform to the notion that, with development, there is a progressive diminution of area covered; they create a progressively sharper articulation of a figure-ground pattern; but they also indicate a further criterion-- laterality.

Each of the categories shows a particular saliency at a particular age level. Thus, among four and six-year-olds, the predominant form of self-touching is bilateral self-stimulation. The children move both hands in unison onto legs, face, mouth, or torso. Among eight and 10-year-olds, finger/hand movements are the salient forms of self-stimulation. The area traversed is more circumscribed, and their hands are sufficiently restrained to allow free traffic for eye-to-eye contact. However, a patterned differentiation in which hands act upon the body is not yet established, nor do we note the deployment of asymmetry in communication. The relatively restrained posture, which is suggested here, seems to be a subdued form of bilateral self-stimulation which had flourished at four and six years of age. Finally, from 12 years of age onward, finger/hand motions persist, albeit at a lower level. Yet, when direct body touching occurs, it is asymmetrical and clearly patterned. The hand acts as agent upon the body as object.

The discovery (and it was a belated one for us) that self- stimulation must be described along lines of laterality, suggests the rather far reaching possibility that representing and focusing activity may take place in different parts of the hemisphere. The observation of lateralized forms of self-touching has led us to an intriguing detour; vis. the exploration of hemispheric dominance in communication. We were fortunate to have recorded the body touching data in terms of preference for left or right hand, although such analysis has not yet been made for object-focused movements. Up through 12 years of age, the left hand is favored--presumably the nondominant hand. The possibility is suggested that representing behavior, in the form of object-focused movements, is carried out by the dominant hemisphere, and focusing behavior is carried out by the nondominant hemisphere.

We have noted earlier that the interference with the maintenance of focal attention creates an internal state of arousal as well as a requirement for the regulation of such arousal. Self-stimulation is but a manifestation of such a state. Can we empirically distinguish the expressive aspects from the regulating aspects, and do these two aspects shift with development? One clue is provided by observations of foot behavior. Foot kick and foot bounce are more clearly manifestations of excitement, and it may be relevant to examine whether such acts co-occur or alternate with self-stimulation. What is to be stressed is that in the earlier ages (four as well as 10-year-olds), the foot activity and self-stimulation occur simultaneously. There appears to be a need for continuous tension discharge, as well as the regulation of attention through soothing and surface stimulation. But at the 14-year-old level, the stimulation tends to become phasic, with foot movements alternating with self-stimulation. We would say that tension discharge alternates with tension reduction via the imposition of patterned self-touching. This phasic aspect of lateral self-stimulation appears to be of great importance in the associative monologue.

In summary, the emerging shifts in the organization of self-stimulation, as they appear during the task of defining a word, can be seen to change along parameters of area covered (from broad to focal), along lines of laterality, and along lines of phasic alternation. These criteria yield patterns of self-stimulation which also make their appearance in different clinical groups. Thus, bilateral self-stimulation was noted in cases of agitated depression where continuing need for defining self-boundaries may be presumed. Finger/hand motions are a prevalent response among those who are vulnerable to interference cues, and use the musculature to stay on the beam. Such movements can be seen in the communication of field-dependent persons under conditions of stress, among chronic schizophrenic patients even under conditions of interpersonal support, as well as congenitally blind individuals. Finally, the well phased-in lateral body touch appears to be an effective adaptation to stress, allowing for the sustained processing of thought. It is a sign of an effective orator or teacher.

THE COORDINATION OF FOCUSING AND REPRESENTING ACTIVITY

Having now described the structuralization of both object- and body-focused movements, a question can be raised concerning their respective onset during response sequence. We addressed ourselves to the issue of onset in three of the age levels: four, 10, and 14. At all three age levels, body touching (as well as foot activity) has its onset prior to verbal definition. This is true whether the form of self-stimulation is bilateral or a highly integrated asymmetrical form of behavior. Only among four-year-olds do object-focused movements occur prior to speech. Thereafter, they always coincide with onset, or occur during the utterance. Indeed, the appearance of object-focused movements in the absence of speech among adults would (except for the language of the deaf) be bizarre behavior.

The differential onset of object- and body-focused activity in the response sequence is quite in keeping with the notion that focusing behavior precedes representing behavior. The possibility arises that effective communication requires not only more speech linked forms of object-focused movements or patterned forms of body-focused movements, but a particular sequential or serial arrangement of the two. This concept is, of course, of great importance for the study of the natural communicative transaction during which representing and focusing are, of necessity, deployed alternately and in sequence.

III   THE INTEGRATION OF REPRESENTING AND FOCUSING STRUCTURES DURING ASSOCIATIVE MONOLOGUE

We shall now consider how the different units of behavior are integrated into a single communicative organization. For this purpose, we shall shift our observations to studies of video recorded interviews in which it is possible to trace the occurrence of kinesic activity as it is embedded in the language product.

It is, of course, a vast step from the definition of a single word in a vocabulary task to an associative monologue. Yet the direction of our expectations concerning the organization of the necessary psychic structures is clearly charted from what has been presented thus far. We have seen in previous sections that verbal representation is facilitated when there is a balance between object- and body-focused activity; that for complex representation to occur, both representing and focusing activity must take place at optimal developmental levels. We shall now consider the particular serial arrangements of such activity. Effective verbalization requires a sequential ordering, where body-focused movements precede object-focused movements and, hence, where focusing precedes representing.

The importance of sequential and purposive arrangements in the deployment of psychic structures as a mark of integrated thinking, has been emphasized by Klein (1965) and Horowitz (in Section 3). What we can look for, in an associative monologue, is a recapitulation of ontogeny. Such a recapitulation is akin to what has been described by Werner & Kaplan as a process of microgenesis (1963). Werner shows that in the establishment of word meaning, it is possible to discern an event sequence which repeats, in condensed form, the successive processes necessary for the organization of communicative speech. He emphasizes the successive deployment of different media of representation, from vague bodily articulation of meanings to linguistic dominance. Werner's account differs from ours in that he states that when linguistic dominance is achieved, "the earlier stage ostensibly dissolves." But what is similar, is the condensed reappearance of an entire evolutionary period taking place in the span of a single utterance. Such a condensation can be interpreted from both the vantage point of information processing and psycho-analytic theory.

From an information processing view, the recapitulation is one which follows the formula: focal attention---> representing. In the infancy observations by both Bruner (1969) and White et al. (1964) cited earlier, we have seen how, during the first few months of life, self-stimulation is closely phased in with the structuring of attention. From the stuckness of hand upon mouth, to the visual discovery of the hands through mutual touch at the midline, we can trace a concomitant shift in the infant's ability to select targets and to exclude extraneous cues. The structuring of attention is co-ordinated with the emergence of intentionality, and there can be no representing without an intention to represent. With this founda-tion, the child moves to prehension of a seen reality and the repre-sentation of an unseen one. This accomplishment of the first year is then recapitulated at many successive levels. It can be observed within the span of a few seconds during an associative flow--the exclusion of the irrelevant (be it from the listener or one's own thoughts), the pursuit of the relevant, seizing upon the object of representing and then confirming it.

From a psychoanalytic viewpoint, the postulated progression fol-lows the formula: confirmation of the sense of self---> representa-tions.[3] Hence, the psychoanalytic view of microgenesis is similar

---

[3]It is recognized that this progression from sense to self to object representation appears at odds with the currently accepted psycho-analytic view of the simultaneous emergence of the two during an early undifferentiated phase (c.f. Hartmann, Jacobsen). It is also opposed to the view of a primary object relationship (Balint). The present view does not deny that the early consolidation of a sense of self (within three months) takes place within the context of a primary object relationship. Moreover, the position suggested here emphasizes the sense of self rather than self-representation. The latter emerges much later, and appropriately deals with what is usu-ally termed secondary narcissism. The distinction between the early development of a sense of self, followed by object representation, is a qualitative one. That is, in the early months, the focus of attention is heavily weighted toward the self, i.e., time spent in sleep or bodily exploration. What we are articulating here is that what emerges at three months or earlier is a primary sense of self involving the distinction between inner and outer, and the cohesive-ness of the body image maturing within the context of an object re-lationship. Yet this primary sense of self does come close to Freud's notion of a primary narcissism.

in structure, but different in content, from the information processing view. The phenomena which psychoanalysis describes are broader
in scope and, moreover, in psychoanalytic theory, there is the attempt
to integrate the experiences evoked by reality with those evoked by
the drives. Thus, the first three months embodies not only a period
involving the conquest of focal attention, but also as both Hoffer
(1949) and Adelson and Fraiberg (1971) have noted, is also a period
of the discovery of the sense of self as a cohesive phenomenological
entity. Most important, this discovery entails the discrimination of
the "me" "not me" together with the taming of bodily excitement. From
the vantage point of drive regulation, the sub-sequence foot kick-->
self-touching suggests that one of the conditions for self-confirmation is the disciplining of bodily excitement. Once there has occurred an approximation of the sense of self, the child can move on
to the representation of object, physical as well as personal. Again,
in an associative monologue during adulthood, as the speaker is faced
with the task of reducing the multiple alternatives, he must tame his
excitement and confirm the cohesiveness of himself as speaker, a confirmation that sets the stage for the representation of objects. In
subtle and subordinated form, the earlier developmental progression
is recapitulated.

The empirical basis for these reflections was provided by our
earlier studies of associative monologue tracing the co-occurrence
of both object- and body-focused movements with formal linguistic
construction (Freedman & Steingart, 1975). We observed that both
discrete body touching and representational movements were highly
correlated with the incidence of complex conditional clauses in
language; that is, those clauses in which the speaker is able to articulate a relational and contingency frame of reference. We asked,
"What are the respective roles of these different motor acts in the
production of this most elaborate language product?" When we shifted
our observations from correlational analyses to sequential tracing
of movements in speech, we discovered a kinesic-linguistic event sequence: discrete body-focused movements occurred during pauses,
prior to clause onset, in the vast majority of instances. Object-
focused movements never occurred prior to clause onset, but rather
occurred in the middle or terminal part of the clause. There appeared to be a consolidating and a delivery motor aspect in language
production. Indeed, it was this observation which suggested the hypothesis that body-focused movement is an attention regulating maneuver.

This initial observation has now been subjected to further study.
Subjects were volunteer college students participating in a study of
monologue and dialogue behavior. In the monologue condition, the
subjects were asked to say whatever came to mind, and to talk for
five minutes. Yet on the basis of test data, the entire sample of
40 subjects could be divided into those termed "symbolizers" and

and "nonsymbolizers" (mentioned earlier), and "focusers" and "non-
focusers" (defined by a measure of field dependency). The subgroup
of subjects who were both focusers and symbolizers consisted of those
young women who were able to produce the most articulate verbal representations of their experiences. We shall briefly outline the kinesic
event sequence of these subjects as an example of an integrated event
structure. The event sequence will first be given a schematic outline
by locating the movements that occur both prior to major pauses and
after them.

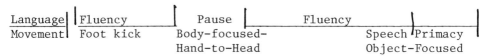

| Language | Fluency | Pause | Fluency | |
| Movement | Foot kick | Body-focused-
Hand-to-Head | Speech Primacy
Object-Focused | |

This event sequence can be viewed not only in horizontal fashion,
as in the above diagram, but in vertical fashion as a ladder. It is
a ladder divided into two parts; one before the pause in which focusing and self-confirmation terminates, and one after the pause in which
representation dominates. At the bottom of the ladder is the foot
kick, an early discharge phenomena, followed by lateral hand-to-head
activity, a motion which may be akin to the hand-to-mouth activity
in Hoffer's (1949) and Bruner's (1969) studies. It is of interest
to note that the freedom to resort to the early hand/head activity
during communication, subordinated in pauses, is prevalent in persons who are able to articulate their imagery vividly and clearly.
It is the motor act during the pause that refreshes (what we call
our Coca Cola phenomenon). At the top of the ladder we can note succinct speech primacy object-focused movements, word-confirming motor
manifestations which sustain the link between image and word.

How do we conceptualize the transition from act to word in the
event sequence just presented? There are three interpretations which
could account for the role of body motions in the evocation of complex verbal representation. These are side effects or epiphenomena,
ideomotor feedback, or self-object confirmation. The side effect interpretation has clearly been discounted in the course of the present
paper. One additional observation can be mentioned which points to
the intrinsic significance of the kinesic acts. When we examined
the correlation of pausing during speech with the complexity of language production, the relationship was insignificant; when we considered the correlation of self-touching during pauses and language,
it was highly significant.

The ideomotor feedback model, offered by Mahl in this volume,
holds that expressive behavior evokes primitive (sensorimotor) memory traces which, in turn, prime verbal representations which are
then brought to consciousness. This is viewed within the context of
a topographical model where motor acts have a connection to the earliest experience with the parental object. Thus, he quite literally
holds that self-touching evokes primary object representations.

Mahl suggests that transitions from motoric expression, to primitive ideation, to verbalization, are continually occurring events in the associative process. One question raised by this model, based on developmental observations, is whether the organism is capable of establishing the kind of symbolic equivalencies at the early level at which it is presumed to take place. Developmental considerations would suggest that where the primary preoccupation is with discrimination of inner and outer and with the organization of attention, the specific representation of an unseen reality cannot as yet be formed.

The interpretation offered here that self- and object-confirmatory maneuvers provide structural but not thematic support for verbal representation, appears to be more parsimonious. Object- and body-focused movements contribute to verbalization by sustaining the differentiation of the self- and object-representations. Without such differentiation, communication is not possible. Without the coenesthetic stimulation supporting the sense of self, images concerning the object world are cut off. Without physical confirmation of thing representations, word representations are not sustained. This interpretation is essentially content free. That is, both through the attainment of focal attention and self-confirmation motorically mediated, the speaker creates the "host condition" favoring the evocation of verbal memory traces. These memory traces, when verbalized, are constantly confirmed through enactive acts (object-focused movements). Yet, the status of the motor act is like that of a catalyst; it evokes vague sensorimotor images, but leaves the verbal operations to more advanced cognitive structures within the person.

This theoretical formulation also has its pragmatic payoff. As we go up the developmental ladder, we can diagnose different kinds of pathology or discontinuity in communication. The most evident distinction is one which emphasizes verbalization failure due to vulnerability to interference, in contrast to a verbalization failure due to difficulties in connecting. In chronic schizophrenia, there is both a known vulnerability to interference and a highly tenuous sense of self; pervasive bilateral self-touching has been observed. In contrast, we might expect, in hysterical or anxiety states, that there would be no primary focusing difficulty, but due to the presence of massive repression, difficulties in connecting image to word results in vague representational gestures. The ladder is even more useful in tracing various kinds of associative discontinuities in the analytic situation. Thus, we can distinguish a drive or impulse disturbance, a focusing disturbance, or a connecting disturbance, as these may be manifest by foot kick, self-stimulation, or object-focused movements. Such observations may contribute meaningfully to the timing of interventions.

POSTSCRIPT

We can now return to the dance which can be witnessed in any recorded communicative sample, but we can view this dance as a

planfully unfolding sequence with known constituents. There is a
focusing component regulating the deployment of attention, and a
representing component regulating the encoding of meaning. Each
is organized hierarchically having its own developmental level.
Each, under optimal conditions, is deployed in sequence so that consolidation of thought precedes representation of meaning. The two
processes may be carried out separately by the two hemispheres;
yet both must act in coordination, for what integrates the two
processes, the two hemispheres, is one organism--one person.

The question can be raised whether the sequential deployment of
foot kick, body-focused, object-focused movements can be accounted
for by the concept of cognitive competence. As cognitive competence
increases, motor discharge becomes less redundant, more purposeful,
more integrated. An answer to this question would be that motor organization is part of cognitive competence. Cognitive competence
is not simply defined by the verbal definition of the word or the
syntax of a phrase. Rather, the ability to achieve this final product requires the continuing harnessing of excitement, confirmation of
self, and the connection of word to image.

Finally, what is the relevance of the structuralization of body
movements, as they have been described, to the transition from the
basic dialogue to the verbal dialogue? It is our belief that such
structuralization is the mediating process which makes a verbal interchange possible. Through the taming of the drives and the confirming of the self, the speaker becomes aware of himself vis-a-vis
the listener. And, through the confirmation of object representation, the speaker makes the meaning of his messages available. In
this sense, a bodily condition for both disembedding and sharing is
created, providing the physical base for negotiating the "anxiety
of influence."

REFERENCES

Adelson, E. & Fraiberg, S. Mouth and hand in the early development
   of blind infants. In James F. Bosma (Ed.), Symposium on oral sensation and perception. Springfield, Illinois: Thomas, 1971.

Barroso, F., Freedman, N., Grand, S., & Van Meel, J. The evocation
   of two types of hand movements in information processing. Manuscript in preparation.

Bloom, H. The anxiety of influence. New Haven: Yale University
   Press, 1973.

Bruner, J. S., Oliver, R. R., & Greenfield, P. M., et al. (Eds.),
   Studies in cognitive growth. New York: John Wiley, 1966.

Bruner, J. S. Eye, hand and mind. In D. Elkind & J. H. Flavell
(Eds.), Studies in cognitive development. New York: Oxford University Press, 1969.

Bucci, W. & Freedman, N. Language and hand: The dimension of referential competence. Manuscript in preparation.

Escalona, S. K. Patterns of infantile experience and the development
process. Psychoanalytic Study of the Child, 1963, 18, 197-244.

Freedman, N. The analysis of movement behavior during the clinical
interview. In A. Siegman & B. Pope (Eds.), Studies in dyadic communication. New York: Pergamon Press, 1971.

Freedman, N., O'Hanlon, J., Oltman, P., & Witkin, H. A. The imprint
of psychological differentiation on kinetic behavior in varying
communicative contexts. Journal of Abnormal Psychology, 1972, 79,
3:239-258.

Freedman, N., Blass, T., Rifkin, A., & Quitkin, F. Body movements
and the verbal encoding of aggressive affect. Journal of Personality & Social Psychology, 1973, 26, 1:72-85.

Freedman, N. & Steingart, I. Kinesic internalization and language
construction. Psychoanalysis & Contemporary Science, Vol. 4, 1975.

Freud, S. (1915a). The unconscious. Standard Edition, Vol. 14.
London: Hogarth Press, 1957.

Grand, S., Freedman, N., Steingart, I., & Buchwald, C. Communicative
behavior in schizophrenia: The relation of adaptive styles to kinetic and linguistic aspects of interview behavior. Journal of Nervous & Mental Disease, 1975, Vol. 161, No. 5, 293-306.

Held, R. & Hein, A. Movement-produced stimulation in the development
of visually guided behavior. Journal of Comparative & Physiological
Psychology, 1963, Vol. 56, No. 5, 872-876.

Hoffer, W. Mouth, hand and ego-integration. The Psychoanalytic Study
of the Child, Vols. 3 4, 49 56. New York: International Universities Press, 1949.

Klein, G. S. On hearing one's own voice. In M. Schur (Ed.), Drives,
affects, and behavior, Vol. 2. New York: International Universities Press, 1965.

Mahl, G. Gestures and body movements in interviews. In J. Shlien
(Ed.), Research in psychotherapy, Vol. 3. Washington, D. C.: American Psychological Association, 1968.

Mehrabian, A. & Williams, M. Nonverbal concomitants of perceived and intended persuasiveness. Journal of Personality & Social Psychology, 1969, 13:37-58.

Miller, A. Verbal satiation and the role of concurrent activity. Journal of Abnormal & Social Psychology, 1963, Vol. 66, No. 3, 206-216.

Piaget, J. The origins of intelligence in children. New York: International Universities Press, 1952.

Rapaport, D. Consciousness: A psychopathological and psychodynamic view. In H. A. Abramson (Ed.), Problems of consciousness. New York: Josiah Macy, Jr. Foundation, 1951.

Rosenfeld, H. M. Instrumental affiliative functions of facial and gestural expressions. Journal of Personality & Social Psychology, 1966, 4:65-72.

Spitz, R. A. Diacritic and coenesthetic organizations: The psychiatric significance of a functional division of the nervous system into a sensory and emotive part. Psychoanalytic Review, 1945, Vol. 32, 146-162.

Spitz, R. A. No and yes. New York: International Universities Press 1957.

Stone, L. The psychoanalytic situation. New York: International Universities Press, 1961.

Van Meel, J., Freedman, N., & Buchwald, C. The organization of object-focused movements during vocabulary definitions in successive age groups. Manuscript in preparation.

Werner, H. & Wapner, S. Sensory-tonic field theory of perception. Journal of Personality, 1949, 18:88-107.

Werner, H. & Kaplan, B. Symbol formation: An organismic-developmental approach to language and the expression of thought. New York: John Wiley, 1963.

White, B. L., Castle, P., & Held, R. Observations on the development of visually-directed reaching. Child Development, 1964, 35:349-364.

Wolff, C. The hand in psychological diagnosis. New York: Philosophical Library, 1952.

THE DEVELOPMENT OF CONVERSATIONAL BEHAVIOR

Allen T. Dittmann

U. S. Office of Education[1]

Washington, D. C.   20202

This paper begins by describing a phenomenon discovered in the laboratory some years ago, outlines some of the reasoning advanced to explain it, reports an extensive follow-up designed to test some of that reasoning, then gives some rather speculative conclusions based on the whole mass of data and the ideas that have been stirred up by it. Briefly, the phenomenon is that young children behave differently in conversations than older children and adults do; the thinking about this has included linguistic, cognitive, and social issues in the development of children at along about the beginning of adolescence.

THE FIRST OBSERVATIONS

The difference between children and adults originally turned up in connection with some psycholinguistic research that D. S. Boomer and I were engaged in. We were studying certain units of speech rhythm that people use to divide up their thoughts and ideas into communicable packages. Speakers need to cast their ideas into such units in order to translate them into words, and listeners need to grasp the units in order to understand what is being said. The unit we first studied is called the Phonemic Clause, after the linguists George L. Trager and Henry Lee Smith (1951). As time has gone on, a somewhat larger unit has also proved useful, one I have called the Final Juncture Unit. While Boomer was studying the speaker's task of encoding, I was concentrating on the listener's task of

---

[1]This study was conducted while the author was in the Laboratory of Psychology, National Institute of Mental Health, Bethesda, Maryland.

understanding or decoding speech. The method was to examine the
distribution of what I called Listener Responses with respect to
the units of rhythm in the ongoing speech being listened to (Dittmann
& Llewellyn, 1967, 1968). Listener Responses consist of head nods
and a number of brief vocalizations that are variants of "M-hm,"
like "Yeah," "I see," and the like, all of which serve as feedback
for the speaker so he can know he is accomplishing his task usefully,
or in other words that he is speaking intelligibly. In the college
students who served as our first subjects, listeners respond in
this way to somewhere around a third of Final Juncture Units in
speakers' rhythmical flow of speech. When we moved on to developmental studies (Dittmann, 1972), we found that children under adolescence respond to about an eighth of such units, and that if we
look only at those just starting school, about half that often. We
discovered another difference, too, one having to do with the timing
of the responses. Adults are almost uncanny in the precision of
their Listener Responses. First, and this is what set us to exploring the responses to begin with, adults insert their Listener Responses almost exclusively at the ends of the rhythm units, almost
never at hesitations within those units. Second, they emit the
responses within milliseconds after the speaker has finished enun-
ciating the unit, in the case of nods sometimes slightly before.
Children, on the other hand, are inclined to be a bit late in responding, so that it is often hard to tell just what part of the
speech they are responding to.

Our first studies were done in a laboratory, and we recorded
the responses first by mechanical means and later by videotape. In
the case of the college students we would have two subjects talking
to each other, with instructions that one of them should carry the
conversational ball for a while, then the other, so that fairly sustained speech was called for by the experimenters. When we found
the very low responsiveness in the first child we recorded, we went
to a nearby private school to find out if he was peculiar in this
respect, or if absence of Listener Response was generally true of
children his age. We were relieved to find that he was not strangely
different from his age-mates, since he was the Boomers' seven-year-
old son. We also found something else in observing a number of conversations on a few visits: there are some circumstances that pull
Listener Responses, where the speaker needs feedback so much that he
will seek out responses if they are not naturally forthcoming. These
are what we described as instructional situations, where immediate
performance is to result. One child might be teaching another a
game they are about to play. The instructing child must know if the
learner is catching on to the successive points he is trying to make
in his explanation. He will look up at the learner to see if there
is a glimmer of understanding, sometimes say, "Mm?" or "Okay?" till
he gets a response. If there isn't any response, he will back off
and try again from another tack. Incidentally, the fact that children

often do respond to these eliciting queries indicates that they are
fully capable of making Listener Responses at fairly early ages.

Armed with this information, we returned to the laboratory to
examine the phenomenon in greater detail. We had children listening
to adults, and children listening to each other. Some of the talk
was relatively free-flowing conversation, and some was instructional.
We weren't able to control this conversation-instruction variable
very well with children for two reasons. One was that adults are
likely to be instructional with children, a point that will come up
later here, and the other that purely conversational talk is hard
for children who are brought to the Clinical Center of the National
Institutes of Health just to sit down and talk. In spite of these
problems, we did learn something from studying the videotapes of
those sessions. First, the rates of response in children, which I
have already referred to, compared with those of adults. Second,
the timing differences, and coupled with those, an interesting sort
of responsiveness that you really need videotaped to see: there
are a number of nods that are so slight that they are probably not
visible to the speaker, and thus cannot serve as feedback for him.
They seem rather to be a sort of automatic production by the listener,
perhaps parallel to the speech-accompanying gesticulations that
Freedman has called object-focused movements. Finally, we found
differences between children's responsiveness to adults and their
responsiveness to other children, and between conversational and
instructional talk, though the sample for this last was too small
to test statistically. One difference we looked for, but did not
find, was that between sexes, but keep sex differences in mind, for
they will come up in an unexpected way in the follow-up data later
on in this report.

PRELIMINARY THEORIZING

After we had collected these first data, we needed to stop and
think about what they meant, so as to know how to plan the next studies. The ideas that came to mind were described in the 1972 article
under the headings of linguistic tie and the social tie. From the
standpoint of linguistics, the Listener Response is at the borderline
between the verbal and the nonverbal. Some responses take verbal
forms, like "Yes" and "I see," while others are somewhat removed
from the purely verbal. The "M-hm" is often just an uncompleted
noise, and the nod seems to be totally nonverbal. In the context
of the other person having just asked a question that admits only
of "yes" or "no" as the answer, however, the nod is a gestural substitute for "yes," just as the head shake serves for "no." There are
some other acts that seem to be Listener Responses, and they are even
less related to the verbal than nods. A few people use an occasional
eyebrow raise for this purpose, and about a seventh of Listener Responses consist of a specific type of smile, one which has a rapid

onset like the ordinary smile, but which also fades rapidly, unlike
other smiles. The timing of all these is the same in regard to the
rhythm structure of the speech being responded to.

I believe that this timing aspect of Listener Responses means
that they are closely related to the encoding-decoding process of
speech, with the chunking mechanism of short-term memory, or in a
word, with the way our neural mechanisms fit in with the nature of
codes. If communication is to be possible, both speaker and listener must share the same code, and must divide up the flow into
comparable chunks, be that flow the neurophysiological processes in
the speaker that we call thoughts and ideas, or the sound waves of
speech that the listener hears and tries to translate back into
thoughts and ideas that hopefully correspond with those the speaker
started out with.

We know that there are a number of manifestations of the chunking process in speakers. Boomer reported in 1965 that pauses are
far more likely to appear at the beginnings of Phonemic Clauses.
A couple of years later, Boomer and Laver found that the most common
types of tongue slip involve misordering words within a single Phonemic Clause. Then Llewellyn and I reported in 1969 that speakers'
body movements are likely to be located at hesitation points in the
rhythm structure of their speech. We have since learned that breathing patterns also correspond to speech rhythm patterns, and in fact,
that speech rhythm seems to drive breathing rhythm far more than you
would expect from looking at tracings of nonspeaking respiration.
Could it be that on the listener's side, part of the reason behind
the occurrence of Listener Responses is that they are a manifestation of the listener's chunking the flow of the speech he hears?
I believe there is reason to conclude precisely this. The exact
timing of adult listeners' responses is not called for by the social
demands of conversation, either in the short latency of the responses
or in the fact that they are inserted at the ends of rhythmical
speech units rather than at hesitations within those units. And, in
view of the wide individual differences we have observed in the frequency of these responses, it would appear that some listeners give
responses more often than speakers need them. We may conclude, then,
that Listener Responses are not produced simply to supply speakers
with needed feedback, but constitute evidence of listeners processing the information of the ongoing speech signal as well.

If children emit fewer Listener Responses than adults, it should
follow from this line of reasoning that they are processing less information than adults, or are processing it less accurately. Indeed,
most adults figure this to be the case when they don't get responses
from children. I have informally observed both parents and teachers
fairly badgering their charges on this account. Think of the many
times we have all heard adults say things like, "Are you listening?"

"Did you hear me?" "Pay attention!" or more innocuously simply adding the soliciting question, "Okay?" after saying something to a
child. The exasperating thing about many children is that after
they have been demanded of by any of these means, they can generally
recite precisely what the adult has just said, and with a tone of
voice indicating a low opinion of the adults pesterings. And in
ways other than the Listener Response, children are just as responsive as adults: in the study reported in 1972, we separated Listener
Responses from what we called Content Responses, like extended comments, questions, and smiles that seemed content-related, and there
was virtually no difference between children and adults in Content
Responses, children even having a slight edge on adults.

From a linguistic standpoint, then, the Listener Response may
well be a language-related accomplishment that is age-related. Just
what age is involved could not be told from our first data, since
we included children of a wide range of ages in our rather small
laboratory sample, and observed only up through the fifth grade in
the school. But before the age of regularly-appearing Listener Responses, there remains the question of whether children really do
process the speech they hear in the same way adults do. The people
who badger are, after all, adults, who may presume a far greater
attention in all their listeners than the children among them possess. Children may actually not take in as much as their parents
and teachers expect them to, and their recitations of what has just
been said may be a dredging up from short-term memory of more than
would have been processed any further without that questioning.

As to the social function of the Listener Response, it gives
the speaker the feedback he needs if he is to continue talking. This
implies that the speaker is talking to a listener, and that the listener is interested in having the speaker continue. In the case of
young children, say before school age, speakers do not talk to each
other in the same sense that adults do. Piaget's description in The
Language and Thought of the Child (1926) tells of the child speaking for the pleasure of speaking, perhaps stimulated by the presence
of someone else, but talking on even if no one is there. Piaget called
this sort of speech egocentric, as indeed it is. Our early observations of children talking to each other showed at least one nonego-
centric aspect of the process: children take turns talking even at
nursery school age, so it looks as if information were being exchanged.
But actually each is relatively oblivious to what the other is saying,
so that two quite separate lines of content can be heard to issue from
two small children. Piaget called this situation collective monologue.
Later on children begin to talk to others, to want them to listen, to
wish to communicate thoughts. As Piaget says, the child in these
instances "speaks from the point of view of his audience" (p.19), a
notion that sounds quite like Mead's (1934) taking the role of the
other. If that were the case, however, why would he not need feedback to confirm the fact that a communication has taken place? My

reasoning when we made those observations was that providing feedback via Listener Responses is more than being able to take the point
of view of the other. It is being able to empathize with the speaker's need for feedback, to give some sort of personal confirmation
to another. Even though the early school-aged child is capable of
engaging in what Piaget called socialized speech, this more personal
giving is still beyond him. Not until preadolescence, in Sullivan's
terms, would such caring about the other for the other's sake, begin
to appear.

These observations brought up another point, one that is perhaps
more mechanical than the empathy referred to just above. Young children talk in short bursts, each speaker turn consisting of one Final
Juncture Unit, or two at the most. Under these circumstances, Listener Responses are superfluous: feedback to help the speaker continue talking is really not needed. Each child's talk is a sort of
running commentary on what he is doing right now, on his immediate
activity. The appropriate response of the listener is to wait his
turn and make a comment on his activity. So on this mechanical
ground alone, perhaps one should not expect many Listener Responses
when children are talking to each other. By the same token, however,
one should expect them when children are listening to adults, because
adults' talk is likely to be longer, but even there, they are infre-
quent.

Finally, we wondered whether the content of the talk made a difference. Perhaps it is only when children begin to talk not so much
about their immediate activity as about more remote topics, or when
the content from one is related to what the other is saying in the
conversation, that children learn what it is to be a speaker who
needs feedback. On all these points we needed more data.

THE FOLLOW-UP STUDY

From this sort of thinking about our observations, a number of
variables presented themselves to be studied systematically, and
they needed to be studied in a more naturalistic setting where their
"true" variation could be observed. First, there was obviously age:
we had not yet learned when adult-type conversation defined along
any dimensions might begin to appear regularly, though we did have
enough information to guess that we should concentrate on late elementary and junior high grades. The second and third variables were
talk to other children versus talk to adults and conversational
versus instructional emphasis. These two would probably be confounded
since talk with adults is likely to contain instruction. Fourth,
there was topic, dichotomized as the immediate activity at hand
versus events removed from the present time or place. Fifth, was
length of talk within speaking turns. Sixth, was number of speaking
turns per conversation. The occurrence of Listener Responses was an
obvious seventh variable, and, finally, the sex composition of the

conversational group, all girls, all boys, or mixed-sex group. All
variables had to be observable and recordable in real time since
videotaping is not feasible in all situations.

Our method was to observe on the periphery of conversations,
making a running record of the Final Juncture Units and speaking
turns in the childrens' talk, categorize the content as immediate
or remote, note whether a child or an adult was talking, indicate
where Listener Responses occurred and who made them, and identify
the protocol by the number, sex, and grade of the conversational
group. Keeping track of this amount of information is not as difficult as it sounds, though it lacks the precision of videotape recording, where records can be viewed again and again. The method
rests on the distinctiveness of the phenomena being recorded. Final
Juncture Units are marked by Phonological features which can be
discerned at distances so great that the words are not "audible."
Changes in speaker turn are easy to identify, and the other variables
are not too great an addition to the task. The method undoubtedly
underestimated the number of Listener Responses, as comparison of
the results with those from the laboratory will show. Behaviors
that are emitted while the observer is looking down at his notes
are obviously lost. The very slight nods that were identified only
by repeated viewings of the videotape in the laboratory setting
add to those.

We concentrated on the oldest grades in the school, the 6th,
7th, and 8th, in line with our guess that the payoff would be located there. It would have been good to have 9th and 10th grades
as well. We first outlined the nature of the project to staff and
teachers. They gave their enthusiastic support, since the problem
is intrinsically interesting to almost everyone. Parents were told
about the study through the school newsletter, and they were encouraged to contact the staff or the researchers if they had any
questions. None did. We then told the children in some detail
what we were doing at the school. In part this was a matter of
informed consent, in part an effort to reduce the "mystery man"
effect. We said we were interested in the "mechanics" of conversation, and how its flow is managed by the participants, as an example of the many unwritten rules of social interaction. We stressed
our disinterest in individuals as such and in the content of the
talk, which we pointed out we could often not hear. We were not se-
cretive about our recording. The notes consisted of little marks
on file cards, which we showed to any children who asked about them.
Children seemed relieved to see our notes, which were a confirmation
of our reassurances, though some may have been a bit disappointed
that our method of recording did not lend itself to gossip. So they
knew quite well what we were up to, and we had an understandable role
in the school. The fact that nothing of their talk got back to staff,
teachers, parents, or other children soon led to an atmosphere of
quite complete relaxation.

We made our observations wherever we judged conversational opportunities to be most likely: when the children were working on
their own, were carrying out projects already assigned, were in
recess, were chatting on the periphery of some organized activity
that did not include everyone at once, like a play rehearsal, were
in periods of relatively free time between activities. In short,
we observed at any appropriate time other than structured group
teaching. Our visits spanned seven months of a school year, and
we made 278 observations on 80 occasions of 344 conversations. We
observed about 3,100 speaking turns consisting of about 5,700 Final
Juncture Units, and saw or heard about 300 Listener Responses.

These sound like large numbers, and they are, but before presenting actual results, I would like to introduce some cautions to
interpretation, because in some ways the numbers are quite small.
First, there is only one classroom in each grade at that school,
so the nature of the group of children in each class, those particular 20 to 30 children, dictates what they do. Second, each class
has one main teacher and the school has a number of specialty teachers. All children spend a lot of time in the specialty rooms
and labs, and those teachers come to the children's rooms as well,
but the main teacher is with the group more than the others are,
so the teacher also introduces influences over which we have no
sampling control. When we think we are talking about age differences,
we are really including some unknown amount of variation from teacher
and some from group. Third, the philosophy of this school is distinctive, and includes ideas about planning for the individual, learning
through experiencing, and group life that leads parents to send their
children there. It may be more heterogeneous than many public schools
with respect to background of parents, but more homogeneous with respect to their orientation to learning, and that may affect the way
conversation is valued, again in some quite unknown way. It was
our impression that the children subscribed to the philosophy of
the school as much as their parents did, for both individuals and
groups were very task-oriented. And they were very loyal to the
school, making for far greater stability than is customary in public
schools: all of the 8th graders had been there since kindergarten,
some since nursery school.

RESULTS OF SYSTEMATIC OBSERVATIONS

The strongest differences in Listener Responses were first between responsiveness of children to other children versus to teachers, and second between grades. There were no overall differences
between groups of different sex composition, though this factor in-
teracted with the others in some surprising ways. The extent of the
two significant main effects was considerable: on the child-teacher
variable, children responded to about 3% of other children's Final
Juncture Units, and to about 11% of those of the teachers. As to
grades, the rates of Listener Responses per Final Juncture Unit were

4% in the 6th and 6% in the 8th. There were no significant interactions between any two of these three variables, but there was a
significant triple interaction, which is shown in Figure 1. The
children are so much more responsive to teachers than to each other
that the figure looks like two graphs laid out on the same grid.
The upper one shows a striking sex difference in responsiveness
to teacher in 6th and 8th grades, with little difference in the 7th.
The groups consisting of boys only, or of both boys and girls, are
very similar: their response rates average about 7% in the 6th and
7th grades, and 16% in the 8th, a jump by a factor of two and a
half. All-girl groups, on the other hand, drop in responsiveness
to teachers between 6th and 7th grades, then maintain that relatively
low level in the 8th. Toward other children, the story is quite different: groups of girls only and of both sexes increase in responsiveness over the three grades, while all-boy groups stay about the
same. The proportional increase in girls' responsiveness to each
other is comparable, if not a bit greater, than the increase of
boys and mixed groups toward teachers over this time, though the
comparison is risky because of the very small proportions.

These trends in the groups of girls seem to be mediated in part,
at least, by their very reaction to the presence of an adult in the
group, whether that adult is participating very much or not. The
all-boy and mixed groups seem to be about equally responsive to
others whether there is a teacher in the conversational group or not.
Groups of girls, however, are much more responsive in the earlier
grades when a teacher is present in the group, and less so in the
8th grade. These strong sex differences make for quite a problem
of interpretation, and I shall return to them later.

Now for some findings about the other variables we included in
our observations. One in which we expected to find a change over
these years was length of speaker turn, as measured by the number
of Final Juncture Units per turn. There were virtually no differences: under practically all conditions in the study there were
about 1.8 units per turn. Apparently the differences in number of
Listener Responses cannot be accounted for by any mechanical factor
like more opportunities for the listener to respond if the speaker
talks longer during his turn. Another variable where we expected
to find differences was length of conversations. On this variable
there were some positive findings, many of them difficult to interpret. Three conditions influenced length of conversation: grade,
sex, and presence versus absence of teacher in the conversational
group. As we might expect, children in the upper grades carry on
longer conversations. Mixed groups have longer conversations than
single-sex groups, and children's conversations are longer when the
teacher is absent from the group. The topic of conversation, that
is, whether it concerned immediate activity versus something more
remote, had no influence on conversational length. There were no
interactions between any pair of the four variables, and, as I said

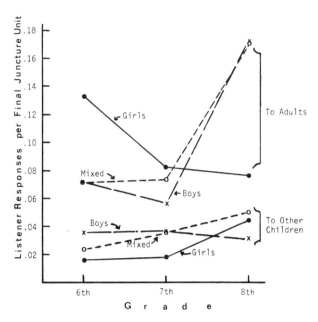

Figure 1.   The interaction of age, sex of conversational group,
and target of response on rate of Listener Response.

before, some uninterpretable triple interactions that might possibly
be attributed to the confounding of teacher and group with grade,
a cautionary problem mentioned above.

One final result.   Recall that we went to observe the children
where they were conversing.   We had no control over what they were
talking about, and did not try to balance the design to represent
topics equally.   We expected an age change on the topic variable.
Younger children, we reasoned, are more action-oriented, and their
talk should therefore be tied more directly to the activities they
were immediately engaged in.   Older children, on the other hand,
should be able to think more abstractly, and therefore would talk
about things more removed from the present in time and space.   But
we found no difference in grade on this variable.   The strongest
difference we did find was in presence versus absence of teacher:
when a teacher was included in the group, almost two thirds of the
conversations were about the immediate activity.   When there was
no teacher, between half and two thirds were about remote topics.
This result should not be surprising in view of the philosophy of
the school and the teachers.   Most of the immediate topics were
about school-related activities, even though they were not necessarily direct "teaching."   These teachers were always on the lookout
for chances to get some educational point across, and brought the

conversations around so that school-type materials could be talked about. The children went along with this direction, because they implicitly agreed that this was a time for school work, especially when a teacher came along to join the group.

DISCUSSION

The most general conclusion from this research is that we have found the time when conversational behavior typical of children begins to turn into conversational behavior typical of adults. The two key clues to this change are the increase in rate of Listener Response and in length of conversations. We have not located the age at which the adult patterns are fully established, because the age range of subjects was restricted. The beginning, however, seems to be about the time of onset of adolescence.

This time in children's lives is one of enormous change in a good many seemingly disparate functions. A change in the domain of conversational patterning, one that spans a number of functions, should therefore be expected. I should like now to trace some of the ways these results fit in with what we know about early adolescence. Let us begin with some facts, then focus on some of those to which the present research is most germane. At the beginning of adolescence there is at once a start of new growth and a consolidation of what has already grown, in each case perhaps more strongly marked than at any other period of life. We pay more attention to the starts than to the stops, because they are so obvious: children shoot up in height and weight and there are all the evidences of sexual maturation; their social horizons expand enormously; their ties to groups are stronger; and, their emotional lives are fraught with the new fears and new excitements over all these changes. At the same time, there is a slow-down of functions that have been growing all along, not a sudden slowing, to be sure, and usually quite invisible, but nonetheless there. In cognitive abilities, there is a crystallization of what has been more flexible before. Second languages are no longer learned spontaneously by the blotter method as they have been earlier, and children injured in the language-relevant areas of the brain after this period can no longer relearn language with the same facility that younger children can. Tests of general ability show smaller increments year by year than they did before. Thinking patterns have incorporated the adult capacity for logical constructions by this time, and there may well be no further qualitative leaps in this domain for the rest of the individual's life.

The data from the present study do not support an examination of all of these quite different progresses and consolidations for what the development of conversational behaviors may tell us about them. And of the linguistic and social ties discussed above, the results of the Follow-up Study have added little about the purely

linguistic. So I shall concentrate here on the social and cognitive.
The text for this discussion will be the work of two theorists,
George Herbert Mead and Harry Stack Sullivan. Mead wrote a good
deal about the development of the self being mediated in large part
by language and communication, but the findings on growth of conversation give only indirect support to this part of his writings, in
that conversation presupposes language. But language as a socially
agreed-upon set of rules that mediates between the individual and
the group exists in a number of contexts other than conversation,
such as formal talk before audiences and writing. The patterns of
conversation that include taking turns and giving feedback to the
speaker are superimposed upon language, and have a set of rules of
their own, apart from the rules of language per se. It is the development of the conversational rules that concerns us here.

In writing about the self, Mead reasoned that it must be considered a social entity. It is an outgrowth of the person's engaging others and being responded to by them, so that one comes
to correct and refine one's acts in advance of actually performing
them, by imagining what those responses might be. This imagining
is what Mead called taking the attitude of the generalized other.
The process is epitomized in the activity of playing organized games.
As one of the players, one knows the rules, that is, knows what one
is supposed to do, one's role in the game. One also knows what the
other players are supposed to do, and is able to take their roles
as well, both when his turn comes to play them as the game progresses
and when he imagines how those others may behave toward him and
toward each other. Each player's role, then, is a product of both
the rules of the game and the players' views of all the others' responses to each move in the game. Thus, the individual must be
able to lose himself in the game and in the various roles it dictates
In the same way, he becomes involved in the rules and roles of the
larger games of community and society, and thereby achieves a self
of his own. Only in this way, says Mead, can the individual become
a person among others. Just when a final integration might come to
pass in the development of the individual is hard to say. Mead was
theorizing about social processes, not conducting empirical research
to yield age norms on social accomplishments. From passing reference
in Mind, Self, and Society (1934) it would seem that the early school
years were involved.

Sullivan also had a social view of the self, one that I believe
is complementary to Mead's. The difference between what Sullivan
called the juvenile and the preadolescent eras in personality development is the important one here. In the juvenile, one learns the
rules of the many games of life, and how to get along with others--
or, to follow Sullivan's emphasis more completely, how to get along
comfortably with oneself while working and learning alongside others.
The child makes many comparisons with others about relative abilities

and skills, but always from what Sullivan calls an extraordinarily
self-centered point of view. On reaching preadolescence, on the
other hand, the child's interest focuses on others in quite a new
way, dramatically marked at first in the relationship to a chum.
What matters to the individual now is no longer exclusively his
own comfort, but rather in addition the feelings of that other
individual, the likes and dislikes, interests and activities they
can share for the sake of being together and enhancing each others'
feelings. Sullivan described this process as the first dawning of
intimacy.

To apply these two Sullivanian stages to Mead's analysis of the
organized game, we should divide the play into two phases: first
getting to know the game, its rules and various roles; and second
becoming involved in it by taking all the roles at once. This
latter becomes possible when the player can understand the other
roles first-hand, as it were, by empathizing with the other players
and what they are up against. Sullivan was more interested in ages
than Mead, but he was no more precise in his estimates. On a single
page he dated preadolescence at the top as somewhere between eight
and one-half and 10 years, and at the bottom as preceding puberty
by a few weeks or a few months! (1954, p. 144)

In the conversation, the rules of the game are to talk, to take
turns, to respond if one is asked, and the like. These are learned
quite early. The adult conversational game has as its purpose communication, and through communication, the purpose of relating to
others. This, I submit, begins only in early adolescence. Two indications that the goal is relatedness come from the findings that
spontaneous Listener Responses increase markedly over the ages
under study here, and that conversations are longer in the older
children. It is my contention that the whole complex of adult
conversation is dependent on having reached the stage of being
able to relate to others in the sense Sullivan called intimacy.

Two variables included in the study gave negative results on
what we had come to define as adult patterns of conversation. One
was length of speaker turn, and the other was topic. Our experience
with adult conversation had been in the laboratory, and our instructions to subjects affected both of these variables. We forced long
turns by asking subjects to hold the floor for fairly long periods
each--not real monologue, but almost. We really do not know how
long their turns might have been in free social situations unen-
cumbered by such instructions. The variable of topic was influenced
as a consequence: subjects chose things they could talk about
for those fairly long turns, and they turned out to be what would
be classified in the present study as remote, trips they had taken,
experiences they had had in college, and the like. If they had
tried to talk about the immediate activity at hand, the topic would
have been that of participating in the study. That topic did occasionally come up, but even then, it was not really the same as two

people in "real life" who might or might not have been engaged in
some "activity" in addition to talking. So strictly speaking, the
situations of the two studies are not comparable, and we cannot
tell if the "negative results" that appear here are really negative.
I have a lingering belief that adults should be expected to take
longer turns and talk about more remote topics than children, but
there is no way of knowing this for sure until adults, too, are
observed in their native habitats just chatting.

The most challenging result obtained here was the wide difference in both length of conversation and responsiveness among the
groups of different sex composition. Current theorizing about the
two sexes at these ages is not very specific, but we do tend to
think of girls as being more socially responsive and adult-oriented
than boys. If we had found either of these to be the case, we
would have nodded wisely and thought nothing further. In fact, for
the first few subjects in the laboratory, it did look as if girls
made "significantly" more Listener Responses, though the difference
was small. The first article (Dittmann, 1972) described the difference as being "in the direction common sense would predict," but in
view of the small size of the effect, nothing further was made of
it--wisely, we learned when we doubled the sample size later and
the difference disappeared. Since we are not precise in our expectations about sex differences, if none had been found in the
Follow-up Study, we would not have thought much about it, certainly
not enough to try to explain away such a "negative finding."

But the way things turned out, that boys and mixed groups are
both more responsive than all-girl groups, and also have longer
conversations, makes it look as if boys were the leaders in social
sophistication, especially in relation to adults, and that doesn't
make sense. I have only a few thoughts to offer in the matter.
First, most of the teachers they came in contact with were women,
and that may have had an effect on these early adolescent children,
the boys being more drawn to them and the girls feeling more competitive. But how should the finding on mixed groups be explained
in these terms? Unfortunately, we did not include in our recording
whether a girl or a boy was doing the talking or who was respond-
ing--that would have been too great a burden on the observers. So
we do not know whether the girls behaved differently when they were
with the boys. We need more data to find this answer.

Some of the problems of girls figuring out their new relationships with boys may certainly have entered here. At about this
age, many girls feel it is not wise to look too bright or alert in
comparison with boys. Boys are apt to be quite competitive, and
girls who want to win them over reason that they should try to
stay out of that competition. Perhaps being responsive to teachers
is an arena for pull-back on the girls' part. Again, we can only
check out that speculation with more data.

ACKNOWLEDGMENTS

This study could not have been carried out without the warm
welcome we received from the staff, children, and parents of Green
Acres School in Rockville, Maryland. From our very first explorations to the more elaborate and systematic scheduling of observations in the Follow-up Study, our flounderings were accommodated
and our refinements of method aided by these dedicated and very
interested people.

Alfred L. Smith, Jr. worked closely with me on the Follow-up
Study while developing one of his own on listening in classroom
instructional situations, the results of which are to be reported
elsewhere. His combined seriousness and good humor, plus his substantive contributions to the method, made the whole enterprise go
more smoothly. He has since collected further observations on conversations in children, taken in a very different setting for comparison.

REFERENCES

Boomer, D. S. Hesitation and grammatical encoding. Language and
    Speech, 1965, 8, 148-158.

Boomer, D. S., & Laver, J. D. M. Slips of the tongue. British
    Journal of Disorders of Communication, 1968, 3, 2-12.

Dittmann, A. T. Developmental factors in conversational behavior.
    Journal of Communication, 1972, 22, 404-423.

Dittmann, A. T., & Llewellyn, L. G. The phonemic clause as a unit
    of speech decoding. Journal of Personality and Social Psychology,
    1967, 6, 341-349.

Dittmann, A. T., & Llewellyn, L. G. Relationship between vocaliza-
    tions and head nods as listener responses. Journal of Personality
    and Social Psychology, 1968, 9, 79-84.

Mead, G. H. Mind, self, and society. Chicago: University of Chi-
    cago Press, 1934.

Piaget, J. The language and thought of the child. (M. Gabain,
    Transl.) London: Routledge & Kegan Paul, 1926.

Sullivan, H. S. The psychiatric interview. H. S. Perry & H. L.
    Gawell (Eds.). New York: Norton, 1954.

Trager, G. L. & Smith, H. L., Jr. An outline of English structure.
    (Studies in Linguistics: Occasional Papers, 3) Norman, Oklahoma:
    Battenberg Press, 1951. (Republished by American Council of
    Learned Societies, New York, 1965.)

ISSUES POSED BY SECTION 2

Jean Schimek

New York University

New York, New York

As the dictionary tells us, communication can refer to "a close or intimate rapport that is sometimes intellectual and often affective" or "a process by which meanings are exchanged between individuals through a common system of symbols (as language, signs, or gestures)." The first meaning seems primary, developmentally earliest and almost synonomous with "object relations." This level of communication is present from the first year of life (see section one) yet remains essential in later development. It can be primarily or exclusively nonverbal, relies heavily on motor and tactile contacts, and is mostly in the service of the gratification of immediate peremptory needs. This kind of communication is a learned "mutual cueing" between two individuals, a patterned way in which a certain behavior in individual A tends to function as a signal or trigger for certain responses in individual B. Such a pattern of consistent signalling is created by and specifically attuned to the concrete uniqueness of the close "object relation" involved--it has only limited generalizability to other situations and persons, and need not involve any conscious communicative intent. By contrast, the second, more advanced mode of communication involves an intentional exchange of meanings, of information represented in symbolic form. It requires a clear differentiation between sender and receiver but does not presuppose any prior close or prolonged relationship between them, unlike the specific mutual cueing of the earlier level. It does require, however, a shared, previously learned, generalized symbolic system, of which language is a prime example. Of course, these two modes of communication are not sharply delineated; there are many intermediate, transitional stages in the developmental sequence from one to the other and some integration of these two modes remains essential for any effective communication--a point which is the underlying assumption in Freedman's and Dittmann's studies.

The papers in this section and in most of the symposium face
the question of the developmental requirements for effective verbal
communication and the relative influence of interpersonal "affective"
factors. Here it may be helpful to make use, in an extended and
modified way, of Chomsky's distinction between linguistic competence
and linguistic performance; I mean the difference between the acquisition of the general rules of language and the individual's actual,
effective use of this capacity, his communicative performance. Linguistic competence is acquired by almost everyone; its necessary pre-
requisites (short of neurological deficit) seem minimal: a certain
amount of human contact and stimulation and some elementary development of self-object differentiation. But the requirements for communicative performance are much more complex and variable. They require, at the very least, a concept of "the other," of the similarities and differences between his and our own communicative code, interests, knowledge and needs--a basic decentering from our own point
of view as the only and absolute frame of reference. It requires
also a wish to communicate, a trust in the efficacy of communication
as leading to some gratification, and a belief in the relative safety
of words over deeds (if the two are not sufficiently differentiated
they become subject to the same conflicts and inhibitions). Thus,
when considering a specific individual or a specific developmental
phase, the problem is not so much the presence or absence of communicative capacity but the range of specific situations, contexts and
partners that shape communicative performance. With these issues,
the vicissitudes of object relations, of self and object representations, of the specific expressions of drives and defenses, acquire
crucial relevance. Much of these issues can be subsumed under the
conveniently broad and somewhat vague concept of empathy.

Kaplan's observations are at the transitional border between
the two basic levels of communication described above. She deals
with aspects of the mother-child dialogue in the second year of life
which are still largely a mutual cueing, though at a time when speech
and clearly intentional communication on the child's part begin to
emerge.

In the regulation of this basic dialogue, the mother's capacity
to know the child's needs and to respond appropriately to them plays
a predominant role. The "empathic" mother must be "specifically attuned to her child's needs" and capable of interpreting various items
of its behavior as anticipatory signals. It is likely that her intuitive sharing of the child's feelings and moods--as a kind of poorly
understood, immediate, sympathetic reaction or affective contagion--
is the essential basis of empathic understanding. But, as Kaplan
points out, this shared feeling reaction in itself is not enough, especially if the mother is simply overwhelmed by it and cannot identify
its source in the child and differentiate it from her other feelings.
The difference between full-fledged affective contagion (and the blur-
ring of self-object boundaries involved) and its use as a tamed, differentiated signal for an empathic response may be somewhat analogous

to the distinction between an anxiety reaction and signal anxiety.

The case of Jane illustrates how a similarity in temperament
and attitudes between mother and child can be an interference with
satisfactory dialogue; the mother has to be sufficiently differentiated from the child in order to be able to transform her global,
over-involved, sympathetic reactions into empathic responses attuned to the child's specific needs. Empathy seems to involve a
constantly shifting balance between sharing and separateness, differentiation and identification, the maintenance of boundaries and
the tolerance for some merging. Empathy is most difficult if we experience the other person as extremely different, unfamiliar and
alien from us. Also implicit in Kaplan's approach is the idea that
the presence of a mother eager and able to promptly anticipate and
gratify a child's every need does not in itself foster differentiation. Empathy requires a sense for the right timing and intensity
of responses, including an intuitive knowledge of when and to what
extent the child can tolerate frustration and delay. This would
seem necessary to make the child increasingly an active partner in
the dialogue, to foster his efforts at intentionally communicating
his needs, initiating gratification and actively influencing his
environment. Part of the process of self-other differentiation is
that the dialogue can and must become more of a give and take, with
the development on the child's side of a "capacity for concern" for
the object as a separate person with its own needs. Without what
Freud called "the frustrating impact of external reality," and what
Piaget conceptualized as the need for accommodation, there can be
little cognitive differentiation or development of a sense of self.
It is interesting to note that different child-rearing ideologies,
depending on culture and period, have different views as to the right
balance of frustration and gratification at different phases of development.

A mother's empathic capacity will not necessarily prevail in
her actual behavior towards the child, under all circumstances and
at all developmental stages. Hope's mother is described as very empathic at a certain stage; but when the child's later development
made demands on her which probably conflicted with her own needs,
her empathy became ineffectual. Similarly, Fay's mother seems capable of empathic understanding, but incapable of using this empathy
in specific areas where her needs and conflicts (for instance, around
oral greed) override her potential awareness of the child's needs.
It is this kind of situation, where an individual's conflicts and
defenses in specific areas prevent him from adaptively using information presumably available to him, which has been the main paradigm
for psychoanalytic explanations. Traditional psychoanalytic theory
has shown little concern for the necessary and sufficient conditions
of the development of the structures that permit the gathering and
communication of relevant knowledge from and to significant others;

it has usually taken this ability for granted and focused on specific
areas of symptomatic interference. Kaplan's illustration of how promising beginnings in the precursors of empathy can disappear at the
following developmental stage, and how apparent deficiencies at one
phase can be compensated at another, points to the limitations of
any linear developmental formulation.

The concept of empathy comes up again in Dittmann's study. He
shows how motoric listener responses are attuned to the rhythm and
structure of the speaker's talk, and how the frequency of these responses tends to increase significantly in the early adolescent years.
Here we have empathic response in the strict sense, as the structured
motoric responsiveness of the listener to the speaker. Dittmann's argument that such responses serve to facilitate the listener's decoding
of speech, and may serve an analogous function to that of the "speech
primacy movements" for the speaker, seems the level of explanation
closest to the data. To what extent this measure can be used as an
index of empathy in the broader sense, as the capacity to take on
and respond to the point of view of a "generalized other," remains
open to question. The fact that the frequence of such responses increases during the same years in which the more mature forms of empathy and dialogue develop is not conclusive; it can at best provide
us with a guiding hypothesis as to some of their meaning and function.
We have no data yet on the influence of these listener responses on
the back and forth of dialogue, on the extent to which the speaker
reacts to them and may be influenced by them. Dittmann has begun to
explore the crucial question of the relationship between these responses and the specific contents of a communication, and that of the
influence of the specific relationship between listener and speaker
on them; but his data are still preliminary and inconclusive, as he
makes clear. He has provided us with a promising objective index
which may be used as an effective tool in the further exploration of
these issues.

Freedman's systematic studies of the structure, functions, and
developmental aspects of body movements during speech illustrate several important issues, which go quite beyond the specific content of
his data. The broadest issue is that of the persistence of earlier
developmental levels and their interaction with later ones. Do they
simply persist, somehow unchanged and frozen, primarily as a potential for regression, as a burden or strain on higher levels of function, as the archaeological metaphors of psychoanalytic theory often
implied? Or do they themselves change and shift their function as
they continue to coexist with later levels? Freedman shows us how
the highest symbolic systems continue to need the support--or at
least are enhanced by--the persistence of the remnants of the earlier
predominantly motoric levels of thought and symbolic representation.
This is possible because these earlier motoric levels keep changing
through development in the direction of an increasing "formular ab-
breviation" or "schematization"; their depictive content is condensed

to a minimum, their intensity reduced until, at the level of speech primacy movements, only some of the "vectorial" and rhythmic aspects of movements remain. The subordination of motoric expression communication to the now dominant verbal system is thus made possible. One can infer, as Freedman does, that object-focused movements help the speaker find the right word for his private imagery and experience. But they also probably contribute to keeping his use of language--as a fixed, impersonal symbolic system--attuned to the specificity and variety of his own experience. For in the transformation of a private code into a public one, of iconic symbols into linguistic signs, there is not only a gain but also a loss of meaning and specificity. Object-focused movements may help to reduce this loss, and give to the speaker, as well as transmit to the listener, the feeling that the speaker says what he means and means what he says. In this respect, it would be interesting to be able to compare body movements with another variable that influences the connotative meaning of spoken language, namely, variations in tone, speed and intensity controlled by the voice.

If object-focused movements deal with the constant balance and oscillation between the private and public aspects of communication codes, body-focused movements seem to relate to oscillations in awareness along the basic self-other axis which underlies all communication. The frequency of such movements increases as a situation or task becomes more stressful or conflicted, and thus some process of tension discharge and tension regulation is involved. Just as object-focused movements, body-focused movements also undergo a developmental structuralization, from global to circumscribed, from continuous and unrelated to speech, to brief pauses occurring before speech clauses, and related in a positive way to syntactic complexity. Thus, depending on the intensity and timing of such movements, they could lead to a withdrawal from communication (as is frequently seen in therapy with psychotic patients), or function as brief emergency measures, and interference in the natural flow of speech but necessary to keep the activity going at all or, at the highest level, as the well-timed "pause that refreshes" and enhances linguistic performance. If further data confirm the suggestion that the distinction between object-focused and body-focused movements has some intrinsic relation to the polarity between the semantic and syntactic sequential aspects of language, a very interesting empirical approach to the general question of the origin of linguistic structures and their relation to sensory motor structures may have been opened.

Body-focused movements do not simply dispose of interfering tension, but provide a specific kind of stimulation, a combination of motor tactile self-stimulation. So, as Freedman suggests, they could be seen as giving a confirmation of the sense of self, a self which is first and foremost a body self, to paraphrase Freud. Why would such self-confirmation, or at least momentary bodily self-awareness, be

part of normal communication? Freedman invokes the interesting idea
of the biphasic functioning of attention, which in order not to become "stuck" and paralyzed has to shift repeatedly from its main outward focus to an internal one. When speaking intently, we usually
project ourselves into the content of the message and undergo some
degree of empathic merging with an actual or imagined listener; our
words may also acquire a life of their own, like the characters in
a novel, as if somewhat out of our control. All this may involve
some temporary loss of a sense of self. Body-focused movements, and
the fleeting inner experiences that may be triggered by them, could
provide a periodic reconfirmation of the self as the author of our
words, as an active agent capable to choice and controlled attention.
Getting back to the level of directly observable data, it would be
interesting to know more about the factors that influence body movements in actual dialogue, particularly the influence of shifts from
denotative secondary process to more primary process communication
including the predominantly emotive and conative uses of language.

     Freedman's studies give a striking illustration of the general
principle that we cannot attribute a specific fixed function to certain behavior (or in clinical terms, to a symptom or character trait),
without considering its changes through development in terms of increasing structuralization and integration within higher levels. The
important notion that earlier developmental levels do not simply disappear (or remain as mere potential for regression) but, through increasing schematization and internalization, remain as integrated
supports for higher levels, may apply to many areas beyond that of
body movements. Such development, for instance, can be seen in the
progression from sympathetic reaction to empathic understanding of
a situation, up to a systematic attempt at understanding someone's
character and history (for instance, as part of the therapeutic process). Such a way of looking at the continued influence of the past
may provide a promising alternative to such psychoanalytic concepts
as binding, neutralization of energy, or regression in the service
of the ego, which do little more than label certain developmental issues. This would apply particularly to the contribution of pre-opera-
tional, "primary process thinking" to higher levels of thought organization, and the persistence of early modes of object relations as necessary to the personal anchoring of more "mature" rational interactions. Lest we get carried away by a view of development as a straigh
march towards differentiation and objectivity (often compensated in
our culture by a cult of the intrinsic virtues of regressive experiences), we may keep in mind Freud's old-fashioned idea that the reality principle is basically only a necessary adaptive modification of
the pleasure principle.

     All three studies in this section share an emphasis on organizing
structures rather than on thematic contents; empathic dialogue, lister
responses and body movements during speech are all regulated by basic

patterns of rhythm, timing and intensity. These structural aspects, as Piaget suggests, may be the common element that sustains the developmental and adaptive continuity between the pre-adapted, rhythmic biological regulation of the earliest interactions between organism and human environment and the acquired effectiveness of the most complex symbolic communicative systems.

SECTION 3
COMMUNICATIVE STRUCTURES
IN PSYCHOPATHOLOGY
AND SENSORY DEFICIT

INTRODUCTION

Psychopathology is not only a disorder of thought but also a
disorder in the transmission of thought. Indeed, the effect of
psychopathology in eroding psychological organization must leave its
imprint on words, gestures, or vocal patterns during human discourse.
Traditionally, emphasis in the study of psychopathology has been
upon the array of cognitive disturbances characteristic of the particular pathological process, with little attention given to the
structure of the communicative act per se. Given the fact, however,
that inferences about cognitive disturbance are frequently based
upon communicated thought, i.e., speech, it becomes imperative to
examine those communicative organizations which enable the trans-
missions of meanings.

Recorded communication samples from distinct clinical populations provide the phenomena upon which this section is based. The
research strategy utilized by the investigators is, of necessity,
naturalistic, and based upon the model of the accident of nature.
The observations are varied, ranging across infantile autism, schizophrenia, and sensory deficit, yet each of the studies converges upon
the relation between communicative organization and the underlying
pathological processes.

Shapiro reports upon his studies of echoic phenomena in autistic children, and proposes that echoing is a primitively structured
effort at social closure activated in a situation in which the limited cognitive capacities of the child do not permit a meaningful exchange. Through such response the autistic child reveals that he does
not understand the speaker, but signals that he has heard him. Whether such an imitative response is a fixation to an early adaptive
mechanism, or whether it constitutes a failure of inhibition, as
Horowitz suggests in his discussion, remains an open issue for further study. In either case, echoing as social closure is but a continuation of those early forms of synchrony described by Spitz, Sander, and Kaplan in the basic dialogue; a communicative object relationship structure which operates prior to the establishment of the
capacity for symbolic meaning.

Steingart's research utilizes the phenomena of language con-

struction. He presents a psychoanalytic interpretation of language
behavior in which linguistic activity is seen as more than simply an
index of cognitive organization. Language construction behavior reflects a speaker's intentions to use his psychic apparatus to express a relative complexity and differentiation of the internal representation of the self and object world. Using both transformational and Piagetian approaches to spontaneous speech in schizophrenic and depressed patients, Steingart shows how the complexity
and articulateness of language construction varies with changes in
clinical state. These shifts in linguistic complexity are seen as
representative of, and dependent upon, the differentiation and complexity of self- and object-representations characteristic of the
particular psychopathology. It is the differentiated experience of
self and other created by such an interchange which becomes implemented in the structure of linguistic units.

Cognitive structures of social closure or of self and object
are not yet sufficient for the delivery of language. Ongoing speech
requires the continuing adjustment and readjustment to inner drives
and tension states. Spoken language is dependent upon internal regulations as well as dyadic regulations. Such regulatory structures
operate both on the psychological and psychophysiological level.
Before a message can be transmitted, it has to be attended to, and
attention requires the regulation of arousal. These views bring the
theory of communication into contact with both the earliest formulations of Freud in The Project and recent psychophysiological concepts.

Grand focuses upon self-stimulation, and sees such phenomena as
compensatory forms of auto-regulation of stimulus nutriment. He
uses his observations of self-stimulating behavior to establish a
link between such activity and the maintenance of optimal levels of
attention for effective language encoding. His observations on the
role of self-stimulation in patients suffering from various "communicative disorders," supports an interpretation of kinesic activity
which is both psychodynamically and neurophysiologically based. The
patterns of communicative behavior differ in the schizophrenic
patient, in the blind, and in those with a transitory linguistic
handicap, yet the principle of auto-regulation is the same. Grand's
contribution is a continuation of the view of the kinesic system as
an essential regulator of ongoing communication.

The view of communicative structures as not only manifestation
of pathology but also as regulators of psychopathology is an important contribution of the papers in this section. Furthermore, the
concept of kinesic self-regulation is novel and has received little
emphasis in communication research. Its significance will reappear
as an important theme for an understanding of the associative process during the psychoanalytic treatment situation, to be taken up
in Section 5.

THE SPEECH ACT: A LINGUISTIC FRAME OF REFERENCE TO STUDY EGO

ADAPTATION OF A PSYCHOTIC CHILD

Theodore Shapiro[1]

New York University

New York, New York 10003

In recent years, infant research and early childhood studies
have focused on the interaction between mother and child as the
relevant unit to be explored in the march of developmental adaptation. This is the vantage point of many psychoanalytically trained
infant investigators (Sander, 1975; Stern, 1971), as well as a number of animal behaviorists (Schneirla, 1960). Mahler's (1975) view
of the separation-individuation process likewise focuses on interactional matrices and postulates "psychic hatching" along with biological maturation. This dominant psychoanalytic view of the problems of infancy also derives, in part, from Hartmann's concept of
"average expectable biological equipment in an average expectable
environment" that also focuses attention on interaction.

While these propositions have yielded rich information about
the psychology of functioning individuals, it tends to omit the effects of the "limitations of the flesh" upon the mental apparatus.
Freud, himself, emphasized these other factors in his early formulations of Actual Neuroses (1895) hypnoid tendencies (1895), constitutional factors in libidinal fixation (1905), the molding effect
of body ego on maturing ego function (1905), and narcissistic ego
distortions (1914). Greenacre's (1952) later insistence on the pre-
disposing effects of intrauterine experiences on later manifestations

[1]The author wishes to express his gratitude to Dr. Lynn Burkes and
Mr. Peter Lucy for their valuable technical assistance in preparing
the data for this manuscript. Dr. Burkes worked on this project as
a fellow in Child Psychiatry contributed to by NIMH fund MHO 7331.
Mr. Lucy worked as a second year medical student. He developed the
reaction time techniques utilized.

of anxiety in the borderline state is an extension of these ideas.
Similarly, the recent deluge of writing by analysts on narcissistic
development is an attempt to deal with the fact that patients who
roughly correspond to these descriptions are seen more frequently
in practice.

The specific solution in theorizing about object-splits, etc.,
I believe, originates in a simple methodological fact that psychoanalysis is an interactional process. The transference is its major tool enabling practitioners to best explore the distortions in
object relations of their patients. However, as a general psychology,
psychoanalysts should not be content with an exclusively object-
relations theory of development. That route has been traveled before by Sullivan (1953). M. Klein (1932) and other classical analysts have always felt these positions to be too fragmentary as a
general approach. While it is plausible that object relations theory
refers to one of the most "human" aspects of our functioning, it is
also the case that a developmentally holistic view requires that
human relations is one, among other behaviors, that rests upon background distortions and limitations of cognitive and other autonomous ego apparatuses.[2]

Reading the literature, with the hope of finding the reasons
for pathology in faulty mothering, has led to as many distortions
as postulating intrinsic ego defects. Moreover, many psychoanalysts
cover themselves for these distortions by shifting from intrapsychic,
to interactional causal statements, and back again as needed. Too
few adopt Winnicott's caution that there is such a thing as "good
enough mothering," and we are not certain as yet which are the "limiting" factors that encroach on the "experience of mothering" versus
"actual mothering." Dyadic studies remain plausible if the hypotheses generated do not automatically exclude nature and nurture
weightings. The research to be described attempts such a task. The
framework is semi-naturalistic and not analytic.

BACKGROUND

I have selected the most deviant children, seen by child psy-
chiatrists, who are without known structural defects of the central
nervous system for study. Autistic or early childhood schizophrenic
children provide a model of severe early behavioral deviance in
which inadequate or "damaged" ego structures may be inferred. However, the interactional matrix is also affected, and careful analysis
of structure of interaction may generate the best hypotheses. Studying language, via the actually deviant speech development of these

---

[2]As practicing psychoanalysts, we usually emphasize the potent effect
of conflict on autonomous functions. I am suggesting that an approach "a tergo" is warranted as well.

children, provides us not only with instrumentality for observing
an aspect of ego functioning, but also offers clues to the elements
necessary for normal development that are not observable when speech
develops smoothly. In the latter instance, we may not see the discontinuities or hierarchic stepwise progression of development because the steps are slurred over. Former work by the author has
shown that autistic and schizophrenic children have a number of disturbances in linguistic processing and coding so that their production appears deviant from the standpoint not only of content, but
structure and context orientation (Shapiro et al.,1975). This paper
will focus on utilizing a framework of "speech acts" (Searle,1969)
in order to examine and understand the communicational significance
of echoing in psychotic children, and from that offer suggestions
regarding its developmental role in normals.

Shapiro, Roberts, and Fish (1970), showed that psychotic children at age four echoed more rigidly than normal two, three or com-
peers at age four. It was even found that a large number of responses of two year olds were newly recoded creative imitations
rather than recorder-like replays. When psychotic children were
studied for grammatical contrast of negation (Shapiro & Kapit, in
press), they proved to be most competent imitators compared to three
year old normal controls who insisted on changing grammatical form
even after instructed not to. Normal five year olds were also good
imitators because they were compliant, but were fully able to produce the most varied grammatical forms when free to do so.

Studying normals, Nelson (1973) showed that children do not
invariably learn nouns-for-things as their first words, as formerly
thought. Rather, there seem to be what she calls "referential"
children whose early corpus (first 50 words) contains a predominance
of nouns, and "expressive" children who do not build their early
vocabulary in that way. The former are more likely to imitate.
Bloom (1974) similarly showed in a naturalistic longitudinal study
of four children, that two were imitators and two were not. She
went on to show that the imitators were as likely to have the same
grammatical forms in their nonimitative utterances as in their imitative ones suggesting that imitation was "progressive," i.e., even
when echoing was a significant behavior, it was a sign of cognitive
or grammatical readiness. This view is in line with Piagetian developmental studies (Sinclair de Zwart, 1969), and contrary to the
view that imitation precedes comprehension and production as indicated by Fraser, Bellugi,and Brown (1963). Propositions endorsing
reinforcement and generalization have been criticized before this
latter work as not fully explaining the rapid onset of creative syntactic forms in small children (Lenneberg, 1967; Bloom, 1970; McNeill,
1970). Fay and Butler (1968) have studied the echoing of non-psy-
chotic, retarded children, and discussed the function of echoing.

One of these suggestions will be expanded in the current paper, and
explored, to understand something about the distorted speech function of psychotic children. Careful experiments by Hermelin and
O'Connor (1970) show that autistic children have an intact auditory
span, but that decoding and association processes are impaired. They
coined the term "echo box memory" to characterize the performance of
these children. Extending this notion, Aurnhammer-Frith (1969)
found the effects of phonological structure to be equal for a group
of eight autistic and a group of eight normal children, but autistic
children were deficient in their appreciation of syntax as presented
in the sequential structure of language. Others (Bartolucci & Albers,
1974; Bartok & Rutter 1974) have similarly showed the inabilities of
these children in syntactic understanding in the specific area of
development of deixis.

Our observations have led us to understand, and the current
paper tests further, the propositions that echoes in young psychotic children represent a device for social closure in a child
whose limited cognitive capacities permit a limited repertoire of
other responses. The index child seems to be saying, "I understand
that I am expected to speak in this social situation, but I neither
understand what is appropriate nor have the wit to do so. However,
I can say something, and that seems to stop you, the interlocator,
from making the same sounds to me." Parenthetically, I believe it
is for this reason that behaviorist techniques, as utilized by Lovaas
(1974), Hewett (1965), etc. have been grabbed-up so readily by many
"therapist-investigators"--not because they produce greater fluency
in language, but the increment in productivity of pat imitative
phrases pleases investigators who count any advance as significant
in what seems to be an uphill battle.

The notion of a speech event as a "speech act" utilizes the
interactional or communicative frame of reference and goes beyond the simply structural view which has been taken in prior studies.
It suggests an ilocutionary intent in an interchange, and a perlocutionary response which says to the initiator of the communication, "I have heard you; I understand you; and I intend to answer
relevantly or irrelevantly in whatever way I am able." While this
interactional model again stresses a two-party system for linguistic
understanding, it leaves open the possibility that the nature of the
response could be analyzed from the standpoint of its functional
pragmatism in a communicative situation. This framework, in conjunction with prior structural models, suggests a number of expectations which can be tested empirically. These expectations will be
explored in the speech sample of a single autistic child of five
years six months, at the time of interviewing. If echoes were but
a simple device for social closure, the following ought to be demonstrated:

1. The total number of responses per unit time of such a child
ought to be greater than the number of responses of a comparable

child at a similar stage. A subhypothesis of this notion is that
if the increased number of responses within the time sample were
due to the "social closure strategy" of echoing, then echoes would
have a more rapid reaction time. Thus, we could compare the reaction time for echoes versus non-echoes, as well as the uniformity
within each subsector of utterances to infer the degree of processing time necessary.

2. Mean length of utterance (MLU) of echoes should be somewhat
longer than the mean length of utterances (MLU) of other responses
of the same child, because intrinsic grammatical coding devices
would be bypassed for echoes and not constrained as much as when the
child is trying to code his own response on the basis of restructuring and matching processes.

3. The echoing ought to occur at points in the interview
where the question asked taxes the child's comprehension, i.e.,
echoing ought to follow demands which are more complex than those
that elicit appropriate acceptable responses.

4. It would be expected that when an echo chain is set into
motion that echoes might cluster, as though the child falls into
a perlocutionary mode that satisfies the interaction, and this
becomes a "sticky set" used beyond the necessity of the moment.

5. The remainder of the corpus of responses of the child ought
to be limited in its variety, suggesting the functional need for so
simple a device as echoing as an intermittent response type when
cognitive-linguistic capacities are stretched beyond available re-
sources.

If we can demonstrate these five points in a sample of speech
of an autistic child, we will have satisfied the hypothesis that
viewing echoing as a speech act offers a sufficient frame of reference to understand an aspect of the limited ego functions of this
psychotic child. This interpretation, then, may be used to suggest
parallel deficits in object relations leading to distorted "child-
mother" or "child-other" interactions. Both of these functional
problems would need be secondary to the limitation of cognitive sub-
structure, and neither would have priority in this child viewed as
typical of a group. It also would be instructive to compare the
speech act of this child to the child with average biological equipment to see how normal language learning facilitates object relations
as well as the reciprocal proposition.

BRIEF HISTORY

Evan was first seen at 4 years 6 months after a speech and hearing evaluation at four. His mother's chief complaint was that he was
withdrawn and had not developed language adequately. He screeched

and spent much of his time at the television set, panicking when
it was turned off, but was not "really" watching it. He was interested in mechanical things, and took a can of coffee or oil to
bed rather than a soft object. He had recently been destructive.
He was coordinated and seemed unaware of danger. Temper tantrums
in which he threw himself on the floor, undressed, and threw things
were elicited at the slightest provocation. He grimaced, played
with his fingers, and occasionally covered his ears and walked on
his toes.

He was the first child of an 18-year-old black mother and a
German born white father. Both were teachers. Evan was full term
(birthweight of 7.7 pounds) and aside from an occipital hematoma,
no birth defects were noted. The hematoma subsided in two months.

The infant was hypotonic but irritable until nine months. He
was described as "colicky," and had difficulty falling asleep at
night unless he was held and rocked, which his mother did. Bedtime
rocking continued until he was 2.6. Evan was breast-fed and began
drinking from a cup at nine months without a transitional bottle.
He began to feed himself at three years of age. He was not yet
bowel trained at time of admission.

No significant medical history was elicited. He sat unaided
at six months, stood at seven months, and walked at 11 months.
He smiled at six weeks, and is described as having made good eye
contact until about 1.6 when he withdrew. However, he was never
considered an affectionate child. He would sit in a corner when
people, other than his parents, were present, and avoided eye contact.

At 2.6, Evan was enrolled in a day care program but was dropped
after three months because he was "not interested." At home, he was
hyperactive but withdrawn and quiet in the nursery. His mother
stopped working to care for Evan and her second child, born when
Evan was 2.10.

Evan's language development included vowel sounds between three
to five months, but no babbling. At 18 months he said a few single
words, e.g. "cookie," "juice," and responded variably to his name.
At two, he pointed at words that his mother was reading to him, and
learned the alphabet and numbers "within a week." His production
was exclusively designations. His vocabularly expanded little between two to three years, and he did not combine words. At three,
he echoed entire sentences, and identified pictures "if he wished
to." While he understood a few simple directions at four, his
parents still thought he might be deaf.

On admission, Evan was described as a handsome, neatly dressed,
tall, well developed, light skinned Negro boy. His facial expression

was bland except for grimacing. His responses were delayed, and
attention was fleeting. He made no overt social overtures and
cried only briefly when his mother left him. When she returned
1-1/2 hours later, he did not look at her, but ran out of the nursery.
At first, he would not sit at the examining table, but was soon able
to be engaged in testing. He adapted to the reversal of the Gesell
formboard (36 months level) and played with the non-animate toys,
ignoring the family dolls. He only scribbled at pencil and paper
tasks. He did not pay attention when his mother encouraged him to
make an "o" and responded, "no" when she asked him to draw a pump-
kin which he apparently had been capable of doing.

He sat in the examiner's rotary chair saying, "take it off, I
get off" and turned around on it. He named items such as "zipper"
and "egg," but would not name "letters." He named his mother's
mouth, but no other parts of the body. He added a few words out of
context with no apparent relevance to the current setting. He comprehended minimally. Some of his speech was unintelligible, he
did not respond to his name and ignored many questions and commands.

He was diagnosed as an early onset psychosis corresponding,
in varying nomenclatures, to early infantile autism or childhood
schizophrenia, autistic type. He improved at the Bellevue Nursey
with milieu, educational, and drug therapy. He made some attachments to nursery personnel and sought them out on occasion to verbalize his wishes and aims. While he continued to spend much of his
time alone, some interaction and eye contact was tolerated; his
attention span increased, and he could persist at assembling a picture puzzle for up to 30 minutes. His affect broadened with better
modulation and less irritability. His language production and comprehension improved. At discharge, his speech was largely intellig-
ible and more spontaneous, but stilted. Much of what he said was as
though speaking out loud to himself, but he also used speech to
communicate needs. His productions usually referred to the current
circumstance, and his vocabulary remained limited. He was discharged
to a specialized treatment center and his mother continues to work
with him.

METHOD

Evan was seen between the ages of four years nine months, and
seven years six months. During the three years, he was audio-taped
ten times for ten-minute stimulated sessions. In addition, special
linguistic testing was instituted from time to time. The examiner
stimulated the child's productive speech by asking simple questions
about objects, picture books, and other play material. A transcript
of the recording was prepared and correlated with an observer's context notes of the interview.

The utterances were classified according to a two dimensional scale of morphological complexity and communicative value (Shapiro & Fish,1969). Communicativeness includes distinctions between non-communicative and communicative speech. The latter encompasses such utterances as simple social greetings, appeal, or wish-oriented speech, as well as complex symbolic speech. Noncommunicative speech includes isolated expressive speech, echoes and utterances with little or no contextual reference. The present study contrasts the echoic and nonechoic responses in terms of MLU, stimulus conditions, and latency of the child's echoing of the examiner's speech compared to the mean latency of all other functional categories of the child's speech. Response latency, for our purposes, is defined as the time intervening the examiner's model sentence or query and the child's utterance.

A duplicate tape of the original recording was made, and a ten-second gap was introduced at the end of each of the child's utterances to facilitate analysis with reaction time equipment. The duplicate tape was played on a Tapesonic deck, the signal from which was fully rectified and demodulated, and then sent to a Bechman Offner polygraph. The tape was also monitored auditorily. The polygraph produced a paper recording which was advanced at a rate of 50 mm. per second. The modified signal caused a pen on the polygraph to produce a peak corresponding to each syllable of recorded speech. The response latencies were obtained by measuring the interval on the polygraph recording between the last peak of the examiner's speech and the first peak of the child's utterance. (The error of the circuitry and polygraph was 1/100 of a second. The intervals on the polygraph recording could be measured to within a milllimeter so the error from this source was two hundredths of a second. Presumably these two sources of error often cancelled each other. In any case, all response latencies are accurate to three hundredths of a second).

Evan progressed in his language development from a MLU of 1.1 to a MLU approximating 2. He always remained highly deviant and echoed frequently. When he was 5.6 years, he had a MLU of 1.78, indicating that many of his utterances were above two words in length, and that he was beginning some syntactic structuring. This sample was selected for study.

RESULTS

Evan produced 139 utterances in the ten-minute period with MLU 1.78., consisting of 58 echoes (41.7%) and 81 nonechoes (58.3%). See Table 1. There were ten prespeech utterances among his nonechoes that were not used to calculate the mean length of utterance (Table 2,A). There were 12 poorly contextualized utterances, 8 appeal utterances, 48 designations, and 3 answers to questions. This sample

Table 1

Ten Minute Speech Sample

Evan (5 years 6 months)

	Echoes	Nonechoes	Total
Number of Utterances	58	81	139
Percent Utterances	41.7	58.3	100%
MLU	1.95	1.67	1.78
Reaction Time Variance(s)	603.54^{*+}	18,467.94 ($5,534.38^{**}$)	

*53 Echoes used for reaction time

**Omitting noncommunicative responses

$^{+}$Mann-Whitney U   p < .00011

was then studied in terms of the four dimensions previously outlined: (1)   Speed of response and total number of responses within
the examination period.   (2)   MLU of echoes was contrasted to nonechoes.   (3)   Analysis was made of which of the interviewer's questions elicitcd echoes and whether they clustered.   (4)   Finally, the
non-echoic responses were analyzed for complexity of syntactic structure and appropriateness of reference.

   1. Evan's 139 responses in ten minutes were compared to the average
frequencies of children formerly studied for echoing behavior during
similar ten minute examinations (Shapiro, Roberts, & Fish, 1970).   A
sample of eight hospitalized psychotic children produced a mean total
number of utterances of 84.6 (range 62-123; only two of these subjects
had more than 100 responses).   A combined sample of 18 normal children
between the ages of 2.0 and 4.9 had a mean number of utterances of 93
(range 72-113).   The group of four-year-olds more closely comparable
to Evan's chronological age showed a mean total number of utterances
of 90.1.   Thus, Evan produces more utterances during the examination
time than his comparison groups of psychotic children and clearly
more than normals.   The overall impression was that Evan's high frequency of echoes accounted for the increased number of responses,
because it appeared that he responded to the examiner with shorter
latency.   To test this hypothesis, the reaction times of echoic and
nonechoic responses were measured separately.   The hypothesis was
further extended that echoic responses would be more uniform in
their latency because varied processing times might be necessary for
other responses as compared to echoes.   The variance of the echoic

sample was S=603.54 while the nonechoes variance was S=18467.94
verifying the greater uniformity of the latency of echoic responses
in this sample. Because of the difference in variance, a t-test was
not used to test the significance of the difference between means.
The nonparametric Mann Whitney U Test was employed. The difference
between the echoic and nonechoic responses was highly significant
(p >.00011). (Because of difficulties in the time sample, 53 of the
58 echoes were used for study or 44.5% of the entire sample.)

2. The mean length of utterance: It was hypothesized that if
the echoes were not processed by the usual encoding, but only subject to a more general constraint on length, that the echoes should
be longer than coded utterances. The MLU of echoes was 1.95, and
the non-echoes, 1.67. However, since MLU does not take into account
syntactic structure or the context in which they are produced, further
hypotheses were tested.

3. Echoes were elicited a total of 58 times during the interview. However, a number of the echoes occurred in bursts ranging
from two to 11 consecutive responses so that 27 of the 58 echoic
responses initiated a group of echoes. That is, there were nine
bursts of echoing which were more than two echoes long, some ranging
as high as eight to 11 times. This observation suggests than when a
child begins echoing, this becomes a temporarily preferred strategy.

For structural analysis, we included some responses which were
not completely congruent echoes because we wanted to test the range
of all imitative responsiveness. Consequently, some productions had
inflectional changes, telegraphic selection, and grammatical transformations which suggest that, at the least, he is on the verge of
grammatical development (Table 2,B).

Structural alterations, however, account for a small percentage of the corpus of echoes (13 of 58). The single perseveration
does not require presumed grammatical knowledge or new words. Correct naming, associated with pointing, is ambiguous as to function
because he is simply repeating what the examiner has said though it
is associated with a concrete environmental object-- again, no restructuring is required. The mitigation was a response to "count
fingers." He repeated verbatum, and proceeded "one, two, three,
four, five." This was an often heard rote sequence for Evan. The
only two utterances classified as echoes that comfortably can be
considered as being at the threshold of new grammatical forms were
the inflected plural change and a negative transformation. When the
examiner said "show me -- touch it." He responded "don't touch it."
However, this also may not be a true negative transformation because
he had often heard the prohibition in just that form. The positive
phrase may have triggered the more often heard negative. At best,
we may say he shows knowledge of the relationship between the two
phrases.

Table 2

Analysis of Echo (Variants) and Nonechoes

Evan (5 years 6 months)

A.	Nonechoes	# Utterances
	Prespeech	10
	Designations	48
	Wish/Command	2
	Answers	3
	Phatic	6
	Poor-Context	12

B.	Structurally Altered Imitations	
	Perseverative	1
	Telegraphic (omits article)	1
	Telegraphic (omits clause, object pronoun, preposition)	6
	Names as points	1
	Inflectional change (pluralizes final S)	1
	Mitigated echo (adds rote counting)	1
	Mitigated phatic	1
	Negative transformation	1

Turning now to the variety of questions that elicited echoes, aside from those where he responded in a phatic way or continued a burst of echoing that had begun, it is evident from the relative complexity of the queries that he may not have comprehended the question. For example, when the examiner asked, "Where is the boat blue? Show me?," he said, "blue" and pointed to the yellow. At another point, the examiner asked, "What kind of book?" He responded "book." After he named a ball, he was asked, "What can you do with the ball?" He answered telegraphically "do ball." Then the examiner said, "Can you throw a ball?" Evan answered "throw a ball." Continuing, the examiner then asked, "Can you bounce a ball?" The child ignored the query, turned the page, looked at another picture, and named a brush. He could then comply when the examiner asked what else was shown and said, "comb," clearly indicating that he could readily name things. Indeed, some 48 of his nonechoic, communicative utterances were designations (Table 2,A).

Further verification for this proposition comes from a burst of echoing that was initiated after he had named an orange. The examiner asked, "What do you do with an orange?" He repeated "orange." The examiner again asked, "What can you do with an orange?" The child said "do orange." The examiner then offered a semi-nonsense query, "Do you throw it?" Evan responded, "throw it." Examiner, "Or eat it?" He responded "eat it." Similarly, later on, when the examiner suggested "let's talk about something else," the child responded "talk something else." These responses suggest that there is limitation in comprehension which, in turn, severely limits the appropriate productive output of this child, and at such junctures, he resorts to echoic behavior.

CONCLUSIONS

A speech act framework permits us to stress the dyadic nature of early language learning rather than the emergence of facility with the code. In that sense it corresponds to what psychoanalysts have recently emphasized in their developmental hypotheses that lean on interactive matrices to study the individuation processes. Jerome Bruner (1974) makes the point that "Grammar originates as a set of rules abstracted from jointly regulated activity which has been codified in the culture of the linguistic community" (p. 7). Bruner sees grammar's emergence, even if naturally latent, as paralleling prior perceptual and attention structures, each of which enables the development of prediction and sentence closure. Action structures usually carried out with the mother i.e. action toward or away from the self, leads to "case grammar forms (agent, action, object) and ultimately in its most sophisticated form to deixis" (the changing referent for a single object where in one instance it is here, and then there, or regarding persons at once I, you, and he). The question that our data asks is, why did Evan not emerge with a normal repertoire, if potentials for grammatical and cognitive structures are part of average biological equipment in humans? Are we to turn to schizophrenogenicity in mothering for explanation? Our exploration of the structure of his interactions does not include his early interactions with mother. However, even with adequate environmental exposure in the nursery, he did not show adequately progressive language development. By contrast, even neglected children in postmarasmic states learn to speak. While institutionalized children may, at times, emerge as affectionless criminals, they seem to know noun from verb, etc. Could one argue for a specific "quality of mothering as yet undefined" to account for autistic language as described? We think not. The deficits seem to penetrate deeply into cognitive structures themselves. A recent report by Simon (1975) goes so far as to localize a substrate deficit in the brain itself.

The interactive developmental view should not force us to propose that all that evolves is a result of that interaction. Rather, the interaction also describes the species of capability of each of the parties. We are not simply as we are acted upon. That would satisfy a behaviorist's paradigm in which all that emerges was once in the environment. Parenthetically, autistic children are much

studied by behaviorists because there seems to be so little in the
way of intervening variables in the black box. On the other hand,
preformist postulates do not tell us how and when language and
speech emerge or what are the limits of the environment that any
given organism will tolerate.

Freud has been attacked from both sides, as a biological matura-
tionalist on the one hand, and an overzealous environmentalist on
the other. However, in actuality, Freud echoed the classicist's
epigram that all of behavior is a combination of "necessity and accident," thus leaving the way open to examine the contribution of
each. Hartmann's adaptational view, likewise, demands study of the
contribution from both sides. Let us see how Evan's behavior reveals
contributions from both sides of our postulated dyad.

Evan can form few grammatical constructions. He has turned toward the most concrete environment reflected in his limited, largely
nominal vocabulary but is stymied in understanding and producing
creative grammatical forms as even normal 30 month old children can.
He echoes when in doubt, and that he does with a uniform reaction
time suggesting the limitations in integrating and encoding for such
a response. He avoids the human environment because he cannot process
what is offered, so he backs off. His echoing is an adaptation to
some dimly recognized need to speak even though he does not understand. A mentally deficient child functions differently. He is retarded across the board, can tolerate close contact and affection,
and use his deficient intelligence to its limits, but the autistic
child has learned to make short shrift of the world because it con-
fuses him. The inability is not outside, but at the experiential
level. Perhaps, mimicking Bruner, his attentional and perceptual
apparatuses are timed differently and are too variable to be a reliable guide to later grammatical development, i.e., the neuroper-
ceptual background of action schemata which are said to underlie
grammatical form may be awry. This still leaves room for etiologi-
cal hedging, but not for hedging in adequate description of structure of behavior. This careful description of behavioral structure
within the framework described permits greater clarity with respect
to designating the direction for our interest while not disrupting
the human context in which development takes place.

Object relations theory and theories of environmental determination are as incomplete a description of the scope of human adaptation
as is Behaviorism. Psychoanalysts who emphasize only these parameters
should remember that they represent but one sector of a possible bevy
of functions and interactions that create "homocommunicandis."

REFERENCES

Aurnhammer-Frith, U. Emphasis and meaning in recall in normal and
  austistic children. Language and Speech, 1969, 12:29-38.

Bartak, L. & Rutter, M. The use of person pronouns for autistic
children. Journal of Autism and Childhood Schizophrenia, 1974,
4:217-222.

Bartolucci, G. & Albers, R. Deictic categories in the language of
autistic children. Journal of Autism and Childhood Schizophrenia,
1974, Vol. 4, No. 2.

Bloom, L. Language development: Form and function in emerging
grammars. Cambridge, Mass.: M.I.T. Press, 1970.

Bloom, L., Hood, L., & Lightbown, P. Imitation in language development: If, when, and why. Cognitive Psychology, 1974, 6:380-420.

Bruner, J. S. The ontogenesis of speech acts. Journal of Child
Lauguage, 1974, 2:1-19, Great Britain.

Fay, W. H., & Butler, B. V. Echolalia, IQ and the developmental di-
chotomy of speech and language-systems. Journal of Speech and
Hearing Research, 1968, 11:365-371.

Fraser, C., Bellugi, U., & Brown, R. Control of grammar in imitation, comprehension and production. Journal of Verbal Learning
and Verbal Behavior, 1963, 2:121-135.

Freud, S. (1895b). On the ground for detaching a particular syndrome from neurasthenia under the description anxiety neurosis.
Standard Edition, 3:87. London: Hogarth Press.

Freud, S. (1905). Three essays on the theory of sexuality. Standard Edition, 7:125-245. London: Hogarth Press, 1953.

Freud, S. (1914c). On narcissism: An introduction. Standard Edition, 14:73-102. London: Hogarth Press, 1957.

Freud, S. & Breuer, J. (1893-5). Studies on hysteria. Standard
Edition, Vol. 2, London: Hogarth Press.

Greenacre, P. The predisposition to anxiety. Part I. In Trauma,
growth and personality. New York: Norton, 1952.

Hermelin, B. & O'Connor, N. Psychological experiments with autistic
children. Oxford, England: Pergamon Press, 1970.

Hewett, F. M. Teaching speech to an autistic child through operant
conditioning. American Journal of Orthopsychiatry, 1965, 35:927-
936.

Klein, M. The psychoanalysis of children. London: Hogarth Press,
1932.

Lenneburg, E. H. Biological foundations of language. New York:
Wiley, 1967.

Lovaas, O. I., Schreidman, L., & Koegel, R. L. A behavior modification approach to the treatment of autistic children. Journal of
Autism and Childhood Schizophrenia, 1974, Vol. 4, p. 131.

Mahler, M., Pine, F, and Bergma, A. The psychological birth of the
human infant. New York: Basic Books, 1975.

McNeill, D. The acquisition of language: The study of developmental
psycholinguistics. New York: Harper and Row, 1970.

Nelson, K. Structure and strategy in learning to talk. Monographs
of the Society for Research in Child Development, 1973, 38: (1-2
Serial #149).

Sander, L. W. Some determinants of temporal organization in the
ecological niche of the newborn. Read at the Annual Meeting of
the American Academy of Child Psychiatry, St. Louis.

Searle, J. R. Speech acts: An essay in the philosophy of language.
London: Cambridge University Press, 1969.

Schneirla, T. C. Instinctive behavior, maturation, experience and
development. In B. Kaplan & S. Wapner (Eds.), Perspectives in
Psychological Theory. New York: International Universities
Press, 1960.

Shapiro, T. Language and ego function of young psychotic children.
In E. J. Anthony (Ed.), Explorations in child psychiatry. New
York: Plenum, 1975.

Shapiro, T. & Fish, B. A method to study language deviation as an
aspect of ego organization in young schizophrenic children. Journal of the American Academy of Child Psychiatry, 1969, Vol. 9,
No. 3.

Shapiro, T., Roberts, A., & Fish, B. Imitation and echoing in young
schizophrenic children. Journal of the American Academy of Child
Psychiatry, 1970, Vol. 9, No. 3.

Shapiro, T. & Kapit, R. Negation in young schizophrenic children.
Journal of Psycholinguistic Research, in press.

Simon, N. Echolalic speech in childhood autism. American Journal
of General Psychiatry, 1975, 32:1439-1446.

Sinclair de-Zwart, H. Developmental psycholinguistics. In D. Elkind
    & J. H. Flavell (Eds.), Studies in cognitive development: Essays
    in honor of Jean Piaget. New York: International Universities
    Press, 1969.

Stern, D. A microanalysis of mother-infant interaction: Behavior
    regulating social contact between a mother and her 3 1/2-month
    old twins. Journal of the American Academy of Child Psychiatry,
    1971, 10:501-517.

Sullivan, H. S. Interpersonal theory of psychiatry. New York:
    Norton, 1953.

A COMPARATIVE PSYCHOPATHOLOGY APPROACH TO LANGUAGE BEHAVIOR

Irving Steingart

Downstate Medical Center

Brooklyn, New York   11203

The mark of the innovative theoretician is the creation of a new language about theoretical structures and processes which brings an explanatory order to events which previously only could be described as disparate, unrelated phenomena. I think one can maintain, at least in a rough fashion, that Freud created at least three such new clinical (as opposed to metapsychological) languages for us which remain vital today. Freud's (1905) topographic theory, with its systems of Conscious, Preconscious, and a dynamic Unconscious, operating within different conditions of conflict with the psychosexual drives, produced such an ordering for neurotic, perverse, and normal sexual behavior. Freud's structural theory, with its systems of Id, Ego, and Superego, operating again within different matrices of conflict, but now with aggressive as well as psychosexual drives, supplemented the topographic theory and expanded this ordering of human behavior. For example, with this new structural theory of the mind, Freud (1923) could explain the interrelations among states of normal grief, melancholia, and mania. The third theory of the mind which supplements the first two is actually the oldest of the three. Freud (1900) called it "the psychic apparatus." I would prefer to call it the "meaning apparatus." It has to do with how an individual comes to represent experiences for himself and acquires signs (especially language) in connection with such representation. Freud needed this theory of the mind, again operating within different psychodynamic contexts, to comprehend, e.g., the interrelations among the nightly dreams of normal individuals and the hallucinations of schizophrenics (1900, 1911b).

All three of these theories of the mind have moved us toward integrations of normal behavior with various kinds of psychopathology. This is something which is true by definition. It is what

we mean by a scientific theory, and the more integration it accompli-
shes the more powerful the theory. It was always Freud's working
method to compare and contrast descriptions of specific psychopath-
ologies and normal behavior on the assumption that such a procedure
would generate general theoretical insights about all behavior. The
research I will describe follows this procedure.

With respect to these three theories I have just described, I
believe that the "psychic apparatus" theory has not been given the
explicit importance due it in the psychoanalytic situation. This
is probably because, in our workings with essentially neurotic
individuals, a certain integrity to the psychic apparatus is taken
for granted. I am in essential agreement with André Green who, in
his recent review of literature about the treatment of schizophrenic
and borderline individuals, states the following:

"It seems to me that the essential function of all these much-decried
variants of classical analysis only aim, in varying the elasticity of
the analytic setting, at searching for and preserving the minimum
conditions for symbolization. Every paper on symbolization in psychotic or prepsychotic structures says the same thing couched in
different terms"[1] ... and

"From this point of view the analyst does not only unveil a hidden
meaning. He constructs a meaning which has never been created before the analytic relationship began" (1975, p. 12).

I would not quite put it as Green does. I would rather say
that we deal here with a life situation in which good enough object relations and adequate drive gratification are inseparable
from an optimal realization of symbols. And, also, I would say
that the analyst constructs new <u>forms</u> or organizations of meaning
out of archaic sorts of symbolization already possessed by the patient. But I am, nonetheless, in essential agreement with Green's
contention that what is in the foreground of the therapeutic problem with such individuals is the integrity of the psychic apparatus
itself.

The paper is organized as follows: First, examples of a procedure for examining psychic apparatus function through a system
for evaluating language behavior which has been used in our laboratory, and established as reliable (Steingart & Freedman, 1972) will

---

[1] I understand that Green, here, uses the term "symbolization" to
mean representational processes and structures in general, together
with those signs (especially linguistic) with which such representation can be expressed, and that Green does not mean by "symbolization"
only that very special type of representation we designate as "primary process."

be presented. As the different types of language behavior which we codify are described, some important findings from psycholinguistic literature which I believe support these kinds of analyses will be reported along the way. Second, some findings about language behavior, thus analyzed, from studies of subjects who suffer different types of psychopathology as well as clinically normal individuals will be presented. Third, an interpretation about our research findings in terms of Freud's psychic apparatus theory of the mind will be observed. And, finally, some possible ways in which these language behavior measures can contribute to research within the psychoanalytic situation will be indicated.

Following are some concrete examples of the way in which language behavior is coded.

Table I presents a major dimension termed Language Function which is subdivided into three categories: Connective Description, Patterned Description, and Patterned Contingency. These subcategories refer to what we can do, and communicate, with language with regard to the organization of reality. These three major categories are grammatically coherent, surface sentence structures which differ from one another in terms of the kind of structural information about experience which is communicated by an individual's choice of language behavior. Thus, the table contains the category Narrative language behavior. Such language behavior, no matter how elaborate, at best only describes connections between representations of experience. Complex Portrayal language behavior consists of surface complex sentences which use grammatical devices to represent some patterned interrelation among experiences. Complex Conditional language behavior also consists of surface sentence structure arrangements which represent a patterned interrelation among experiences, but now with a causal, deductive, or purposive framework via the selection of appropriate grammatical devices.

These differences in linguistic activity represent a clear line of development in the functional organization of language behavior. At first, language functions only to represent successive, or additive, "frames" of experience relatively unrelated to one another. This changes into more complex, patterned interrelations among experiences but these are still only descriptive portrayals of experience. And, finally, language can function so as to communicate a structure of some type of causal, deductive, or purposive (i.e., conditional or contingency) matrix which is applied to immediate experience. Such a categorization of language behavior is responsive to the question of how a person selects or uses grammatical skills for the communication of an organization of reality. It derives from seminal observations conducted by Piaget (1923) which have been supported by recent, more rigorously designed developmental studies of language development (e.g., Hunt, 1970; Loban, 1963).

Table 1   Long and Short Sentence Examples of Different Types of Language Behavior Obtained from Clinically Normal and Patient Subjects Grammatical Elaboration

Language Function	Conjoining Transformations	Embedding Transformations
Connective Description	**Narrative Language Behavior** _Long_ /("People got together) (and they talked) (and there were right wing people and left wing people and black people and white people")/ 22 words – 3 clauses _Short_ /("That is the whole trouble")/ 5 words – 1 clause	
Patterned Description	**Contiguous Conditional** _Long_ /("I'll fight it with all my might")/ /("See? In that way I won't get myself down and out) ... (That down and out feeling I used to have")/ two sentence total 27 words 3 clauses _Short_ /("Nobody would listen to them") (and (So they went out ...) (and busted some windows")/ two sentence total 13 words 3 clauses	**Complex Portrayal Language Behavior** _Long_ /("I felt) (especially upon hearing the tape again)... (that the music had been taken out of our hands) ... (that it was just happening")/ 26 words – 4 clauses _Short_ /("I feel it's a viscious cycle")/ 6 words – 2 clauses
Patterned Contingency		**Conditional Language Behavior** _Long_ /("If I don't go to school this ... summer) (I'll probably go down) (to visit them) (since I haven't been um)... ((you know)) very far south in the United States")/ 28 words – 5 clauses _Short_ /("They were velvet")(because it was winter time")/ 8 words – 2 clauses

At the top of Table I are the terms "conjoining transformations" and "embedding transformations." There is solid observational footing about how language behavior actually does change with age with respect to "conjoining" versus "embedding" transformations. Sentence elaboration via coordination devices, which can be compared roughly to deep structures affected by Chomsky's "conjoining transformations" (Lyons, 1968), shows in surface structure as compound sentences and is something which "...seems to be learned relatively early" (Hunt, 1970). Sixth graders can accomplish such sentence elaboration via coordination with a skill equal to that of a superior adult. Another finding is that even superior adults do not produce more _full_ dependent clause formations per main clause than do eighth graders, which can be referred roughly to deep structures affected by Chomsky's "embedding transformations" (Lyons, 1968), and shows in surface structures as complex sentences. What does distinguish the superior adult's grammatical skill--and what really accounts for significant increases in the amount of information "packaged" into longer surface sentences--is the skillful way in which the superior adult can delete verbal material into a variety of less than full clause formations, including subclausal forms such as prepositional phrases.

Any really extended elaboration of what is called Narrative language behavior will involve the manifestation in surface language structure of conjoining transformations, with or without deletions of redundant subject or predicate information. One, thus, can utter what we call a Simple Narrative sentence--"That is the whole trouble" which is a single, independent clause. Or, one can create a "chain" of such independent clauses--"People got together and they talked and there were right wing people and left wing people and black people and white people." You can perhaps imagine a railroad train with more and more box cars being added. Or, if you shut your eyes, and imagine a young, preschool child talking excitedly about a visit to the circus, you might begin to hear Narrative language behavior: "I went to the circus and saw the clowns and the elephants and the tigers, etc., etc...."

You will notice that Complex Portrayal language behavior is identified with embedding transformations which are manifest in surface language structure. You might, at this moment, try to imagine embedding transformations as an arrangement of "Chinese boxes," one sentence, so to say, inside the other. Consider the following sentence: "I felt that it was just happening." This sentence already contains a major clause "I felt," and a dependent clause "that it was just happening." This embedding of a major and dependent clause already takes us a step beyond the simple connection of independent clauses just described in Narrative language behavior. The major and independent clause convey a patterned interrelation between two sorts of information, one major, which asserts an experience has taken place, and one minor, which "doubles

back" upon the main clause and describes something about this experience. I can elaborate this sentence still further by inter-
polating between these two clauses we have just described, two
additional pieces of information, in the form of two more dependent
clauses, which also serve to qualify the major assertion that an
experience has taken place. Thus, we get the complete sentence:
"I felt especially upon hearing the tape again (Insertion 1) that
the music had been taken out of our hands (Insertion 2) that it was
just happening." Thus, we end up in surface language structure with
what is traditionally called a complex sentence, which indeed describes some complex patterned interrelation among experiences. But
surface complex sentences can show other, even further kinds of com-
plications of embedding operations. For example, a clause can be
inserted between the subject and predicate constituents of another
clause, as in this sentence: "This paper, which I wrote, is now
read." In our scoring system, when a surface sentence contains examples of both conjoining and embedding transformations, the embedding transformations take precedence in terms of how the sentence is
scored.

Obviously, both Complex Portrayal and what is called Complex
Conditional language behavior share the characteristic of having
embedding transformations evident in their surface construction.
The important difference between these two kinds of more complex
language behavior has to do with an individual's choice of grammatical devices. In one instance, Complex Portrayal language, complex sentences function to structure some type of description of
experiences. The sentences of Complex Conditional behavior go beyond a description of experiences and interrelate some kind of purposive, causal, or deductive contingency relationship among experiences. Thus, an example of Complex Conditional language behavior
would be as is indicated in the Table: "If I don't go to school
this summer, I'll probably go down to visit them, since I haven't
been, you know, very far south in the United States." The word
"since" is used here as a conjunction (rather than preposition)
and, together with the other conjunctive term "if," interrelates
all this complex sentence information according to some relational,
contingency ideas of purpose and reason. There is sense of syllogism
about such complex sentence formations, a kind of "if-then" deductive
flavor. But notice how the logically or formally necessary term
"then" actually is left out of the sentence. And notice also the
presence of a less than complete clause formation ("to visit them")
with the subject term ("I") implied but omitted. It is this kind
of deletional activity which especially characterizes the development of syntactic skills (e.g., Hunt, 1970; O'Donnell, 1967).

Such contingency structuring of experience with language behavior can be expressed in another way, which we call Contiguous
Conditional language behavior, and such language behavior cannot be
directly identified with the presence of either conjoining or embedding transformations in surface structure. Following is an

example of what we call Contiguous Conditional language behavior:
"I will fight it with all my might. See? In that way I won't get
myself down and out, that down and out feeling I used to have." In
this particular example, a patient has used the demonstrative ad-
jective "that" to refer back to the first sentence and establish a
contingency matrix. These two contiguous sentences clearly do not
represent a descriptive, connective string of Narrative behavior, or
even the patterned description of Portrayal language. They are interrelated with each other according to some relational, contingency
idea of cause and effect, although this is not accomplished through
a traditional complex sentence. In the second example of Contiguous
Conditional language the word "so" clearly is used as an illative
(inference making) conjunction to establish a similar contingency.

Our first way of examining the vicissitudes of language behavior
in psychopathology, with this coding procedure, was to examine the
language behavior of a single patient whose clinical state underwent
cyclical change (Steingart & Freedman, 1972). Perhaps the most fa-
mous example of cyclic changes in clinical state we have in psychopathology are those from mania to depression. But another kind of
cyclic change we meet upon in psychopathology is the patient whose
clinical state undergoes change from a persecutory paranoid condition, to psychotic depression, and back again. Our first data will
be about such a patient. Our cyclic patient is a married woman, in
her early thirties. The data derive from 10-minute portions of each
of four therapy sessions. Each of these four therapy sessions coin-
cides with a distant clinical state, according to descriptive chart
notes written by the patient's therapist, and an independent evaluation of these notes made by us.

In Figure I, our data is presented in percentages, showing the
incidence of clause output for each type of language behavior, per
state, per entire 10-minute segment, relative to the entire grammatical output of the patient for each language sample. In a graph form
we have combined all types of Narrative language behavior as well as
both types of Conditional language.

The most important point to be made in this Figure is that Conditional and Narrative language behavior show definite and opposite
shapes which distinguish the four clinical states. Narrative behavior makes an inverted "V" shape. Both depressed states show more
Narrative language than both paranoid conditions. Conditional language behavior is like a "V" shape due to the fact that both paranoid states show more Conditional language compared to both depressed
states. Thus, Narrative and Conditional language behavior are completely nonoverlapping for our cyclic patient's depressed and paranoid states.

We next proceeded to evaluate the statistical significance of
these interstate differences. These four 10-minute segments were

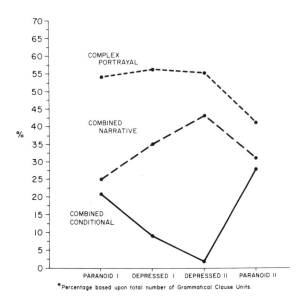

Figure 1   Cyclic Patient.   *Percentage of types of language
behavior for three clinical states.

each subdivided into five 2-minute intervals. This produced ten
2-minute interval language scores for each of the combined depressive and paranoid states. Tests of significance then were applied
to the mean interval percentage scores for these clinical states
as shown in Table 2.

Only mean differences which reach a $\underline{p}$ of .15, or less, are
shown, and it is Narrative and Conditional language behavior which
discriminates between the patient's depressed and paranoid states.
This kind of two-minute interval examination also shows that the
language behavior characteristic of each clinical state is not the
result of some "bunching" up; that is, it is characteristic of the
entire language sample. We also established that such language behavior was not just characteristic of psychopathology. It occurred
as much for language which was manifestly free of persecutory, delusional, or depressive content (Steingart & Freedman, 1972). We
could also demonstrate that there was no systematic relationship
between type of clinical state and amount of language produced by
the patient, nor any systematic relationship between clinical state
and types of therapist intervention (Steingart & Freedman, 1972).
These considerations led us to the conclusion that these different
types of language behavior we have identified bear an intrinsic relation to type of clinical state.

But a question that still can be raised is why the Narrative
language behavior difference does not reach ordinarily accepted

Table 2

Mean Percentage Interval Scores for Two Language
Behavior Measures by Clinical State for Cyclic Patient

Language Behavior Measures	Clinical States		t value (two-tailed) Paranoid vs. Depressed
	Paranoid	Depressed	
N*	10	10	
Narrative	.28	.39	1.66 p < .15
Conditional	.23	.06	3.53 p < .01

*Number of two-minute intervals for each clinical state

levels of statistical significance (p only < .15). We were interested
in this question. You may recall from Figure I that while the patient's second paranoid state showed less Narrative language than
either of her two depressed states, it also showed more Narrative
language than her first paranoid condition. A close reading of the
10-minute segment for this second paranoid state of our cyclic patient convinced us that paranoia was less evident in this session
compared to her first paranoid state. Consequently, we instructed
a staff psychologist who was utterly unaware of the purpose of this
research, to evaluate the tapes of both paranoid states of our cyclic patient. She was asked to compare these two sessions with respect to both paranoid delusional and depressive content. Both
quantitative ratings and qualitative summary descriptions were obtained for each of the two paranoid states. The second of the paranoid states, indeed, was described by this psychologist as more of
an admixture with depression.

A second study of comparative psychopathology investigates
further this variable aspect of paranoid experience, but this time
within the context of chronic schizophrenia (Grand, Freedman, et al.,
1973). Sixteen male, chronic schizophrenic patients were selected
from a large sample of patients originally treated and studied over
ten years ago at the Psychopharmacology Clinic at Kings County Hospital. Originally these patients were subjects for a study to predict

hospitalization proneness among chronic, psychiatric patients (Freedman, Rosen, et al., 1967). Each of these sixteen, recalled, chronic schizophrenic subjects was involved in a ten-minute open-ended, unstructured interview designed to explore the patient's current activities, social relations, and feeling states with interviewer interaction only for purposes of clarification of what the patient said.

Two groups of eight chronic schizophrenics each were identified as either socially isolated or socially belligerent on the basis of psychiatric and psychologic assessments, as well as social history obtained from a family member. Also, psychiatric rating scales filled out for each patient at the beginning of the original research project makes clear that other psychopathology parallels the social behavior differences between the two groups.[2] One group of rating scale items, called "paranoid thinking," weighted such descriptions as ideas of reference, ideas of influence, suspiciousness, and so forth. Another group of rating scale items called "schizophrenic thinking" weighted such descriptions as irrelevance of speech, stereotypic speech content, etc.. One can find, only among the socially belligerent, chronic patients, cases in which the rating of paranoid thinking was more than twice as much as schizophrenic thought, and the reverse is only found among our socially withdrawn, isolated chronic schizophrenics. From this, and other examinations of this psychiatric rating scale data, we concluded that the group characterized by social belligerence showed features of relative unsystematized, paranoid activity in the context of chronic schizophrenia, compared with our other group of patients, who showed social isolation and cognitive disturbance characteristic of classical schizophrenia. One, of course, is immediately reminded of Freud's (1911b) early conviction about the different kinds of significance which attach to these different psychotic features. A Hollingshead and Redlich Index of Social Position (1958) was applied to these two groups of patients to assess level of education, job status, and so forth, and no significant difference was present.

The analysis of the language behavior of the samples of these two groups of chronic schizophrenics is depicted in Table 3. All of these patients were placed on placebo one week prior to the collection of these samples.

The results indicate, again, that a persecutory paranoid state of consciousness, even as part of a mix of chronic schizophrenia, is still associated with differences in language behavior consistent with the findings of our cyclic patient. The chronic schizophrenics designated as socially belligerent, whom we consider to be individuals who also possess unsystematized paranoid activity, have significantly more Conditional language behavior, whereas our more socially isolated

[2]I am grateful to Professors David Engelhardt and Reuben Margolis for making this data available to me.

Table 3

Mean Percentage Scores for Different Types of Language
Behavior and Mean Total Clause Output for Socially
Isolated and Socially Belligerent Chronic Schizophrenics

Language Behavior	N = 8 Withdrawn (Schiz.)	N = 8 Belligerent (Paranoid)	t-value (two-tailed)
Fragmented*	.06	.05	N.S.
Simple Narrative	.29	.19	2.22 p < .05
Elaborated Narrative	.10	.11	N.S.
Complex Portrayal	.54	.52	N.S.
Combined Conditional	.07	.18	2.67 p < .02
Total Clause Output**	162	197	N.S.

*The percentage of Fragmented language is based upon total speech
output, including both grammatical and ungrammatical utterances.
The percentages of Narrative and Complex language sum to 100%
since they are based on grammatical utterances only.

**10-minute sample.

group of chronic schizophrenics show significantly more Simple Narrative language behavior. In the next chapter, Dr. Stanley Grand will
discuss other aspects of this data which relate such differences in
language behavior to certain types of variability in the motor behavior of these same chronic, schizophrenic subjects. Notice again
that there is no difference in total grammatical clause output. Nor
is there any difference between these two groups in another category
of language behavior which is called Fragmented language. These are
utterances which appear as grammatically incomplete sentences in
speech. For example, a sentence subject term might be introduced
and never predicated; or a word or a phrase may be stated which is
not obviously a subject term, but the utterance can not readily be
related to any subject term in its immediate vicinity. There was,
incidentally, no difference in Fragmented language for any of the
changes in clinical state of our cyclic patient.

A third and final study of comparative psychopathology, involves
clinically normal subjects. The language behavior of field-independent
and field-dependent, successful female college students, matched for
verbal I.Q., was examined in Dialogue and two kinds of Monologue
communication conditions. The complete description and results of

this study have been published elsewhere and include important differences between field-independent and field-dependent subjects in
the Monologue conditions (Steingart, Freedman, et al., 1975).   But
here we will focus on certain identical effects upon types of language
behavior, and language output, for all these clinically normal subjects which were produced by the change in communication situation
from Dialogue to what was called Warm Monologue.   In the Dialogue
situation, the subject was presented with an interviewer who explained some of the functions of the equipment in the recording room,
and who tried to make the subject as comfortable as possible.   The
interviewer then inquired into several areas of the subject's life,
her major interest and hopes, social activities, and dating patterns.
The interviewer deliberately avoided probing into conflict areas.
His attitude might best be described as reflecting a sustained,
shared, focused attention on whatever the subject said, like the
interviewer with our chronic schizophrenic subjects.   This attitude
was reflected in his nonverbal behavior, e.g., nodding in agreement
and leaning toward the subject.   This positive nonverbal attitude
was continued into the Monologue situation, which was introduced with
the following instructions to the subject: "I would like you to talk
for five minutes.   I would like you to talk about something that is
personally meaningful to you.   I shall not interrupt you.   Just talk
until the time is up."   This constituted what we termed a warm Monologue communication situation.   The data to be described is presented
in Table 4.

Inasmuch as subjects had more opportunity to speak in Monologue,
it is perhaps to be expected that all of our subjects, both field
independent and field dependent, would increase their clause output
in Monologue.   The more important finding has to do with the relative
percentages of Narrative and Conditional language behavior, which
have, so to speak, exchanged places in the transition from Dialogue
to Monologue communication for all of these subjects.   There was, incidentally, no differences in Fragmented language within our clinically normal subjects, as was true for our chronic schizophrenics,
and for the variations in clinical state of our cyclic patient.

The relative prevalences of Narrative and Conditional language,
which characterized the difference between the psychotic depressed
versus paranoid states of our cyclic patient, as well as the difference between our more schizophrenic versus our more paranoid chronic
patients, is here reproduced for our clinically normal subjects.   In
other words, what is brought about by endogenous, psychotic depressive, schizophrenic, and paranoid psychopathology, is replicated in
clinically normal subjects by a change from Dialogue to Monologue
communication.   Is there a meaning we can give this comparative
psychopathology of language behavior which is relevant to psychoanalytic theory?

Table 4

Mean Percentage Scores for Different Types of Language Behavior
and Mean Total Clause Output for Clinically Normal Subjects in
Dialogue and Monologue Communication

Type of Language Behavior	Communication Situation N = 14		t	p (two-tailed)
	Dialogue	Monologue		
Combined Narrative	.19	.35	5.13	<.001
Complex Portrayal	.43	.45	.30	N.S.
Combined Conditional	.38	.20	3.90	<.01
Clause Output*	86.94	111.12	2.92	<.02

*5-minute sample

A way to begin to answer this question is afforded by some
further research (Grand, Steingart et al., 1975). Grand was able
to obtain certain additional data for 10 of the 16 chronic schizophrenic and paranoid subjects described earlier. Five of these 10
chronic patients previously had been identified as socially belligerent and relatively more paranoid, whereas the remaining five subjects previously had been identified as socially isolated and ex-
hibiting schizophrenic signs of thought disturbance. Grand examined
correlations between the language behavior of these 10 chronic schizophrenic and paranoid subjects and their performance on the venerable
Stroop Color-Word Test (1935). But a significant difference was
found to exist on the Hollingshead and Redlich Index of Social Position (1958) between these two smaller groups of five chronic patients.
The Stroop Color-Word Test involves reading skill which certainly
could be influenced by Index variables, such as education and type
of work, so it became important to control, by partial correlation,
any such effects which might obscure the influence of type of psychopathology itself.

The Stroop Color-Word Test consists of three 9 X 11 inch cards,
A, B, and C. Card A (called word-naming) contains the color-names
red, green, yellow, and blue printed 100 times in random order in
black ink and arranged in ten lines of ten words per line. Card B
(called color-naming) contains the colors red, green, yellow, and
blue, printed in asterisks equal in number to the number of letters
in the words, and again arranged in ten lines of ten units per line
following the same pattern as Card A. Card C (called the conflict
card) consists of the same arrangement of colors, but this time they

are printed as color-names incongruent to the color of the ink (e. g., the ink color red appears in the words blue, green, and yellow, but never in the word red). Speed of reading color-names on Card A, and speed of naming the colored inks on Cards B and C, comprise the scores for task performance. An interference measure is derived from the scores on Cards B and C by means of the formula: $\frac{C-B}{B}$. The numerator of this fraction represents a residual time, over and above simple color encoding time, and reflects the extra reading time required due to the addition of incongruous word names on Card C. The denominator of this fraction takes such extra reading time in relation to color-naming time, and thus this ratio score corrects for individual differences in speed of color-naming.

Details of the interesting results of this study have been published elsewhere (Grand, Steingart et al., 1975), but I want to cite certain results which have to do with the correlations Grand found to exist between Total Narrative and Total Conditional language behavior and two types of Stroop reading times. Total Narrative language behavior is significantly and positively correlated with the amount of time a subject needed to read Card A, i.e., simply read the list of words which named different colors. On the other hand, this same Narrative language behavior was significantly and negatively related with the interference measure which involved a comparison between reading times on Card B and how long it took a subject to read Card C, the conflict card. The correlations for Total Conditional language and these same two reading times were reversed, and also significant. Thus, a subject relatively high in Conditional language could read the color names on Card A relatively quickly. But this same subject experienced significantly more interference with Card C. We assume it took such a subject a longer time to read Card C because he found it harder to inhibit a response to utter the word on Card C, whereas he was required to name the color of the ink with which the word was typed. Thus, paradoxically, those more paranoid, chronic schizophrenic subjects who demonstrated relatively superior language skill and function, through more production of Conditional language behavior, are also more handicapped in a situation which requires a kind of turning away from language in favor of the immediacy of color registration in consciousness. Chronic, more withdrawn, schizophrenic subjects, who demonstrated relatively impoverished language skill and function through more production of Narrative language behavior, found it easier to ignore language in this way. This is an irony perhaps, but not really a paradox. In fact, these Stroop-Test findings were predicted. George Klein (1970) has reported that obsessive-compulsive, clinically normal subjects show similar Stroop Test Color-Word interference performance compared to more hysteric normals, and I suspect similar differences in language behavior would have been found between these same two groups.

I believe we can consider that the conscious registration of a Stroop Test patch of color is akin to what Freud had in mind when he spoke about a "thing cathexis," and that the naming of this color is what Freud meant by "word cathexis" (e.g., 1915a). For further, direct support of such an interpretation, I can now cite other, predicted Stroop Test findings which dealt, exactly, with time required to name colors (i.e., Card B performance). A significant, positive correlation exists between the amount of Narrative language behavior--which you will recall characterizes our more socially isolated, chronic schizophrenics--and the amount of time required to verbally encode colors. A negative, significant correlation exists between amount of Conditional language--characteristic of our more paranoid, socially belligerent, chronic schizophrenics--and time required to name colors. Thus, I believe Freud would have found all of these Stroop Test findings quite compatible with the application of his concepts of "thing" versus "word" cathexis to comparative psychopathology (e.g., 1915a).

These concepts of "thing" versus "word" cathexis were essential constructs for Freud's theory of a "psychic apparatus." Above all, Freud came to this theory of the working of the mind from his study of dreams. Then, in characteristic innovative fashion, he generalized these concepts to explain phenomena as diverse as schizophrenic hallucinations and the normal development of consciousness. But Freud's important contribution to cognition theory hardly lay in any discovery by him of dreams. His revolutionary insight about cognition revealed to him by his study of dreams was this: While a person experiences himself as <u>perceiving qualities</u> in a dream, he is actually <u>thinking</u>-- and that a latent, more abstract thought can be discovered by the technique of free association. Thus, Freud (1900) was led to a construct of a "psychic apparatus" which can show "progression" and "regression." It is a psychological construct which posits the existence of a kind of ensemble of what Freud called "thought structures." This continuum of thought, in part, is conceptualized along a range which moves from developmentally immature picture or thing- like representations to representations which are very abstract, and as such can only be expressed by language. It is important to point out that Freud did <u>not</u> equate the thing-like picture representation end of this continuum with any notion of primary process thinking. He was quite clear about how dream formation consists of two separate, interrelated aspects. In one aspect, the abstract dream thought first must become "capable of being represented" (1900, p. 390)--one might say decomposed--into thing-like pictures by regression in the psychic apparatus. After such an abstract form of thought is represented in pictures, Freud said, the primary processes of condensation and displacement can then make use of such picture representation for dream construction which enables this abstract thought to escape censorship. This is possible, Freud said: " ... because in every langauge concrete terms, in consequence of the history of their development, are richer in associations than conceptual ones" (1900, p. 340).

However, I do not believe that Freud's use of such a succint term as "word cathexis" does justice to his own belief that the relational properties of mature thought are made possible by language. Already, in his early work The Interpretation of Dreams, Freud describes how language facilitates the creation of a "new series of qualities or attributes" (1900, p. 617). What are these new qualities or attributes? Eleven years later (1911a) Freud indicated how thoughts pertaining to "relations between the object impressions" (p. 16) especially become capable of being represented by the acquisition of language. This latter point Freud makes perhaps most explicit in his paper the "Unconscious" (1915a): " ...thought proceeds in systems so far remote from the original perceptual residuals that they have no longer retained anything of the qualities of those residuals, and, in order to become conscious, need to be reinforced by new qualities ... by being evoked with words, cathexis can be provided with quality even when they represent only relations between presentations of objects and are thus unable to derive any quality from perceptions. Such relations, which become comprehensible only through words, form a major part of our thought processes" (p. 202). Word cathexis, Freud stated in this same paper, thus brings about a " ... higher physical organization ..." (p.202).

But Freud, despite his own keen appreciation about the relational properties of mature, abstract thought, continued to use a term like "word cathexis." However, such an emphasis upon this term "word" does not convey any appreciation for the syntactic skills which occur with such abstract, relational thought. Perhaps he meant to use the term "word cathexis" as a kind of short hand for "language," and thus intended to indicate the acquisition of both semantics and syntax. But I do not think so. I think what really fascinated Freud about language was, indeed, certain kinds of words. Or, better stated, how a latent dynamic meaning could be found for certain words which belong to a class called by linguistics contentatives (e.g., Brown, 1973). Contentatives are nouns, adjectives, and verbs. Many such words are signs for ideas which do make ready, direct, concrete reference to persons, objects, actions, and attributes which possess vivid qualities--and thus lend themselves to dynamic interpretations, via free associations, when they appear in the manifest content of a dream or the language of a schizophrenic. Conjunctions, which enable complex sentences, are included in another class of words which linguists call functors (e.g., Brown, 1973). Functors do not make reference in any such simple direct way to objects. You cannot, say, point to an inference-making conjunction in the same way you can point to a house, or the color red. Functors, unlike contentatives, serve to identify important grammatical sentence structures and functions. Thus, if one wishes to continue to talk about economic quantities, it would be better to talk about a cathexis not of words but of a "something" which makes possible the formation of an incredible, to all intents and purposes, limitless variety of sentences. And this "something" which can produce sentences apparently involves meaning structures which enable, from the beginning, functional integrations of grammar and semantics to an extent not previously suspected (e.g., Brown, 1973).

I already have mentioned how developmental research makes clear that what characterizes superior language behavior is the syntactically skillful production of longer complex sentences--which then, especially, can perform the function of Conditional language to express the structure of contingency relationships. We have found a congruence between such developmental research and our comparative psychopathology data with adults depicted in Figure II.

This Figure indicates that our clinically normal subjects produce only one type of sentence--a Conditional sentence--which is more complex (longer) than that uttered by our chronic schizophrenics. There is no difference in the average sentence length of either Portrayal or Narrative language between our clinically normal and chronic schizophrenic subjects. It is for this reason that it is only among our clinically normal subjects that their average Conditional sentence length significantly exceeds the average complexity (length) of their Portrayal sentences. Our clinically normal and chronic schizophrenic subjects are the same in that the average sentence length of both their Conditional and Portrayal sentences significantly exceeds the length of their Narrative sentences.[3]

Of course, any comparison of language behavior between our normal and schizophrenic subjects is hazardous in view of many uncontrolled factors such as sex, age, verbal intelligence, etc. But I can at least point to another finding, and at least consider certain implications of the total patterning of our findings for the use of language as a measurement device to investigate comparative psychopathology. The additional finding is that it is not only the average length of Conditional sentences which distinguishes our normals from schizophrenics. The percentage clause output of Conditional language--a measure of how often such language is spoken--also distinguishes the two groups. A comparison of Tables 3 and 4 shows that our normal subjects uttered three times as much Conditional language in half the dialogue time compared to our schizophrenics.

---

[3]Related findings, incidentally, exist for the different states of our cyclic patient. Significant differences exist between the length of Conditional versus Portrayal sentences in the cyclic patient's paranoid states. But no such differences exist in her depressed states. This is because her Conditional sentences became shorter, and equal to her Portrayal sentence language length, which did not vary with her clinical state.

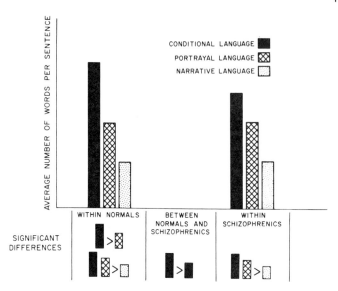

Figure 2   Comparisons of conditional, portrayal, and narrative
sentence length differences for normals and schizophrenic
subjects in dialogue communication.

In order to draw out the implications of our findings for language as a measurement device, I first have to make explicit something only implied in Figure II. This is, that there is no difference in average sentence length for any of our three types of language behavior within our normals (Field-Independent versus Field-
Dependent), or within our schizophrenics (Isolated versus Belligerent). This is what enabled us to consider our normals and schizophrenics as total groups when we examined their sentence complexity.
Now it is clear that it is only Narrative versus Conditional language
differences in percentage clause output which distinguishes within
our chronic schizophrenics, not how long the sentences produced.
The opposite is true of our clinically normal subjects. I mentioned
earlier that differences in percentage clause output for Narrative
versus Conditional language did not distinguish between our field-
independent and field-dependent subjects, either in Dialogue or
Monologue communication. I have just added that average sentence
length differences also did not discriminate between our field-independent and field-dependent clinically normal subjects in Dialogue.
But now I can add that we have found that sentence length differences do distinguish between field-independent and field-dependent
clinically normal subjects in their Monologue communication (Steingart, Freedman, et al., 1975).

All of this suggests that to examine how two types of marginally
adjusted chronic schizophrenia affect the complexity (length) of

these three different types of sentences is like an attempt to discover a difference between very poor black and white people in
terms of how many courses they consume as a function of whether
they are eating breakfast, lunch, or dinner. Sentence complexity
simply is too demanding, too fine a measure, to discriminate within
such severe psychopathology. An attempt to examine how field-independent versus field-dependent types of normals affect the percentage clause output for these three different kinds of language
behavior is like an attempt to discover a difference between very
rich black and white people in terms of how often they eat three
meals a day. Sheer language output, which does not take into account linguistic complexity, is too gross a measure for our clinically normal subjects. The complexity (length) of sentence formation is necessary as a more demanding measure in order to discriminate language behavior within these clinically normal subjects.
And, at least for the extreme types of verbally superior, clinically normal subjects we studied, even sentence length complexity
becomes a meaningful measure only in a condition of relatively unstructured, Monologue communication.

     Now, there is a further, and final, step I would like to take
by way of an interpretation of our language behavior measures. But
I do not mean by a "further and final" interpretation that I now
will offer an explanation for this language behavior which necessi-
tates Freud's formulations about psychic energy. This explanation
can "stand on its own feet." Here, I simply and only regard "thing
cathexis" versus "word cathexis" to be psychological, polar constructs that define points (regions) on some meaning apparatus, and
this apparatus, throughout, consists of conceptual structures of
one form or another. This does not sound different from Freud's
construct of a psychic apparatus with its ensemble of thought structures. But two points need to be clarified.

     First, Freud's concept of a "thing cathexis" can be misunder-
stood to mean the philosopher's "thing-in-itself," something "out
there" with its particular, unique qualities which somehow becomes
copied directly and veridically in the mind like a camera takes
pictures. I stress that "thing cathexis" already implicates conceptualizing activity and thus the production of some type of conceptual structure. In fact, I think it useful to consider that
Freud's "thing cathexis" constitutes a thought structure which
Piaget (1951) calls a "pre-concept." And remember, Freud did not
say that adult regression to this ontologically earlier formation
of the psychic apparatus is what is meant by the primary processes.
Such regression enables (but does not inevitably instigate) primary processes. The defining contents of a pre-concept are always
some impelling quality (action) attributes. The pre-concept does
not possess the stability of a mature conceptual structure (what
Piaget calls "mobile equilibrium"), and because of this it can lend

itself to dynamic associative content via the primary processes of
displacement and condensation. Point number two has to do with
Freud's term "word cathexis," which I think blurs what must remain,
conceptually, functionally related but separate phenomena of thought
and language. Research conducted with deaf-mute children (e.g.,
Furth, 1964) reveals the acquisition of relatively mature conceptual
thought structure with only slight retardation compared to normals,
even though these children possess little or no language comprehension or production of any sort. Skills with sentence construction
programs may be considered a necessary springboard for certain special types of still more abstract symbolic logic. But language itself is not a sufficient cause for even such an advance in representation which must build upon earlier established conceptual structures (Piaget, 1967).

Now, I come directly to this other explanation for the variability in language behavior which I have described. This is, that these
changes in language construction programs can become determined by an
individual's intentions with respect to self-object representation.
If one's organization of consciousness is such that rather fundamental contingency ideas are structured and employed in lengthy, complicated sentences, then one lives in a particular kind of world
(consciousness). Language has a special significance because only
certain special integrations of grammar and semantics will enable
the communication of such abstract, contingency ideas to another.
But, then, I think it reasonable to consider that such an emphasis upon language structured, contingency reality, in communication with
another, must also extend to the representation of this same communicative object relationship. If I speak to you with a great deal of
Conditional language behavior, structuring my experience for you on
a contingency basis and interrelating many ideas in a lengthy, complicated surface sentence, it is not just a world in general I thus
linguistically represent which is so different and distantiated
from more immediate "thing" or picture-like representation. I suggest that the representation of my object relationship with you also
is so structured in my consciousness. This can be thought of as a
variable of linguistic differentiation. It is a variable which, at
least for adults, must be considered as something different from,
but may be importantly related to and subserve, the psychoanalytic
construct of self- object-differentiation. It tells us something
about an individual's distance from those more thing or picture-
like qualities which are always potentially available for a more
immediate kind of representation of an object relationship.

But now, our use and knowledge of comparative psychopathology
can especially return us dividends. We do consider that a persecutory paranoid organization of consciousness involves heightened
differentiation between self- and object-representations. We can
see how complex sentences utilized for lengthy Conditional structures

would subserve such self-object differentiation. Language behavior
which emphasizes, and communicates to another, complex reasons,
causes, purposes, etc. about one's experiences treats the other as
someone who cannot be expected, or experienced, on some <u>direct</u>,
<u>empathic</u> <u>basis</u> to fully understand the speaker. This can be most
easily and sharply contrasted with Narrative language behavior.
The relatively simpler sentence construction programs of Narrative
language behavior preclude any communication to the listener of any
complex contingency basis for one's experience. This, I suggest,
may be used to express an intention to treat and experience the
other as someone who is expected to understand the speaker on such
a more direct, empathic basis. In this way, we can understand the
increase in Narrative language produced by clinically normal subjects in Monologue communication. In Monologue communication, the
object-representation serves only in the role of the listener.
As such, only as a listener, the object can be represented psychologically as less differentiated from the speaker. Consequently,
intentions to communicate explanations, inferences, or purposes
about one's experiences, such as would be expressed in Complex Conditional language, are reduced in Monologue communication while
Narrative language would increase. In this way, we can also understand an increase in Narrative language as a consequence of the de-
differentiation in self- object-representation which we consider to
be evidenced in schizophrenic and psychotic depressive forms of
consciousness.

Our findings about how language behavior can change from Dialogue to Monologue, with our clinically normal subjects, leads to
the possibility that these same measures may have relevance for
research within the psychoanalytic situation. For example, these
same measures can perhaps be used to assess process during the analytic hour, i.e., progression and regression in the psychic apparatus (Freud, 1900). If so, then the vicissitudes of such psychic
apparatus functioning could be systematically related to topographic
and structural considerations (assessed by some other means).

Another use of these measures in the psychoanalytic situation
lies in the complex area of the nature of the therapist-patient relationship. Certainly, we believe that the productive empathy an
analyst can experience for a patient is something real for both people, and thus somehow transmitted, and that without it treatment
must suffer. Such real, productive empathy probably is transmitted
in a variety of ways--linguistic, paralinguistic, and nonlinguistic--
and the transmission modality likely possesses differential significance for different kinds of people. I suggest that these language
construction measures may be capable of pointing to certain optimal
patterns of concordant and complimentary language exchange between
therapist and patient, and that these patterns may be relevant to a
judgment (by some other means) about the extent to which productive

empathy is evident in a particular treatment session. I have used the terms "concordant" and "complimentary." These are terms introduced by Deutch (1926), and especially developed by Racker (1968), to describe two types of identifications made by an analyst with the patient which mediate productive empathy: "Concordant" means an identification made with the patient as subject; "complimentary" means an identification made with an object representation possessed by the patient. A certain spontaneous patterning of sameness and difference in language construction, between patient and analyst, may be one important modality for empathy transmission. And such empathy transmission may be especially important for borderline and psychotic patients, about whom we believe that sensitive therapeutic response to the status of the psychic apparatus itself is the critical treatment issue (Green, 1975).

REFERENCES

Brown, R. A first language: The early stages. Cambridge, Mass.: Harvard University Press, 1973.

Deutch, H. (1926). Occult processes occurring during psychoanalysis. In Devereux (Ed.), Psychoanalysis and the occult. New York: International Universities Press, 1953.

Freedman, N., Rosen, B., Engelhardt, D. M., & Margolis, R. Prediction of psychiatric hospitalization. 1. The measurement of hospital proneness. Journal of Abnormal Psychology, 1967, 72:468-477.

Freud, S. (1900). The interpretation of dreams. Standard Edition, 4 and 5. London: Hogarth Press, 1953.

Freud, S. (1905). Three essays on the theory of sexuality. Standard Edition, 7:125-245. London: Hogarth Press, 1953.

Freud, S. (1911a). Formulations on the two principles of mental functioning. Standard Edition, 12:218-226. London: Hogarth Press, 1958.

Freud, S. (1911b). Psycho-analytic notes on an autobiographical account of a case of paranoia (Dementia Paranoides). Standard Edition, 14:166-204. London: Hogarth Press, 1958.

Freud, S. (1915a). The unconscious. Standard Edition, 14:166-204. London: Hogarth Press, 1957.

Freud, S. (1923). The ego and the id. Standard Edition, 19:12-66. London: Hogarth Press, 1961.

Furth, H. G.   Research with the deaf: Implications for language
and cognition.   Psychological Bulletin, 1964, 62:145-164.

Grand, S., Freedman, N., & Steingart, I.   A study of the representation of objects in schizophrenia.   Journal of the American Psychoanalytic Association, 1973, 21:2, 399-434.

Grand, S., Steingart, I., Freedman, N., & Buchwald, C.   The organization of language behavior and cognitive performance in chronic
schizophrenia.   Journal of Abnormal Psychology, 1975, 84, 621-628.

Green, A.   The analyst, symbolization and absence in the analytic
setting.   (On changes in analytic practice and analytic experiences.)
International Journal of Psychology, 1975, 56, Part 1, 1-19.

Hollingshead, A. B. & Redlich, F. C.   Social class and mental illness.
New York: John Wiley, 1958.

Hunt, K. W.   Syntactic maturity in school children and adults.   Monograph of the Society for Research in Child Development, 1970, 35,
No. 1.

Klein, G.   Perception, motives, and personality.   New York: Alfred
Knopf, 1970.

Loban, W. B.   The language of elementary school children.   National
Council of Teachers English Report No. 1, 1963.

Lyons, S.   Introduction to theoretical linguistics.   London: Cambridge Universities Press, 1968.

O'Donnell, R. C., Griffin, W. J., & Norris, R. C.   Syntax of kindergarten and elementary school children: A transformational analysis.   National Council of Teachers of English Research Report No.
8, 1967.

Piaget, J.   (1923).   The language and thought of the young child.
New York: Meridian Books, 1955.

Piaget, J.   (1945).   Play, dreams, and imitation in childhood.
New York: Norton, 1951.

Piaget, J.   Six psychological studies.   New York: Random House, 1967.

Racker, H.   Transference and countertransference.   New York: International Universities Press, 1968.

Steingart, I. & Freedman, N. A language construction approach for
the examination of self-object representation in varying clinical
states. In Robert R. Holt & Emanuel Peterfreund (Eds.), Psychoanalysis & Contemporary Science, Vol. 1. New York: The Macmillan
Co., London: Collier-Macmillan, Ltd., 1972.

Steingart, I., Freedman, N., Grand, S., Buchwald, C., & Margolis, R.
Personality organization and language behavior: The imprint of
psychological differentiation on language behavior in varying
communication conditions. Journal of Psycholinguistic Research,
1975, Vol. 4, No. 3, 241-255.

Stroop, J. R. Studies of interference in serial verbal reactions.
Journal of Experimental Psychology, 1935, 18:643-661.

This research has been supported by Grant No. MH-14383 from the
United States Public Health Service, National Institute of Mental
Health.

ON HAND MOVEMENTS DURING SPEECH: STUDIES OF THE ROLE OF SELF-

STIMULATION IN COMMUNICATION UNDER CONDITIONS OF PSYCHOPATHOLOGY,

SENSORY DEFICIT, AND BILINGUALISM

Stanley Grand

Downstate Medical Center

Brooklyn, New York 11203

I would like to describe a particular line of research which I and my colleagues at the Clinical Behavior Research Unit have been engaged in over the past few years. This research has been concerned with hand movements accompanying the speech of those who, for various reasons, experience disruptions in their communicative contact with others. These studies have been conducted within the context of a larger research program which aims at understanding the function of kinesic behavior during speech. A basic assumption underlying this program has been that hand movements which accompany speech, quite apart from their intrinsic communicative value for the listener, play an important supportive and regulating role in the organization and coding of thought for the speaker himself. Our focus upon those who experience disruption in communicative contact was chosen as a way of testing this assumption.

Let us begin by considering verbal communication, and particularly, Freud's view of the function of words in the evolution of essentially human behavior. In 1893, Freud wrote "the man who first flung a word of abuse at his enemy instead of a spear was the founder of civilization" (p. 36).[1] Two main issues are highlighted by this comment: first, that words evolve out of a matrix of overt actions, and are, indeed, a symbolic representation of these actions; and second, that words provide inhibitory control over the direct discharge of impulse into action. These themes were to reappear in many forms throughout Freud's writing, but were most succinctly stated in his 1911 paper on the Two Principles of Mental Functioning where he suggested that thinking "is essentially an experimental

---

[1]Freud actually attributed this statement to an unidentified British author. (See editor's note on page 36, S. E. III).

kind of acting accompanied by displacement of relatively small quantities of cathexis together with less expenditure of them" (p. 221).

Thus words, as surrogates for action, enable a tremendous advance in psychic organization through their capacity to mentally
represent and control action in the service of reality adaptation.
Implicit in this view is the notion that verbalization entails the
interweaving of both ideational and motoric processes--what George
Klein (1970) called "ideo-motor structures." Indeed, Klein (1965)
pointed out that Freud actually proposed a model for such an interweaving in the Project (1895). There, Freud reminded us that the
primary function of the vocal apparatus was originally the diffuse
vocal-motor discharge of tension accumulation. Under the impact of
the requirement for reality adapted action, diffuse vocal-motor
discharge gradually came under the modulating direction of words
which provided for effective vocal-motor discharge in speech. Thus,
speech came to carry the double burden of conveying meaning and
regulating optimal levels of tension discharge. It is this double
aspect of words which we, along with Klein (1965), assume to be
reflected in the communicative act of speaking.

Earlier, in this volume, my colleague Dr. Norbert Freedman
presented our conceptual frame of reference for understanding hand
movement behavior which highlights the role of the hands in supporting this dual function of representation and control which words
provide. That is, Dr. Freedman demonstrated, through data drawn
from developmental and language processing studies, that the movements of the hands, upon or at some distance from the body surface,
may be enlisted to support and sustain the link between an image and
its verbal referent, as well as to facilitate the flow of ideas
by regulating tensional states through patterned self-stimulation.
We have come to call these two strands of hand movement accompaniments to speech object-focused and body-focused activity, respectively.

In the present paper, I will focus upon the role of hand movements in providing self-produced cues, or feedback, which may have
a regulating function in communicated speech. The data to be presented are derived from groups of subjects drawn from populations
which function, during the course of their daily lives, under conditions which limit or disrupt their contact with the environment;
that is, those who, for reasons of psychopathology, sensory impairment, or linguistic curtailment, live in relative isolation from the
supportive stimulation provided by environmental contact. While
each form of relative isolation may endow the communicative process
with qualitatively distinct characteristics which are, in and of
themselves, of interest to the communication researcher, our interest
here lies in the role that hand movements may play in compensating
for such limitations. Our working assumption is that self-stimulating

feedback from the hands may provide regulatory cues for the speaker
when the external information array ordinarily useful in this respect is curtailed.

This assumption derives from contemporary psychoanalytic theorizing (Hartmann, 1939; Rapaport, 1958; Miller, 1962; Klein, 1965;
Holt, 1965) which emphasizes the importance of optimal levels of
stimulation for effective ego functioning. Rapaport (1958) termed
such stimulation "nutriment" (Piaget, 1936), which he believed was
crucially important for the development and differentiation of ego
structure. Klein (1965) extended this view to include the nutriment which derived from self-produced stimulations, or feedback,
and highlighted the role which such stimulation played in effective secondary process communication. Recent experimental literature amply demonstrates such a view (e.g., Yates, 1963; etc.), and
Klein (1965) and others (Holzman et al., 1966) have confirmed it
with respect to the auditory returns from one's own speech.

It is in this sense that we view the movement behavior which
accompanies speech to be an important source of feedback, or re-
afferentation, to use Von Holst's term (1954), providing nutriment which aids in maintaining the effective structuring of communicated thought. Movement behavior during discourse is self-stimulating. In a way similar to that of the auditory returns from one's
own voice (Klein et al., 1970; Holzman et al., 1966), hand movements
accompanying speech provide self-produced cues which aid the speaker
in the effectiveness of his intention to communicate to others. The
visual, proprioceptive, and kinesthetic stimulation supplied by hand
movement can be an important adjunct to the vocal confirmation of
whether or not one's communication has matched what one intends to
say. Movement of the hands during discourse may not only illustrate,
augment, or substitute for the verbal articulation of thought (Ekman &
Friesen, 1969, 1972), but in its self-stimulating role may also facilitate or inhibit the verbal flow (Dittmann, 1970), as well as maintain
the focus of attention upon what one intends to say (Grand et al.,
1975). Such a role for hand movement behavior during speech has its
roots in the earliest eye, hand, and mouth coordinations of the 3-month
old child (Bruner, 1969), which serve as his first attempts to coordinate his inner tensions with a purposeful mastery of the external world.
The subsequent linkage of hand movement to speech reflects, in our
view, an abridgement and subordination of such early self-initiated
action sequences in the evolution and development of verbal thought
as experimental action (Freud, 1911).[2] In short, movement behavior
which accompanies speech can provide feedback, which itself is a
motoric regulator and stimulus to further thought.

_____

[2]Gordon Hewes (1975) has reviewed the evidence that gestures preceded
language philogenetically, and suggests the possibility that at some
point in human evolution the two systems were co-active, providing redundancy in representation.

I   HAND MOVEMENT BEHAVIOR IN CHRONIC ISOLATED AND CHRONIC BELLIGER-
ENT SCHIZOPHRENIC PATIENTS

I would like to begin with a study which my colleagues and I
conducted several years ago (Grand et al., 1973, 1975) in which we
looked at the hand movement behavior accompanying the speech of a
group of chronically isolated schizophrenic patients. Isolation
in schizophrenia was of particular interest to us in the following
way. It has by now been relatively well established that there is
a relation between social isolation and high levels of basal arousal
in schizophrenic patients (Venables, 1963, 1964). Further, an attention regulating impairment has been noted by some in this disorder (Silverman, 1964; Venables, 1964; Spohn et al., 1970) which
appears to be related either to some form of central integrative
defect (Holzman, 1970) or to an impairment in the normal selectivity of attention (Spohn et al., 1970). Since high arousal has the
effect of narrowing attention (Easterbrook, 1959) and thereby gating
out stimulation, it would appear that arousal serves to reduce the
stimulus load. Furthermore, since social isolation also reduces
stimulus input, both mechanisms screen out stimulation which might
otherwise be overwhelming for certain schizophrenic patients to integrate.[3] That is, high arousal and isolation in schizophrenia appear to serve as adaptive stabilizing strategies which reduce the
stimulus load to manageable proportions. What little experimental
data exists with respect to this issue highlights the temporarily
salutary effects of isolation upon symptom expression. For example,
studies of schizophrenic and psychotic patients subject to sensory
isolation all report decreases in symptom levels during short periods
of reduced stimulus input (Azima & Cramer, 1956; Harris, 1959;
Schechter et al., 1969).

In light of such considerations, we wondered how isolated patients would differ from nonisolated patients in dealing with the
heightened stimulation of an interview situation requiring communication and social contact with an interviewer. At the least, we
would expect that the automatic and characteristic stimulus gating
mechanisms of these isolated patients would be subject to great
stress. Might we then observe compensatory efforts to bolster the
stressed gating mechanisms? For example, would isolated patients
differ from nonisolated patients in the degree to which they engage
in stereotypic and repetitive self-stimulating behavior, a type of
behavior already observed by Adams (1967) to be a way of increasing
his catatonic patient's vigilance toward the threat of social involvement? Might such self-stimulation provide what Holt (1965) has
termed "tonic support" for cortical integration, or, in the language
of ego psychology, "nutriment" for maintaining effective attention
regulating structures?

----

[3]Whether this gating mechanism acts like a filter (Broadbent, 1958), (
simply like an attentuator (Treisman, 1964) of incoming stimulation, (

Our speculation about what to expect from our isolated as compared to nonisolated schizophrenic patients was that they would ex-
hibit relatively greater use of body-focused movements accompanying
their speech during the stressful interview experience. Body-focused
movement, as opposed to other sorts, would provide maximal somesthe-
tic input, which, in terms of the way we understand such input to
operate, should narrow attention to the most adaptively relevant interview cues.

We compared a group of eight chronically isolated patients with
a group of eight similarly chronic schizophrenic patients who exhibited a contrasting style of social adaptation--that is, an oppo-
sitional and belligerent stance in their social interactions. While
this style was perhaps equally maladaptive in terms of social behavior, it nevertheless brought these patients into more frequent contact, suggesting a greater tolerance for more intense stimulation
from the environment. The two groups of patients were similar with
respect to education, socio-economic position, length of illness,
and several psychological measures, such as Rorschach F+%, Porteus
Maze performance, and a measure of social role obtained from the
T.A.T. Belligerent patients differed from isolated patients only
in respect to showing a higher level of manifest anxiety on the
Taylor scale. All patients were placed on placebo one week prior
to our study.

The major trends in our analysis of hand movements which accompanied the speech of Isolated and Belligerent patients during a
10-minute video taped interview segment are presented in Figure 1.
The data clearly support our hypothesis that Isolated patients would
engage in self-stimulating body-focused movements to a greater extent than nonisolated patients. The difference in the amount of
continuous body touching was significant at the .02 level. Furthermore, a significant positive correlation of .54 (p< .01) was obtained
between the amount of continuous body touching and patients' scores
on the index of "Solitariness"[4] by which we measured their degree of
social isolation. The rates of object-focused movements were exceedingly low and not different from one another.

---

on the other hand as a "response filter" (Deutch & Deutch, 1963), is
left open here. It goes beyond the scope of this paper to consider
the exact mechanism of attention deployment or its central or peripheral status.

[4]The Index of "Solitariness" used in this study is a subscale of the
Hospital Proneness Scale developed by Freedman et al., (1967) to predict hospitalization proneness in schizophrenic patients. Briefly,
this scale measures responses of the patient's relatives describing
the patient as seeking to be out of communication with others, but
not as sulking or pouting. Thus, statements such as "He stays in
bed all day"; "She didn't talk, just watched TV," would be coded as
evidence of solitariness.

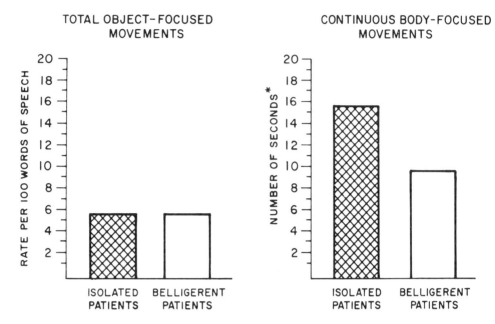

Figure 1   Rate of Object-Focused movements per 100 words of speech, and duration of Continuous Body-Focused activity observed during a 10-minute segment of video taped interview conducted with Isolated and Belligerent schizophrenic patients.
*Time scores transformed by $\sqrt{X + .5}$.

What kinds of body-focused activity did our Isolated patients utilize? Our system for coding hand movements distinguishes several types of body-focused activity. Table 1 shows the relative saliencie of types of movements for our patients. Looking at the bottom half of this table among the subcategories of continuous body touching, finger-to-hand activity significantly distinguishes Isolated from Belligerent patients. Direct and indirect body-touching is about equal in our two groups. Finger-to-hand activity is the least patterned of our continuous body touching categories, consisting of one hand acting upon the other in bilateral, repetitive, nondirected fashion. Direct and indirect body touching is more patterned in the sense that the hand acts, usually in unilateral, directed fashion, upon some particular body part as if to caress or soothe it. Thus, these data suggest that Isolation in our patients is associated with the least patterned continuous self-stimulating activity.

By contrast, and unexpectedly, the data revealed that Belligerence was associated with the most patterned body-touching activity. That is, Belligerent patients exhibited significantly more discrete,

Table 1

Means and S.D.s of Object-Focused and Body-Focused Activity Scores
During Interview[1] for Isolated and Belligerent Schizophrenic Patients

Kinetic Behavior	Isolated N = 8		Belligerent N = 8		t-value (two-tailed)
	X̄	SD	X̄	SD	
A. Object-Focused[2]					
(1) Speech Primacy	4.64	3.11	3.44	2.42	N.S.
(2) Representational	.86	.96	1.75	1.47	N.S.
(3) Nonrepresentational	.46	.32	.69	.47	N.S.
B. Body-Focused[3]					
(1) Total Continuous Body-Focused	16.50	3.98	9.66	5.95	2.70 p < .02
(a) Finger-to-Hand	12.15	8.20	5.79	5.20	1.85 p < .10
(b) Direct and Indirect	6.24	6.85	5.63	6.40	N.S.
(2) Discrete Body-Focused	8.38	6.02	14.25	7.08	1.78 p < .10

[1]A 10-minute communication sample.

[2]Rates per 100 words of speech.

[3]Number of seconds transformed by $\sqrt{X + .5}$.

noncontinuous body-focused hand movements than did Isolated patients.
In our system of coding, discrete body touching is brief (under 3
sec.), focused, and instrumental, as in scratching or picking at
the body surface, and is clearly phased-in with the speech flow insofar as such movements tend to occur during pauses in speech. Previous work with normals has shown that such movements mainly occur
either prior to sentence onset, or early in the sentence. Perhaps
discrete movements have something to do with planning the sentence,
or, as Dittmann (1970) suggests, may aid in decision making about
lexical and syntactic aspects of speech.

This latter fortuitous finding piqued our curiosity about the
kinds of language used by our Isolated and Belligerent patients.
Specifically, we wondered whether the two forms of body touching
would be associated with different kinds of language organization.
If the compensatory feedback from continuous finger-to-hand body
touching is indeed adaptive, in that it helps narrow the focus of
attention, we speculated that the language product associated with
such movement ought to be relatively simple and straightforward.
By contrast, if discrete body touching is related to sentence planning, then such hand movements ought to be related to the articulation of more elaborate or complex ideas in communication.

A way of testing these speculations was available to us in the system of language analysis developed by our colleague Dr. Irving Steingart, and described in his paper. I will not review this system of analysis here, but will simply say that the assessment of language codes which he developed gives us an estimate of the relative degree of functional complexity of an individual's language product. Utilizing this system of language analysis, we computed the percentages of each type of language utilized by our Isolated and Belligerent patients and correlated these percentages with both of our body touching measures. As we suspected, a significant correlation of .56 (p <.05) emerged between finger-to-hand activity and the most simple form of Narrative language (i.e., a form which utilizes simple, discrete, independent clauses). Support for the hypothesis that discrete body touching would prime a more complex form of language is given by a significant correlation of .53 (p <.05) between discrete body touching and a complex conditional form of language organization which articulates patterned interrelations among experiences through the use of grammatical devices which link these experiences into a causal, deductive, or purposive matrix.

Our speculation about these forms of body touching, then, is that they provide feedback which aids in the articulation of different organizations of language behavior. When excessive distraction through sensory overload occurs, as in the Isolated schizophrenic patients, continuous and repetitive rubbing of one hand upon the other helps filter the overload by narrowing attention. Apparently, this facilitates the articulation of simple chunks of information to be communicated. When interference from stimulus overload is not an issue, and more complex ideas are being readied for communication, Discrete hand movement may help to release these complex organizations into speech.

An alternative interpretation of these data might be that the body touching we observed is simply an overflow reaction to stress, and not compensatory as we have suggested. There are three reasons we think this not to be the case. First, a stress reaction would surely be indexed by fragmentation of language, as Mahl and his colleagues (1963) have amply demonstrated. We found relatively little language fragmentation in either of our samples of patients. Second, it will be recalled that it was our Belligerent patients who were mos subject to stress, as indexed by their high Taylor Manifest Anxiety Scores, and it was these patients who produced the most patterned and discrete body touching as well as the most complex, functionally organized language behavior, both of which are inconsistent with stress discharge reactions. Finally, we correlated the Manifest Anxiety Scores with each of the discriminating Body Touching and language measures and were not surprised to find that the MAS scores were uncorrelated with these measures. For these reasons, we were encouraged in our conviction that hand movement during speech provides compensatory self-produced "nutriment" for the priming and support of formal organizations of communicated thought.

II   HAND MOVEMENT BEHAVIOR IN THE CONGENITALLY BLIND

I would like to turn next to a study conducted in our laboratory with a group of relatively normal, though congenitally blind
subjects. This population provides a unique opportunity for observing the effects of massive sensory curtailment upon the use of the
hands for compensatory self-stimulation during communicative discourse. Indeed, the total unresponsiveness of the blind infant to
visual stimulation has been seen to underlie a number of motoric
manifestations serving a compensatory function. For example, it has
been suggested that the body rocking and blindisms observed in the
congenitally blind infant are specific motoric compensatory devices
for lack of adequate stimulation from the environment (Ribble, 1943;
Keeler, 1958; Scott, 1969). Furthermore, the establishment of the
onset of blindisms at about 3-5 months, a time roughly at which
reaching for external objects appears in normally sighted children,
reflects, as David Freedman and his colleagues (1970) suggest, a
link between such blindisms and the use of the body as a replacement
for appropriately stimulating external objects upon which drive tension can be discharged and mastery can be experienced. Thus, among
the blind, thought, as well as communication, should bear the strong
imprint of early sensori-motor schemata (Piaget, 1936) derived from
self-stimulation of the body and its surfaces. Indeed, Scott (1969)
suggests that the reproduction of an image for the blind is the reproduction of motoric touch sequences or schemata, a point dramatically
illustrated by Dahl (1965) in the case of Helen Keller. Dahl suggested that the motor acts with which Miss Keller signalled her needs
and wants to others, were in large measure, motor components of the
wished for, and hallucinatorily vivid, gratifying object representation itself, "a repetition of a component of a previous experience
of satisfaction" (p. 537). Therefore, we view the hand movement
accompaniments of speech in the blind as an important source of
data for our study of the role of movement in thought processing,
as well as its role in providing essential nutriment for sustaining
communicative structure.

In our selection of subjects for this study, we were careful
to screen for serious psychological as well as physical and neurological handicaps. The final sample consisted of 10 congenitally
blind students between the ages of 17 and 21 years, enrolled in a
training program at the Industrial Home for the Blind in Queens,
New York. The cause of blindness in all Ss was diagnosed as retrolental fibroplasia. All Ss were of normal intelligence, and none
showed any signs of CNS impairment due to a history of prematurity
and over supply of oxygen while in the incubator.

In considering the kinds of hand movement behavior that one
ought to expect in congenitally blind subjects, we were heavily influenced by the fact of the absence of early visual feedback obtained normally from eye-hand-mouth coordination (Bruner, 1969),

and its role in establishing differentiated self- and object-schemata (e.g., Hoffer, 1949). We therefore expected that those movements which take place at a distance from the body surface, providing information to a listener through enactment, will be severely curtailed in the congenitally blind due to the failure in early infancy to obtain visual feedback cues, or nutriment, for the establishment of such motor structures. On the other hand, we expected that there would occur a heightening of the use of the body for feedback information, and hence, an upsurge of those forms of movement behavior which take the body as object. The primacy of early body touching, particularly hand-mouth touching (Hoffer, 1949) for the establishment of "touch sequences or schemata" (Scott, 1969), has been amply demonstrated for normal infants (Gesell et al., 1960), and for the blind, especially in the work of Fraiberg and her colleagues (Adelson & Fraiberg, 1971). Of crucial importance for the blind is the establishment of hand upon hand touching at the midline, a form of movement which, if not present by the fifth or sixth month of life, results in developmental deviations (Adelson & Fraiberg, 1971). We expected, then, that since hand upon hand touching was particularly important in the establishment of early sensori-motor schema, such movement would continue to be of primary importance in communicative behavior, and in the conceptual organization and integration of reality as well.

In order to have a basis for evaluating forms of communication behavior in the blind, we compared the data obtained in this study with the data obtained from a group of 24 sighted college students in a previous study (Freedman et al., 1972). The college sample was comparable in age and socio-economic status. Evaluation of overall word fluency scores obtained from the Christensen-Guilford Word Fluency Test (1959) for the groups of blind and normal college students indicated that there was no significant difference in fluency between the two groups.

Turning to the data, we were not surprised to find that in our population of congenitally blind Ss there were virtually no object-focused hand movements. By contrast, there was virtually constant body-focused motor activity accompanying the speech of these Ss. This activity consisted of various forms of body-focused activity, including continuous finger-to-hand and continuous direct and indirect body touching activity. However, some of the body touching activity observed was unscorable with our present system of analysis, since it consisted of a type of movement on the body surface which combined aspects of both discrete, that is brief and instrumental body touching, and a form of punctuating movements on the body surface which were phased into the rhythm of the speech flow. It was as if these Ss used their body surface in a way similar to the way normally sighted Ss use their hands in space, to punctuate and emphasize the content of their speech. The development of an appropriate category for codifying such movements is a task for future work

The remainder of the body-focused activity which was scorable by our assessment procedures is presented in Table 2 where we compare the prevalence and quality of body-focused activity in the blind and normally sighted college students during a five-minute monologue segment of the interview tape.

Two observations stand out in this table. The first deals with the sheer quantity of self-stimulation. Considering the total body-focused activity score (finger-to-hand plus direct and indirect body touching), we note not only that there is much more of such activity among the blind, but that the scores are exceedingly high. Converting the transformed time scores into real time would show that blind Ss spent an average of 230 out of 300 sec. in some form of self-stimulation whereas among the sighted Ss the corresponding time spent would amount to about 100 sec.

The second observation pertains to the form of preferred self-stimulation. The higher rate of body-focused activity among the blind than sighted Ss is almost entirely accounted for by the high rate of finger-to-hand activity.

Recalling that finger-to-hand activity also distinguished our Isolated from our Belligerent schizophrenic patients, and there appeared to support a most simply narrative type of language organization, we wondered about the way that finger-to-hand activity might support communication in the blind. Based upon our understanding of the role of the hands in schema formation for the blind, it seemed reasonable to expect that this form of self-stimulation might support more complexly organized forms of linguistic communication in normal, relatively competent, albeit blind symbolizers.

As a way of exploring this question, we correlated our blind Ss' scores for finger-to-hand activity with Steingart's measures of linguistic complexity. The results of this correlational analysis revealed a highly significant, and positive correlation of .86 p < .01, between finger-to-hand activity and Complex Portrayal language, a type of language which articulates a patterned interrelation among experiences, but which does so only descriptively, without a conditional or contingency framework. Thus, as we expected, the relation between finger-to-hand activity and Complex Portrayal language in the blind, contrasted with the kinesic-linguistic relationship observed in the sample of socially isolated schizophrenic patients.

The developmental history of the blind is important for the understanding of these contrasting findings. For example, it has been suggested by Adelson and Fraiberg (1971) that "the crucial adaptive task for the blind infant is the freeing of the hand from the mouth for pursuit of the complex integrative work of perception .... In the absence of vision, it is the hand that must create

Table 2

Means and Standard Deviations of Continuous Body-Focused Activity

Scores* During Monologue in Congenitally Blind and Sighted Ss

Kinesic Behavior	Congenitally Blind Students, N = 10		Sighted College Students, N = 24		t (two-tailed)
	$\overline{X}$	SD	$\overline{X}$	SD	
Total Body-Focused Activity	15.28	5.19	10.11	5.48	2.59 p < .02
Finger-to-Hand	11.46	7.35	6.59	5.82	2.05 p < .05
Direct and Indirect	6.07	6.86	5.68	4.99	.19

*Time scores per 5-minute communication sample transformed by formula $\sqrt{X + .5}$.

the bridge between the body self and the world of objects" (p. 420). We have already indicated that these authors deem the occurrence of hand-to-hand contact at the midline, at approximately four months, crucial for normal development in the blind. Apparently, hand-to-hand contact at the midline substitutes, in the blind child, for the kind of stimulus nutriment important to the development of focal attention, which vision provides for the normal child (Bruner, 1969). Lacking visual cues, the blind infant appears to rely upon bilateral self-stimulation of hand upon hand at the midline to provide focus and direction to thought and action. Extrapolating from these considerations, we suggest that communicative demands made upon blind Ss trigger hand-to-hand self-stimulation as a way of compensating for the relative lack of attention directing feedback from the listener which is ordinarily available to the sighted through what Dittmann has earlier in this book called the "listener response" (i.e., head nods, facial expression, etc.)—a response which guides the form and direction of the speaker's communication. That is, hand-to-hand stimulation in the blind would be a motoric substitute for the type of visual nutriment which serves to focus attention upon those listener cues which regulate the communicative flow. This suggests that in the blind the feedback from bilateral stimulation of the hands serves to keep thought on track by heightening the speaker's attention to what he is saying.

Returning now to the contrasting way such self-stimulating feedback supports relatively simple Narrative language in the schizophrenic patients and Complex Portrayal language in the blind, we would like to suggest that this contrast highlights the fact that feedback from continuous hand-to-hand activity aids in focusing attention upon whatever language programs are characteristically useful to these groups for dealing with the interview stress. Whether feedback from the hands could modify such programs in the direction of more or less complexity is an empirical matter requiring future experimental studies.

III HAND MOVEMENT BEHAVIOR AND BILINGUAL COMMUNICATION

I would like now to turn briefly to a study currently being
conducted at our center by Dr. Luis Marcos who is attempting to explore the relationship between hand movement behavior and verbal
encoding in a group of subordinate bilingual Ss; that is, normal
bilinguals for whom language competence is relatively poorer in the
second language. Quite apart from the important and basic issues
of how information is stored and transferred from one linguistic
system to another (Kolers, 1971) in such people, the phenomenology
of communicating in a nondominant language system is of interest to
us here insofar as it suggests problems for the speaker in regard
to the informational returns from hearing himself speak in a not
too well commanded language. Klein (1965) has reminded us of the
importance of the feedback from one's own speech in establishing
an "average expectable" communicative environment, and he has demonstrated (Klein & Wolitzky, 1970) the disrupting effects upon
thought itself of depriving one of such important informational returns. Klein (1965) suggests that "the afference of one's own
speech is a critical factor in maintaining reality oriented communicated thought--that is, thought conveyed through speech. If
vocalization is to be effective, its success should, like that of
all self-produced stimulation, depend partly upon the informational
feedback to the speaker himself" (p. 326). The study of delayed
feedback from one's own speech, has amply demonstrated this fact
(Yates, 1963).

It is in this sense that we turn to the study of subordinate
bilinguals communicating in both their dominant and nondominant
languages. Communicating in a "foreign" language represents a condition of disrupted feedback, both from self-produced vocalization
cues, as well as from the response from the environment. The stress
of speaking in a "foreign" language consists, in large measure, of
the disruption of the auditory "reports," to use Freud's term of the
Project (1895), of familiar semantic, syntactic, and phonetic attributes of the mother tongue. From our point of view, it should also
have consequence in respect to compensatory self-generated hand
movements to aid in overcoming such stress. We expected, then, that
those movements which could aid the specific task of overcoming lexical, grammatical, and articulatory difficulties ought to increase
when speaking in the nondominant language system. That is, our hunch
was that object-focused movements rather than body-focused movements
would increase under the communicative stress of speaking in a foreign
language. This, simply because the difficulties inherent in speaking
a foreign language primarily involve problems of translation and retrieval rather than those concerned with the focusing of attention.
Thus, movements which take place at some distance from the body surface, providing visual and proprioceptive feedback, might prime or activate relatively weakly organized schema or linguistic structures of
the second language system. In this regard, one is reminded of one of
Weisenburg and McBride's (1935) aphasic patients who could read the

word EARTH after making circular movements with his hand, or of
another's ability to say the word SCISSORS only after wriggling his
fingers back and forth as in cutting.

    The data which I will report were obtained by Dr. Marcos in
pilot work. As such, it is preliminary data which must await confirmation in the major study itself. However, both the magnitude
of effects and their consistency across all Ss indicate that the
findings in this study will most likely be confirmed in the final
sample.

    Eight adult subordinate bilinguals served as subjects in this
preliminary study. There were four men and four women ranging in
age between 24 to 41 years. Four of the eight bilinguals had English as their primary language, and Spanish as their secondary language. The remaining four S's primary language was Spanish, and
English was their secondary language. Language dominance, which
was assessed by an extensive battery of language dominance scales,
confirmed that for both English and Spanish bilinguals, their primary language was indeed their dominant, most highly commanded one.
This was true for each of the eight subjects.

    The video taped material from which our hand movement data were
obtained consisted of a 10-minute segment during which each S was
asked to speak for five minutes on an abstract topic, and five minutes on a concrete topic. Ss did this in each of their two languages,
counterbalanced appropriately for first and second language, and
concrete and abstract topic. In the present report, we are not considering the concrete-abstract breakdown of the data, and will only
report total 10-minute segment scores for hand movement categories
in the primary and secondary languages.

    Table 3 shows the mean scores for our hand movement categories
pooled over the groups of English-Spanish and Spanish-English bilinguals. The most striking aspect of this table is the fact that, as
we expected, speaking in the second language produced an increase in
all forms of object-focused hand movements. The total rate of object-
focused movements almost doubles when shifting from communication in
the first to the second language. Inspection of the component categories of object-focused movements reveals that the major significant
increases occur in relation to those speech primacy punctuating movements which appear to emphasize the articulatory flow of the speech,
that is, those movements which are phased in with the rhythm of
speech, providing emphasis on its beat quality. The subject appears
to be measuring his speech with his hand, perhaps as an aid to emphasizing the articulatory aspects of the foreign language. In addition, a highly significant difference between the mean rates of
nonrepresentational speech failure movements occurs when shifting
from first to second language. This appears to be the opposite side
of the coin, since such movements, which have a groping quality, occur when word finding falters, and may reflect the speaker's effort,

Table 3

Means and Standard Deviations of Object- and Body-Focused Activity

Scores in The First and Second Languages of English-Spanish and

Spanish-English Bilinguals in Monologue Communication[1]

Kinesic Behavior	1st Language		2nd Language		t (two-tailed)
	$\bar{X}$	SD	$\bar{X}$	SD	N = 8
A. Total Object-Focused[2]	17.49	14.76	31.51	17.50	4.31 p < .01
I Speech Primacy					
(a) Punctuating	7.26	8.53	14.64	12.73	3.47 p < .01
(b) Minor Qualifiers	7.10	7.65	11.38	11.17	1.35 N.S.
II Motor Primacy					
(a) Representational	2.77	2.84	3.99	2.80	1.19 N.S.
(b) Nonrepresentational	.36	.34	1.50	.89	4.27 p < .01
1 - Speech Failure	.15	.23	.93	.71	2.99 p < .05
2 - Pointing	.21	.28	.57	.50	2.04 N.S.
B. Body-Focused[3]					
I Total Continuous Body-Focused	12.60	6.15	10.29	7.18	2.47 p < .05
(a) Finger-to-Hand	11.48	7.45	8.49	7.94	1.78 N.S.
(b) Direct and Indirect	2.60	2.43	4.34	2.47	1.22 N.S.
II Discrete Body-Focused	10.75	7.44	8.12	6.12	1.21 N.S.

[1]Ten-minute interview segment.

[2]Rate per 100 words of speech.

[3]Seconds transformed by $\sqrt{X + .5}$.

albeit often nonsuccessful, to retrieve words or ideas. While those
categories of movement which are associated with the representational
or qualifying aspects of movement (e.g., minor qualifiers and representational movements) also increase in the second language, they
do not reach acceptable levels of significance.[5]

---

[5]Dr. Felix Barroso has suggested that one probably ought not to expect that representational activity will increase in the second language since the primary obstacle to coding in the second language is
not object finding but word finding. It follows from this suggestion
that hand movements may be useful in regard to the study of object
relations. That is, hand movements may be important signposts of
the degree to which objects are conserved intrapsychically. If so,
this would help explain the paucity of object-focused movements noted
in the communication of our schizophrenic patients.

Thus, while all object-focused movements increase in the second language, the major effect of hand movement in this pilot study was revealed in the effort to express and to retrieve words from memory storage. We believe that such movements operate via visual and kinesthetic feedback loops to either confirm, through emphasis, the appropriateness of one's articulations, or prime the weakly organized language system. They may serve functions similar to the functions served by the auditory feedback from vocalization qualities; that is, as corrective feedback for emphasis, and editing, and as a stimulus to prime retrieval operations in verbal encoding.

Turning to the bottom portion of Table 3, we see a surprising reversal of effect with respect to body-focused movements. Here the major trend is for such movement to occur with relatively greater duration during communication in the first language. This is particularly evident in the significant difference between first and second language in the duration of total continuous body-focused movements. While this finding was not expected, we might speculate that it, too, reflects the greater emphasis on verbal encoding in the second language. That is, given the heightened use of hands as an aid to word finding and articulation in the second language, less time can be directed toward movements at the body surface. An alternate (and perhaps more intersting) hypothesis about this finding is that when speaking one's primary language, where word finding and articulation are relatively easy, associations spread out and stimulate distracting trains of thought. In this case, again, touching the body in a continuous and repetitive fashion would serve to focus attention upon the ideas to be conveyed to the listener. Such a view would be consistent with the oft-noted clinical observation that speaking in one's mother tongue, as opposed to a second language, is associated with a lowering of resistance to remembering and working through early life experiences (Greenson, 1950; Krapf, 1955).

IMPLICATIONS

In concluding this presentation, I would like to draw several implications from these studies which focus upon the significance of the motor apparatus for effective thought processing. Klein (1965), in discussing the relation between vocalization and speech, suggested that "in directly involving the motor apparatus for the emission of sounds, speech goes beyond words by enlarging the means of coding thoughts and of conveying the affect and motive organizers of behavior (p. 329). Our data suggest that not only speech, but the hand movements that accompany it, participate in thought processing. This participation consists, most probably, in two interrelated but distinguishable functions. One is perhaps a precondition for the other in that it fulfills the prerequisite of focusing attention so that ideas can be articulated in a relatively organized way. The other provides for the motoric enrichment of the symbolic code through its abridged (re) enactment, or through the emphasizing and qualifying operations of hand movement.

In our view, the upsurge of continuous body touching, and particularly the touching of one hand with the other, observed among our isolated schizophrenic patients and our congenitally blind subjects, reflects the attention focusing function of hand movements. We have suggested here that the socially isolating experiences of the emotionally withdrawn schizophrenic patient and the sensory isolation of the congenitally blind subject result in profound deprivations of stimulus nutriment which underlie the need for compensatory self-stimulation. Both forms of deprivation provide ideal conditions for the inward turning of attention with its concomitant focusing upon the world of personal experience. The necessity to communicate to another, that is, to redirect attention from one's inner world to an object in the external environment, imposes a condition which requires the establishment and continuous reinforcement of the boundaries between the self and others (Feder, 1952; DesLauriers, 1962). As Lilly (1956) and others (Solomon et al., 1961; Miller, 1962) report, under conditions of stimulus deprivation, compensatory self-stimulation serves as a comforting, constant safeguard against the loss of reality contact. It is our view that the continuous rubbing of the body surface with the hands during discourse sustains the boundaries between self and object, and thereby enhances the capacity for maintaining the focus of attention on cues in the "external" world. One might speculate here that the blindisms noted among three-month old congenitally blind infants may serve a similar function by providing repetitive proprioceptive inflow which focuses attention in the absence of the normal visual organizers of cortical activity. The absence of self-induced stimulation, not only among the blind (Adelson & Fraiberg, 1971), but also among those subjected to extreme environmental deprivation (Freedman, 1971), often lead to severely deviant patterns of autistic development. Thus, quite apart from whatever drive gratification may be obtained from self-stimulation (Hotter, 1959), evidence for an integrative, attention regulating role of feedback from self-stimulation of the body, is highlighted by these data.

The second way that hand movements may enrich the coding of thought is suggested by our data from the bilingual study. Speaking in a second language, apart from lexical and syntactic problems, raises certain difficulties contingent upon the disruption of familiar accoustical feedback from one's own voice. Not only are there differences in grammatical construction and word usage in the second language, but the auditory returns from the voice, which provide

on-line monitoring of what and how one is speaking, are also relatively unfamiliar to the speaker himself. Interestingly, it is,
we believe, in respect to just those unfamiliar aspects of second
language communication that compensatory hand movements occur in
our data. That is, the categories of punctuating and speech failure
movements showed significant increments when shifting from first to
second language. It is as though the hands are engaged in a steady
effort to find, shape, and emphasize the vocal patterns involved in
the articulation of relatively unfamiliar words. In a sense, it is
as if the speaker was turning up the volume of his speech by high-
lighting its vocal characteristics. Punctuating movements seem to
behave like the voice itself does when auditory feedback is occluded
(Klein & Wolitzky, 1970), i.e., the voice volume goes up. We would
suggest that punctuating and speech failure movements, in our bilinguals' speech segments, compensate for a subjective sense of both
failing to adequately articulate a message for a listener, as well
as failing to adequately match some inner sense of the correct articulation of the words for the speaker himself. That is, the hands
are invoked in the effort to overcome the discrepancy between the
internal representation of the word spoken, and the feedback from
one's own voice in the articulation of this mental representation.[6]
In this way, hand movements which accompany speech may support the
link between an image of the word and its verbal articulation.

    All this leads, then, to a final implication which we believe
follows from our data. That is, that movements which accompany
speech play a role in the process of bringing mental contents to
awareness. Freud, in his Project for a Scientific Psychology (1895)
and elsewhere (1900), outlined an important theory of the relation
between attention and verbal thought processes which we feel is
relevant to this point. For Freud, in order for verbal thought to
achieve conscious status, it had to attract attention. However,
since attention was only attracted by indications of sensory quality,
thought had to be connected to motor innervations resulting from
speech and sound presentations. Thus, word images provided the indication of quality which attract attention to thought. The view
which we would like to suggest is that movements of the hands upon,
and at some distance from the body surface, during speech, provide
additional qualities of sensory and ideo-motor experience which are
linked to this attention regulating role of speech. Data generated
at our center have suggested that while the role of some forms of
such additional support is reduced as the linguistic system comes
to dominate communication, it may re-emerge under conditions which
disrupt the normal inflow of stimulus properties from the environment. Just as raising the level of one's voice serves as a compensatory feedback mechanism for keeping thought on track when auditory

---

[6]This "closed loop" or servomechanism model of error correcting feedback is well known in engineering and computor technology, and was
proposed as a comprehensive model for human behavior by Miller, Galanter & Pribram (1960).

returns are occluded in vocal isolation studies, the repetitive rubbing of the body surface or the emphatic or depictive movement of the hand at some distance from the body surface, serve as a compensatory self-generated feedback mechanism to insure the directedness of one's thinking when visual, auditory, and/or social cues are relatively absent. Our focus upon the importance of the link between sensory, ideational, and motoric components of the verbalization process hopefully provides a meaningful vantage point from which to observe and understand communicative behavior.

REFERENCES

Adelson, E. & Fraiberg, S. Mouth and hand in the early development of blind infants. In James F. Bosma (Ed.), Symposium on oral sensation and perception. Springfield, Illinois: Thomas, 1971.

Azima, H. & Cramer, Fern J. Effects of the decrease in sensory variability on body schema. Canadian Journal of Psychiatry, 1956, 1, 1:59.

Broadbent, D. E. Perception and communication. London: Pergamon Press, 1958.

Bruner, J. S., Oliver, R. R., Greenfield, P. M., et al. (Eds.), Studies in cognitive growth. New York: John Wiley, 1966.

Christensen, P. R. & Guilford, J. P. Manual for the Christensen-Guilford Fluency Tests. Beverly Hills: Sheridan, 1959.

Dahl, H. Observations on a "natural experiment"--Helen Keller. Journal of the American Psychoanalytic Association, 1965, 13 :533-550.

Des Lauriers, A. M. The experience of reality in childhood schizophrenia. New York: International Universities Press, 1962.

Deutch, J. A. & Deutch, D. Attention: Some theoretical considerations. Psychological Review, 1963, 70:80-90.

Dittmann, A. T. The body movement speech rhythm relationship as a cue to speech encoding. In A. W. Siegman & B. Pope (Eds.), Studies in dyadic communication. New York: Pergamon Press, 1970.

Easterbrook, J. A. The effect of emotion on cue utilization and the organization of behavior. Psychological Review, 1959, 66:183-200.

Ekman, P. & Friesen, W. V. The repertoire of nonverbal behavior: Categories, origins, usage, and coding. Semiotica, 1969, 1(1), 49-98.

218   S. GRAND

Ekman, P. & Friesen, W. V. Nonverbal behavior and psychopathology. In R. J. Friedman and M. M. Katz (Eds.), The psychology of depression: Contemporary theory and research. The Govt. Printing Office, 1972.

Federn, P. Ego psychology and the psychosis. New York: Basic Books, 1952.

Freedman, D. A., Fox-Kolende, Betty J., & Brown, S. L. A multihandicapped rubella baby. Journal of the American Academy of Child Psychiatry, 1970, 9:298-317.

Freedman, D. A. Congenital and perinatal sensory deprivation: Some studies in early development. American Journal of Psychiatry, 1971, 127:1539-1545.

Freedman, N., Rosen, B., Engelhardt, D. M., & Margolis, R. Prediction of psychiatric hospitalization: 1. The measurement of hospital proneness. Journal of Abnormal Psychology, 1967, 72:468-477.

Freedman, N., O'Hanlon, J., Oltman, P., & Witkin, H. A. The imprint of psychological differentiation on kinetic behavior in varying communicative contexts. Journal of Abnormal Psychology, 1972, 79:239-258.

Freud, S. (1893). On the psychical mechanism of hysterical phenomena: Preliminary communication. Standard Edition, Vol. III. London: Hogarth Press, 1962.

Freud, S. (1895). Project for a scientific psychology. Standard Edition, Vol. I. London: Hogarth Press, 1966.

Freud, S. (1900). The interpretation of dreams. Standard Edition, Vol. IV & V. London: Hogarth Press, 1953.

Freud, S. (1911). Formulations regarding the two principles of mental functioning. Standard Edition, Vol. XII. London: Hogarth Press, 1958.

Gesell, A. & Armatruda, S. Developmental diagnosis. (2nd ed.) New York: Hoeber, 1960.

Grand, S., Freedman, N., & Steingart, I. A study of the representation of objects in schizophrenia. Journal of the American Psychoanalytic Association, 1973, 21,2:399-434.

Grand, S., Freedman, N., Steingart, I., & Buchwald, C. Communicative behavior in schizophrenia: The relation of adaptive styles to kinetic and linguistic aspects of interview behavior. Journal of Nervous and Mental Disease, 1975, 161,5:293-306.

Greenson, R. R. The mother tongue and the mother. International Journal of Psychoanalysis, 1950, 31:18–23.

Harris, A. Sensory deprivation in schizophrenia. Journal of Mental Science, 1959, 105, 235.

Hartmann, H. (1939). Ego psychology and the problem of adaptation. New York: International Universities Press, 1958.

Hewes, G. W. The current status of the gestural theory of language origin. Paper presented at N. Y. Academy of Science Conference on Origins and Evolution of Language and Speech. New York, September, 1975.

Hoffer, W. Mouth, hand, and ego integration. Psychoanalytic Study of the Child, 3/4, 1949.

Holst, E. von. Relations between the central nervous system and the peripheral organs. British Journal of Animal Behavior, 1954, 2:89–94.

Holt, R. R. Ego autonomy re-evaluated. International Journal of Psychoanalysis, 1965, 46:151–167.

Holzman, P. S. Perceptual dysfunction in the schizophrenic syndrome. In R. Cancro (Ed.), The schizophrenic reactions. New York: Brunner/Mazel, 1970.

Holzman, P. S., Rousey, C., & Snyder, C. On listening to one's own voice: Effects on psychophysiological responses and free associations. Journal of Personality & Social Psychology, 1966, 4:432–441.

Keeler, W. R. Autistic patterns and defective communication in blind children with retrolental fibroplasia. In P. Hoch and J. Zubin (Eds.), Psychopathology of communication, 1958.

Klein, G. S. On hearing one's own voice: An aspect of cognitive control in spoken thought. In M. Shur (Ed.), Drives, affects, behavior. Vol. 2, 1965.

Klein, G. S. Peremptory ideation: Structure and force in motivated ideas. In G. S. Klein (Ed.), Perception, motives, and personality. New York: Knopf, 1970.

Klein, G. S. & Wolitzky, D. Vocal isolation: The effects of occluding auditory feedback from one's own voice. Journal of Abnormal Psychology, 1970, 75:50–56.

Kolers, P. A. Bilingualism and information processing. In Scientific American (Ed.), Contemporary Psychology. San Francisco, Calif.: W. H. Freeman, 1971.

Krapf, E. E. The choice of language in polyglot psychoanalysis. Psychoanalytic Quarterly, 1955, 24:343-357.

Lilly, J. C. Mental effects of reduction of ordinary levels of physical stimuli on intact healthy persons. Psychiatry Research Report, No. 5, A.P.A., 1-9, 1956.

Mahl, G. The lexical and linguistic levels in the expression of emotions. In Peter H. Knapp (Ed.), Expression of the emotions in man. New York: International Universities Press, 1963.

Miller, G. A., Galanter, E., & Pribram, K. H. Plans and the structure of behavior. New York: Holt, Rinehart & Winston, 1960.

Miller, S. C. Ego autonomy in sensory deprivation, isolation and stress. International Journal of Psychoanalysis, 1962, 43:1-20.

Piaget, J. (1936). The origins of intelligence in children. (2nd ed.) New York: International Universities Press, 1952.

Rapaport, D. The theory of ego autonomy: A generalization. Bulletin of the Menninger Clinic, 1958, 22:13-35.

Ribble, M. A. The rights of infants; early psychological needs and their satisfaction. New York: Columbia Press, 1943.

Rosenzweig, N. Sensory deprivation and schizophrenia: Some clinical and theoretical similarities. American Journal of Psychiatry, 1959, Vol. 116, 326.

Schechter, M. D., Shurley, J. T., Sexauer, J. D., & Toussieng, P. C. Perceptual isolation therapy, a new experimental approach in the treatment of children using infantile autistic defenses. Journal of the American Academy of Child Psychiatry, 1969, 8:97-139.

Scott, R. A. The socialization of blind children. In D. A. Goslin (Ed.), Handbook of socialization theory and research. Chicago: Rand-McNally, 1969.

Silverman, J. The problem of attention in research and theory in schizophrenia. Psychological Review, 1964, 71:352-379.

Solomon, P., Kubzansky, P. E., Leiderman, P. H., Mendelson, J. H., Trumbull, R., & Wexler, D. (Eds.), Sensory deprivation. Cambridge, Mass.: Harvard University Press, 1961.

Spohn, H. E., Thetford, P. E., & Cancro, R.   Attention, psycho-
physiology, and scanning in the schizophrenic syndrome.   In R.
Cancro (Ed.), The schizophrenic reactions.   New York: Brunner/
Mazel, 1970.

Treisman, A. M.   The effect of irrelevant material on the effi-
ciency of selective listening.   American Journal of Psychology,
1964, 77:533-546.

Venables, P. H.   Selectivity of attention, withdrawal, and cortical
activation.   Archives of General Psychiatry, 1963, 9:74-78.

Venables, P. H.   Input dysfunction in schizophrenia.   In B. Meyer
(Ed.), Progress in experimental personality research, Vol. 1.
New York: Academic Press, 1964.

Weisenberg, T. & McBride, K. E.   Aphasia.   New York Commonwealth
Fund, 1935.

Yates, A. J.   Delayed auditory feedback.   Psychological Bulletin,
1963, 60:213-232.

This research has been supported by Grant No. MH-14383 from the
United States Public Health Service, National Institute of Mental
Health.

ISSUES POSED BY SECTION 3

Mardi J. Horowitz

University of California, San Francisco

San Francisco, California 94143

A common theme in the three contributions to this section is an attempt to shed light on the cognitive processes and/or structures that sustain or lead to the erosion of verbal communications. I shall review the main findings of each of the three contributors as they pertain to this particular theme, and then discuss the general theoretical model itself.

Theodore Shapiro focuses on the communicative significance of echoing in psychotic children. He suggests that the echoes function as a device to achieve social closure for a child who has limited cognitive capacity and only a limited available repertoire of other responses. We can infer from these findings that even though there is not normal progression in the cognitive structures that underlie language production, the child is able to establish a relationship. Avoidances of the human environment tend to occur when the child cannot cognitively process what is offered and has to back off.

The echoing is seen as an adaptation to some dimly recognized need to speak even though he does not understand what has been spoken to him. The findings that support this hypothesis about the nature of the echoing response are those of less reaction time before echoing responses than nonechoing responses, and echoes that are of greater length than the nonechoes. The echoes also seemed to occur in clusters. It appeared that when the child was limited in comprehending what was spoken, he tended to resort more frequently to echoic behavior. The cognitive structure that might be relatively absent in the autistic child would be seen as an inner model not only of self and object relationships, in terms of patterned sequences of appropriate responses, but also in the ability to decipher language, order conceptual responses, and assemble these into the action sequences necessary for appropriate speech.

223

In the absence of these more mature cognitive structures, the
child would be seen as using a more primitive one, in which there is
retention of imagery of what has been heard, an imitative model of
the relationship between self and other, and a relative short circuit-
ing of this imitative model into speech production. Repetition of the
use of this relatively primitive system of cognitive processes and
cognitive structure would make it a habit pattern to be used whenever
there was a sense of threat or stress on a relationship. In other
words, the child would learn that he could reduce the situation of
threat by production of echoes because these echoes had the semblance
of conversation.

Irving Steingart reviews methods of categorizing communicated
language from relatively simple descriptions to very complex packages
of information. The more complex the package of information, the
more the sender is relying on his own cognitive ability to organize
that information in complex codes, and an equivalent ability on the
part of the listener to amplify the received information with an inner model of structural complexity. The minimal structural complexity is not only a cognitive structure, which might be called the self
and object relationship or the core interpersonal relationship, but a
variety of "if statements" that would describe various contingencies
for this relationship. Granted that both persons have such a cognitive structure, they can engage in the cognitive process of developing, transmitting, receiving, decoding, and responding to information
packaged in very parsimonious units.

In the study of a single patient, Steingart then showed that
the most complex language occurred more frequently when that person
was in a paranoid state, whereas the most simple narrative language
was used during states when that patient was relatively depressed.
This corresponds to a clinical formulation of the patient and of these
particular psychopathological states. That is, in the paranoid states
the operant cognitive structure is a relationship between self and object in which the object is seen as having various threatening motives
The depressed state is seen as one in which the person also has self
and object cognitive models, but in which the person is less concerned
with the object, because he is expecting himself only to be hopeless
and helpless in relation to it. The self and object core cognitive
structure, in many ways firmer (however irrational) in the paranoid
state of the same patient, would dictate a more complex language ability, while the relative despair of the more depressive state, associated with whatever physiological changes might limit cognitive processing capacity, would tend to lead the patient toward emitting less
complex language or toward an erosion of the capacity for complex
language behavior.

In the second study described by Steingart, 16 chronic schizophrenic patients were divided into two groups of eight; those socially
isolated and those socially belligerent. The belligerent patients,

who were felt to have unsystematized paranoid activity, had significantly more of the complex language, that is the conditional language
behavior, while the socially isolated group showed significantly
more narrative language behavior. The third study involved normal
subjects who were involved in both dialogue and monologue conditions,
and the findings there were that narrative behavior was more prevalent in the monologue condition, and more complex language was found
in the dialogue condition. The findings from both of these studies,
again, are consistent with the hypothesis that when there is an activation of a cognitive structure involving self and object relationships, the person will not only try to produce more complex language
about the conditional relations between himself and another person,
but also will be enabled by the situation to use more complicated
language. Conversely, the more the person has his attention turned
inwards, is actually isolated or is feeling isolated, the less the
need and also the ability to emit complicated language behavior.
This, incidentally, has an implication for psychotherapy; persons
are more able to engage in complex thought processes when they are
involved in an interpersonal communicative process than they are when
they are thinking alone in a "monologue" condition.

In the presentation by Stanley Grand, there was attention to
the correlation between hand movements and accompanying speech. Once
again, there is the assumption that there is a cognitive structure,
having to do with the coherence and stability of self-representations as well as self and object representations, that underlies
the ability to develop high level cognitive processes required for
complex communications. Grand goes on to develop the idea of stimulus nutriment as a support for the activation and maintenance of
these coherent cognitive structures. The hand stroking and self-
stimulating efforts would be seen as a way of supplying the supportive
nutriment of a coherent self-representation, when such self-representations were under threat of fragmentation or some kind of internal
discord.

The eight isolated patients were compared with the similar eight
belligerent patients. The isolated patients had more seconds of continuous body-focused movements than the belligerent patients. There
was also a significant positive correlation of 0.54 between continuous body touching totals and that particular patient's score on the
index of his isolation. In general, the results were seen as supporting the idea that self-stimulation may be helpful in narrowing
the focus of attention, which would affect the underlying cognitive
structure of self-representation, in that its maintenance would support the cognitive processing of information and sustain language in
situations of stress.

There was then a report on the study of blind subjects in whom
virtually no object-focused hand movements were found. In contrast,

there was almost continuous body-focused motor activity. This
would support the hypothesis that the modality of touch replaces
the modality of sight to maintain an inner cognitive model of the
self.

The author then predicted that object-focused movements rather
than body-focused movements would increase under the communicative
stress of speaking in a foreign language. This prediction was based
on the assumption that object-focused movements were used as punctua-
tions, and that there might be the need for relatively more cognitive
process support because of the relative weakness of organizational
grammar with a second language. The findings supported this prediction. This, then, provided a contrast in that the self-focused
body movements are seen as supporting what is basically a cognitive
structure, the self-representation, whereas the object-focused movements in this case not only supported the cognitive structure of the
current self and object relationship, but also function in support of
the organizational system or grammar.

I have repeated some of the findings within the three papers,
in order to state the coherent theory presented by this group. The
production of verbal speech in a communicative context is based on
certain cognitive processes and cognitive structures. The cognitive
process that is necessary is organizational capacity for setting up
the fundamental concepts as well as the ordering of words themselves.
A fundamental cognitive structure is an inner model of the relatedness
between self and object, but this in turn probably depends on the integrity and coherence of the immediate self-representation. In states
where there is brittleness, fragility, splitting, or multiplicity of
self-representations, or the same multiplicity or fragmentation of
self and object core schemata, there will be impairment in the person'
ability to use high level communicative verbal skills. This erosion
of the basic cognitive processes and cognitive structures that underlie communication may occur as a result of either situational stress,
enduring forms of psychopathology, or handicaps of the basic sensations that lead to coherent development of self and object relationships and communicative capacities.

In what follows now, I will consider more closely the systems
for processing information, both within the mind as forms of cognitive processing, and in expression as forms of communication of information. I shall then reconsider selective aspects of these three
sets of studies as they pertain to this model.

Modes of Information Processing

I have reviewed elsewhere how various theoreticians have conceptualized differentiated modes for the schematization, representation, and expression of information (Horowitz, 1970). These systems
can roughly be catalogued into three sets; the lexical system that

codes information primarily in <u>words</u>, those that code information in <u>images</u> related to the various sensory modalities, and those that <u>enact</u> information. These systems for the codification, representation, and expression of information are interrelated and any given set of information is translated from one system to another. The enactive system is involved not only in motoric behaviors of action, but also in the trial actions involved in gesture, expression, and many movements or tension. The image systems are multiple, corresponding to the various senses; the auditory and visual systems, however, are the ones most prominent in thought. Visual image formation is predominant in dreams, daydreams, and problem solving thought in visual-spatial terms. Lexical thought progresses primarily in terms of word meanings, with a dropping away of the sensory or iconic qualities.

Each system would have its won intrinsic organizational properties, although the acquisition of new organizational properties for any system would be applicable to information processing in the other systems as well. Table 1 gives an example of this type of concept.

Communicative behavior can be separated into these systems, as in the study that correlated expressions in the lexical format of speech with the enactive format of hand movements. The conscious processing of information can also be studied by gaining reports of mental representations. The schematization of information, however, which is sometimes called cognitive structure, can only be deduced from studies of mental representation and communication.

The assumption of schematization is necessary, as Rapaport has pointed out (1957), in order to explain continuities of experience and capacity over time. Some form of schematization is necessary in order to interpret incoming information derived from perception. And some kind of schematization is necessary to think and plan responses in a way that maintains the coherence of a personality and a relationship with another person or a group over time. These schematizations are both formats for cognitive organization, such as suggested by Chomsky (1966) for the generative grammar that underlies the lexical system, and psychological, as formulated in the growing body of psychoanalytic theory on self and object relationships.

When incoming information cannot be completely integrated or interpreted, it is stored in the form of active memory. This form of memory is often called short-term memory, although in special circumstances such as after traumatic perceptions, the registrations endure for such a long period that the term "active" rather than short seems preferable. This type of memory seems to have an intrinsic property of repeated representation until it is terminated by the completion of cognitive processing (Horowitz, 1976).

Table 1

An Outline of Modes of Representation

Mode	Subsystems	Sample Organizational Tendencies	Sample Statement	Sample of Complex Units of Represented Information
ENACTIVE	Skeletal neuro-musculature Visceral neuro-musculature	By directionality and force, by operational end-products	x does this	Gestures Facial expressions Postures
IMAGE	Tactile-kines-thetic Olfactory-gus-tatory Visual Auditory	By simultaneous occurrence, spatial relationships, concrete categorization of similarities and differences	X is like this, X is like Y, X is here and Y is there, X and Y happen together, X does this to Y	Introjects Fantasies Body images Relationship between objects
LEXICAL	(different languages?)	By sequentiality and linear structure, by abstract categorization	$\dfrac{\text{If X and Y then}}{\text{Z because X + Y}} \longleftrightarrow Z$	Phrases or sentences, Stories and histories

Now, with this very brief pre-statement of terms and fragments, and a model of information processing, I would like to return to a discussion of selected aspects of the papers presented, in order to clarify the issues in connecting data from the study in content analysis of communication with theories about cognitive process and cognitive structure.

As already mentioned, Dr. Shapiro presented the hypothesis that echoes are a device for social closure. Now we may consider what other alternative hypotheses might explain his data. Dr. Shapiro alluded to the alternative hypothesis that echoes are an especially heightened primitive function, or a primitive function that has not gained developmentally appropriate inhibition. One such primitive function is the repetition of incoming stimuli stored in active memory. Even this primitive function, however, requires a translation from the auditory system of representation to the enactive system required for the movements of speech. There can, however, be a relative short-circuiting of the longer route of cognitive processing. That is, the incoming stimuli is registered as words, but the meanings of the words are not interpreted, appraised, and followed by problem solving thought and decisions, leading finally to translation of the relatively lexical ideas into the enactive forms required for speech.

In other words, the ordinary response to a question requires the juxtaposition and organization of multiple cognitive processes, and disruption anywhere along the line would prevent appropriate responses. The echo is a simple act in comparison, even though it is also a composite of multiple cognitive operations. One hypothesis states that autistic children have not developed the capacity for the higher order cognitive functions and so use adaptively more primitive routes. An alternative hypothesis, not necessarily contradictory to the first hypothesis, is that the autistic child has not learned to inhibit a primitive function or "short-circuit," and tends to use it more under situations of stress.

The findings of the study support the first hypothesis, but they do not contradict the second hypothesis. If the echo was an uninhibited primitive function, we would also expect a shorter reaction time to precede it. We would also not be surprised that the echoes were longer utterances than the nonechoes, provided that, as we suppose, the utterance of the experimenter tends to be several words long. That is, the experimenter probably does not say "yes" and "no," words likely to be used by the child in nonechoic responses. The second hypothesis would also lead to expectations of the increase in echoic responses under stress. And we would expect a clustering of the echoic responses because of the set of regulatory controls over the primitive cognitive functions. That is, if they were set at a level of either facilitation or relative disinhibition, they would tend to occur again and again. The results, in short, do not distinguish between these hypotheses. They may indeed be complimentary

because of the integrative functions of the mind, even in states of
psychopathology.

Experimental results, as is true throughout this area of research, do not lead to a definitive rejection of alternative hypotheses. Rather, it is characteristic of this area of investigation,
that hypotheses are additive and complimentary, and it is simply a
matter of which ones are hierarchically more important in explaining a given phenomenon. Unlike chemistry and physics, we will seldom
reject hypotheses as never being operative. Developing this type of
model, however, does lead us to the generation of further experiments
that might gradually lead to a clarification. Because of the nature
of our subject matter, our models must always have multiple variables,
and our experiments must gradually increase the number of variables in
volved.

For example, if one is studying the concept of social closure,
there must be studies not only relating the context to the verbal
responses, but relating other means of conservation of intimacy for
providing interpersonal distance. These would include videotapes
with measures of length of time in eye-to-eye gaze or face-to-face
contact, as well as the manipulation of interpersonal distances.
How would addition of such measures effect the alternative hypotheses suggested above? If only hypothesis two was correct, that is,
if the echoic responses were due basically to the nonacquisition of
inhibition of primitive imitative processes, and if the active adaptive use to accomplish social closure was not added to such an effect, then one would not expect a conservation of intimacy effect. If
there is a conservation of intimacy effect, one would expect not only
the findings about echoes, but also meaningful changes in gaze, facial
or body turning, and manipulation of interpersonal distances to accomplish social closure. That is, when the child needed to accomplish
social closure, he would tend to both echo and to nod, look meaningfully at or touch the investigator.

I would like to repeat that I make these remarks to indicate the
necessity of recognizing that theoretical development in this area
will always require consideration of multiple variables, and will
mean that experiments cannot be single definitive designs. One will
either have to do many brief experiments with limited variables, or
very complex experiments with multiple variables. I believe one of
the strengths of this research group is their recognition of this
feature, and the added value of their many relatively simple experiments.

I now turn to Dr. Steingart's presentation. Let me review for
you briefly the highlight for me of what he said. He talked about
linguistic characteristics, and I will talk only about those found
significant across a series of studies; the differences between conditional language and narrative language. The simple, more primitive

less challenging narrative language was significantly more common
in one patient when she was in depressive states than when she was
in paranoid states. It was significantly more common in those isolated and more depressive chronic schizophrenic patients than in the
belligerent quasi-paranoid patients, and it occurred in normal women
significantly more frequently in a monologue condition than in a
dialogue condition.

It was suggested that one explanation of this at the theoretical
level is the degree of coherence of the person's current inner schemata of his self and object representations. I find it useful to
separate self-coherence concepts as a parallel line of development
to dyadic structure development of a self and object representational
network, as suggested by Kohut (1971). In the belligerent and paranoid states, and in the dialogue situation, you expect that the subject is concerned with the relationship between self and other. In
the depressed monologue and isolated states, the person is concerned
with himself and less concerned with the relationship between the self
and the other. In the self-concerned state the person will tend to
process more in the way of unfinished memories and fantasies, as suggested by Singer (1966), and when described, these will tend to have
a narrative or story-line quality. In the belligerent, paranoid
state or in the act of just talking to another person, you expect
more statements that are complicated boundary remarks about interpersonal contingencies, such as "If you don't say something, I'm
going to stop talking to you" and "they're really out to get me because they know I have the secrets of the atomic bomb" and so forth.

Now, what is Dr. Steingart up to in this series of studies? He
is not using speech to study psychosis as psychopathology. And he
is not really using psychosis to study speech. He uses both the
psychotic state and speech recordings to study and make inferences
about cognitive structure and process. As pointed out above, he
uses multiple variables across a matrix from words to observed patterns of social behavior to study inner structure of self and object
schemata and self schemata. As such, self and self-object schematizations are often coded or represented in the form of imagery representation. It would be useful to extend his experiments into the
visual sphere. The same subjects could emit pictorial information as
well as lexical information. That is difficult because most people
refuse to draw. But they could be put in guided imagery circumstances
where they describe verbally a flow of visual imagery.

These imagery products could then be scored to see if in the
depressed isolated monologue condition, people are more likely to
report imagery primarily of the self, and in the other conditions,
primarily of the self and object in dyadic relationship. Or it can
be done the other way. They can use a TAT type of projective test
with some pictures showing a single person situation (such as in por-
traits) and in others, a dyadic situation. They would keep the

affective expression constant across configurations. Would descriptions of these variable schematic stimuli lead to differences in the language structure? One could also videotape these subjects for their body touching and object focused touching as they describe their responses. One would, in this way, get all three modes of expression and representation into one experimental paradigm, a complex multi-variable paradigm as suggested by theory.

To turn to Dr. Grand's presentation, he compared the eight isolated, quasi-depressed patients, and eight belligerent, quasi-paranoid patients and found significantly more continuous body touching and significantly more discrete body touching in the isolated patients. I want to go back and compare that with the earlier study of body touching, where there was more object focused body touching in the less disturbed situation.

One hypothesis about body touching is that the sensation and act stabilizes inner self-schematic boundaries. However, it can also symbolically be a self and object schematization. For example, the finger to hand approximations can symbolically have the finger as the self and the hand as the object or vice versa. Again, this is an alternative view that need not be contradictory. But there is an alternative hypothesis which Dr. Grand mentioned, which is that body touching is an overflow reaction to stress. Now there's some support for that alternative hypothesis, as in animal ecology observations where grooming responses occur when action plans are stymied (as when mating behavior or fighting behavior is stimulated in complex ways, where the animal doesn't know what to do and, rather than do nothing, may begin to groom itself even though it's inappropriate). Dr. Grand rejected this hypothesis because in these subjects there was no fragmentation of language. That does not necessarily disprove the alternative hypothesis, because an overflow behavior that reduces tension could also lead to a reduction of stress and, therefore, no fragmentation of language.

As before, he could add other modalities for additional information. He could also add the visual modalities and then see how the language behavior, the social behavior, and the visual output goes. I think he would thus find additional support for his hypothesis.

REFERENCES

Chomsky, N. Aspects of the theory of syntax. Cambridge: M.I.T. Press, 1966.

Horowitz, M. J. Stress response syndromes. New York: Aronson, 1976

Horowitz, M. J. Image formation and cognition. New York: Appleton-
Century-Crofts, 1970.

Kohut, H. The analysis of the self. New York: International Universities Press, 1971.

Rapaport, D. Cognitive Structures. In J. Bruner (Ed.), Contemporary approaches to cognition. Cambridge: Harvard University
Press, 1957.

Singer, J. Daydreaming. New York: Random House, 1966.

SECTION 4
THE ROLE OF UNCONSCIOUS
AND DRIVE PROCESSES
AS DETERMINANTS OF
COMMUNICATIVE STRUCTURES

INTRODUCTION

In the history of psychoanalytic thought, probably the most powerful concept developed by Freud is that of a dynamic unconscious. This refers to a system of symbolic representation operating outside of awareness, repressed yet actively exerting its influence on ongoing transactions. The dynamic unconscious functions on the principle of psychic determinism, which refers to the impact on behavior of an idea, image, or memory trace, likely rooted in infancy. Considering the importance of these conceptions to psychoanalytic thinking, a description of manifest communication which does not evaluate the impact of the dynamic unconscious would be incomplete. The papers in this section address this powerful regulator of the communicative process.

The objective studies of unconscious processes presented in this section rely not on naturalistic or developmental observations, as we have encountered thus far in this volume, but on laboratory experimentation. Bringing "the unconscious" into the laboratory confronts the investigator with a fundamental methodological issue: how to record the registration of a stimulus far below the threshold of awareness, and then to trace its impact on conscious intentional communication. The two papers in this section reflect the current state of the art in addressing this issue.

Studies of subliminal inputs to the psychic apparatus have intrigued analytic investigators for almost as long as the notion of psychic apparatus has intrigued psychoanalysts. Indeed, Poetzl's studies of brief stimulus input were singled out by Freud in his dream book as holding great promise for the study of unconscious processes. The model for such studies was already suggested by Freud in Section C of Chapter VII of the dream book, where he took up the issue of the psychical instigators of dreams left over from daytime activity. There, Freud suggested that the unconscious appears to effect a transference onto recent preconscious ideas that are either indifferent and have no attention paid to them, or which have been rejected and have had attention quickly withdrawn from them. Poetzl's work indicated that portions of pictures, shown to subjects who were asked to draw them, were apparently not consciously attended to

235

during the initial tachistoscopic exposure, but found their way into
the dreams of the night, and appeared in disguised form. Consciously
attended portions of the pictures were not found in the dreams.

In the years since Poetzl's pioneering work, investigators have
introduced greater methodological sophistication and control into
their studies of subliminal inputs. Shevrin's work is a good example
of this. Shevrin documents the psychophysiological presence of processes operating beneath the level of awareness, activated by stimuli
presented at speeds too fast to be discriminated consciously. His
method is novel in that he shows the impact of subliminal stimulation
on brain function by means of the average evoked potential. The correlation between such neurophysiological registration and verbal response goes a long way toward demonstrating the mind-brain link.
Shevrin then proceeds to argue for the continuity of psychological
phenomena ranging across the spectrum of consciousness, and trans-
lates the model of his own research to a model of communication in
psychoanalysis.

Shevrin's work is basic in that it documents unconscious registration and its relation to verbal response. Silverman goes one step
further. He seeks to identify the conflictual nature of unconscious
meanings, and traces their impact on "pathological communication."
Like Shevrin, Silverman works with a method of tachistoscopic subliminal stimulation. However, he uses a range of psychodynamically relevant stimulus material so that he is able to observe and predict the
consequences flowing from the content of the message. The stimulus
content manipulated in the studies is invariably rooted in earliest
phases of the individual's biography. Thus, Silverman is in a position to evaluate the importance of the regulation of early biograph-
ical representation on symptom formation. Hence, his work constitutes
a test of those notions concerning the unconscious which contain
images of infancy, but which, in turn, exert their influence on the
pathological communication during adulthood.

There are many methodological issues raised by these papers, and
Knapp covers most of them. Two outstanding issues should be stressed
One is the gap remaining in our understanding of the mind-brain relationship in terms of temporal sequencing. How is it possible for a
stimulus, presented in lexical form at 1/100 of a second, to be translated from verbal to imagistic form, and retranslated into verbal
response, all within fractions of seconds? Another issue is clinical. Granted the demonstration of subliminal activation, how powerful an influence is it, not in the laboratory, but in the production
of actual pathology? A full understanding of such issues requires the
integration of laboratory work, and the communicative regulations presented earlier in this book. Section 5, which examines communication
in the psychoanalytic situation, is an effort in the direction of such
an integration.

EXPERIMENTAL DATA ON THE EFFECTS OF UNCONSCIOUS FANTASY ON COMMUNI-

CATIVE BEHAVIOR

Lloyd H. Silverman

New York University

New York, New York 10003

I

In this paper I will present data from an experimental research program of 12 years standing that bear on the influence of unconscious fantasy on communicative behavior. The program was intended to serve two functions. First, it was to provide demonstrations, within the context of tightly controlled laboratory experimentation, of the validity of a key aspect of psychoanalytic theory: that unconscious fantasies can play a powerful role in motivating people. In this function, it challenges those within the fields of psychology and psychiatry who have disputed or ignored this and related psychoanalytic postulates. Second, in addressing the "psychoanalytic community," it attempts to demonstrate that data derived through laboratory experiments can play an important role in the development of psychoanalytic theory. As I have detailed elsewhere (Silverman, 1975a), this development cannot rely solely on evidence from the psychoanalytic treatment situation, but requires many other kinds of data as well; and for the optimal development of the psychodynamic aspects of psychoanalytic theory, data from laboratory experimentation is the most crucial. Here, the two approaches, clinical and experimental can be viewed as complementary in that each has inherent limitations that need be offset by the strengths of the other.[1]

---

[1] In the development of the genetic aspects of the clinical theory, in parallel to the above, observational studies of children and parent-child interactions can be viewed as the complement to the data that emerge in the psychoanalytic situation.

With regard to the laboratory-experimental approach, its principal limitations are its artificiality and its tendency to produce data
of such small magnitude, and lasting for such a limited time, that
they seem irrelevant to real life. But within the context of clinical data that point in the same direction, one can feel considerably
more comfortable accepting the relevance of such laboratory data and
viewing them as emanating from a true analogue of a real-life event.
Conversely, the main limitations of the clinical situation for theory
development in the psychodynamic realm relate to what can be termed
problems in exercising investigatory controls. I am referring here
to the impossibility of holding constant all variables but the particular one the clinician wants to zero in on, and the infeasibility of
utilizing "control interventions." The principal handicap this imposes is in terms of it frequently preventing a reasonably certain
judgment as to whether one aspect of a psychodynamic sequence has
caused another—whether it is a result of the second—or whether both
are the result of some third aspect. Experimental interventions, on
the other hand, do allow for choosing among particular cause-effect
sequences (cf. Silverman, 1975a).

II

The concept of the unconscious fantasy, since the early writings
of Freud, has appeared numerous times in the psychoanalytic literature. However, it has only been within the past two decades that it
has been given detailed and systematic treatment, with major papers
devoted to the subject by Beres (1962), Sandler and Nagera (1963), and
Arlow (1969). In the current paper, I will define "unconscious fantasy" as an organized and structured configuration of unconscious
thoughts and images, motivated (to varying degrees) by libidinal and
aggressive wishes, anxieties, defensive operations, and adaptive
strivings. When a behavior suddenly emerges, intensifies, diminishes
or disappears that is not explicable as a reaction to some conscious
perception, memory, anticipation, or other cognition, the activation
of some unconscious fantasy (or some element thereof) can be seen as
causative. While any kind of behavior can be influenced by such a
fantasy, it is for those behaviors we term "psychopathological" that
its influence is most in evidence. There have been many citations
in the psychoanalytic clinical literature implicating unconscious
fantasies in psychopathology. Most typically, reference has been made
to fantasies that generate symptoms—e.g., the womb fantasy that Lewin
(1935) has described as expressed in claustrophobia. But it also is
to be noted, though this less often has been made explicit, that the
activation of an unconscious fantasy can lead to the dissipation of
a symptom and thus serve an adaptive function. Consider, for example
a woman whose pathology centers around her wish for a phallus. The
birth of a child may well stimulate an unconscious fantasy that this
wish has been fulfilled, thus leading to an abatement or reduction in
symptomatology. This paper will address itself to both the adapta-
tion-interfering and adaptation-enhancing effects of unconscious fantasy on communicative behavior.

III

In the early 1960's, a method termed "subliminal psychodynamic
activation" was developed which allowed for the experimental study of
the effects of unconscious fantasy on psychopathology. Utilizing, as
a starting point, the demonstrations of subliminal registration in
Fisher's pioneering studies and those later investigations stimulated
by Fisher's work (summarized in Pine, 1964), this new type of investigation attempted to utilize the phenomenon of subliminal registration
for stimulating unconscious fantasies so that a systematic, precise,
and controlled appraisal could be made of their influence on behavior.
Over 20 published reports have now appeared in the psychological and
psychiatric literature (summarized in Silverman, 1971, 1975b) documenting the success of this method in achieving its aim, and several
discussions of the implications of these findings for psychoanalytic
theory have been presented (Silverman, 1967, 1970, 1972, 1975a,
1976).

The following is a description of the experimental design that
has been utilized in these studies. Subjects are seen individually
for an experimental session on one day and a control session on
another with their order counterbalanced. The first session begins
with the experimenter briefly explaining to the subject the purpose
of the study in which he is being asked to participate, and his co-
operation is sought. Then the tasks that will be administered so
that the subject's psychopathology can be assessed are described, and
the subject is told that several times during these tasks he will be
asked to view flickers of light through an eyepiece of a machine (a
tachistoscope). He further is told that at the end of the experiment
he will be fully informed about these flickers and the purpose that
they serve. Then the session proper begins with a "baseline" measure
obtained of the subject's propensity for whatever pathological manifestations are being studied. This is followed by the subject being
asked to look into the tachistoscope and to describe the flickers of
light that appear. There follow four exposures of either a stimulus
with content related to an unconscious fantasy (the experimental
session), or a stimulus with (relatively) neutral content (the control session). Each exposure is for a four millisecond duration.
There is then a reassessment of the pathology for a determination
of how the subject has been affected by the particular stimulus that
had been subliminally exposed.

The procedure for the other session is identical to that described except that a different stimulus is exposed between the baseline and the reassessment task series. Subjects who are exposed to
a stimulus with content related to an unconscious fantasy in the first
session are shown the neutral stimulus in the later session and vice
versa. In each session, the experimenter who works the tachistoscope
and administers the assessment procedures is "blind" to which one of
the stimuli is being exposed. Since the subject also is unaware of

the stimulus (it being subliminal), the procedure can be described
as "double blind" in the same sense as in drug studies where neither
the patient nor the person administering the capsule knows whether a
drug or a placebo is being ingested. The evaluation of pathological
manifestations is carried out blindly also.

IV

The results of two types of studies which demonstrate the effect
of unconscious fantasy on communicative behavior will now be cited.
The first type involved investigations in which stimuli were chosen
for stirring up a libidinal or aggressive wish element of a fantasy
which clinical evidence has suggested is psychodynamically relevant
for individuals with a particular symptom. The prediction in these
studies was that this stimulation (compared with subliminal neutral
stimulation) would lead to symptom exacerbation; and in studies
on almost thirty groups of subjects, this prediction has been borne
out. The findings from two kinds of subjects, schizophrenics and
stutterers, are relevant to the current topic--the effects of unconscious fantasy on communicative behavior.

Turning first to the studies of the schizophrenics, our interest has been in investigating the unconscious fantasy element that
is psychodynamically relevant to the gross disturbances in communicative behavior that schizophrenics can manifest. These disturbances
come under two headings. One refers to the schizophrenic's actual
verbalizations, i.e., the degree to which his verbal responses (on
such tests as the Rorschach and Word Association) are characterized
by condensations in thinking, illogic, peculiar ideas, and other
characteristics that betray what generally is referred to as the
"thought disorder" of the schizophrenic. The second type of disturbance involves pathological nonverbal behavior reflecting what Freedman and his colleagues (e.g.1975) have referred to as "body-focused"
(rather than "object-focused") motoric expressions. Included here
are a wide variety of behaviors ranging from inappropriate laughter
and bizarre body movements at one extreme, to such mild anxiety manifestations as drumming one's fingers on the table at the other.

The experimental design described above has been utilized in
15 studies of schizophrenics (total N > 500), eleven of which have
been carried out in our laboratory (summarized in Silverman, 1971),
and four others done elsewhere as replications of our work (Buchholz,
1968; Lomangino, 1969; Litwack, 1972; Leiter, 1973). In each of
these studies, the subliminal presentation of oral-aggressive content has produced an intensification of one of both kinds of communicative disturbances described above that was not in evidence after

subliminal neutral stimulation.[2]

Are the communicative difficulties of schizophrenics specifically linked to oral-aggressive fantasies, or are other kinds of wish-
related fantasies, aggressive and libidinal, also implicated? Here,
two kinds of data are relevant. One line of evidence emerged from a
study by Lomangino (1969) which was carried out both as an independent
replication of our findings and to determine if the aggressive fantasy
implicated in schizophrenic pathology has, specifically, an "oral
component." The schizophrenic sample in this study was divided into
four subgroups, each of which was exposed to a different aggressive
stimulus. For one subgroup, the stimulus consisted of the verbal
message CANNIBAL EATS PERSON; for another, a picture showing such a
scene; for a third, the verbal message MURDERER STABS VICTIM; and
for a fourth, a pictorial depiction of this. When the effects of
these stimuli were compared with the effects of neutral subliminal
stimulation, Lomangino found that only for the first two subgroups
did the aggressive condition intensify disturbance. These results,
thus, point to the specific importance of the oral component in the
aggressive fantasy as a pathogenic element in the schizophrenic's
communicative disturbances.

The second type of relevant data emerged from four studies in
which the effects of stimuli designed to stir up oral-aggressive
fantasies were compared not only with neutral stimulation but with
the stimulation of libidinal fantasies as well (Silverman & Silverman, 1967; S. E. Silverman, 1969; Silverman et al. 1969; Silverman,

---

[2]In these various experiments, a large number of _different_ oral-
aggressive and neutral stimuli have been utilized ranging from pictures of animals (e.g., a lion roaring vs. a bird flying), to pictures
of humans (e.g., a snarling man holding a dagger vs. a man holding a
newspaper), to verbal messages (e.g. CANNIBAL EATS PERSON vs. PEOPLE
ARE WALKING). All told, nine different oral-aggressive stimuli have
been used and eleven different neutral stimuli, and in each pairing
it was the former that has produced more pathology exacerbation.

It also should be noted that in several of the studies of the
schizophrenics, and in a number of studies of other kinds of patients
as well, there also has been a third condition in which the same fantasy-related stimulus, which when presented subliminally intensified
symptomology, was also presented supraliminally. Typically under this
condition, the fantasy-related stimulus has _not_ affected symptomology.
For a discussion of why this is the case and why the subliminal presentation of fantasy-related stimuli is the method of choice for the
laboratory study of the aspects of psychoanalytic theory under discussion here, see Silverman (1972).

Bronstein & Mendelsohn, 1976). In these, various libidinal content
were introduced: oral-receptive, voyeuristic, homosexual, and incestu-
ous; yet, a consistent finding emerged. In all instances, the verbal
communicative disturbance of the subjects, while significantly affected by the (oral) aggressive condition, was not at all affected
by any of the libidinal conditions. Thus, for schizophrenic disturbances in verbal communication--disturbances which are generally viewed
as reflective of their underlying thought disorder--a specific link
to oral-aggressive fantasies can be said to have been demonstrated.
Other kinds of conflictual fantasies leave this kind of disturbance
unaffected, even though, clinically, they have been linked to other
kinds of symptoms.

The last point made above bearing on specificity has been
demonstrated experimentally in our laboratory in three of the studies
already cited. In one of these (Silverman, Bronstein & Mendelsohn,
1976), the incest stimulus, while leaving the verbal communicative
distrubances of schizophrenics unaffected, significantly intensified
the homoerotic orientation of nonpatient male homosexuals. And in
the other two investigations (Silverman & Silverman, 1967; S. E.
Silverman, 1969), the "other effects" of the libidinal stimuli were
found in schizophrenics themselves. That is, while only the oral-
aggressive stimuli affected disturbances in their verbal communication
libidinal stimuli (in these instances involving voyeuristic and homosexual content) intensified nonverbal communicative disturbances of
various kinds. In toto, these findings offer strong support for the
proposition that the communicative disturbances of schizophrenics
are linked to specific unconscious fantasies, a finding which challenges various assumptions within, as well as outside of, the psychoanalytic community (see Silverman, 1975a for detailed discussion).

V

Can the disruptive effects of unconscious fantasy on communicative behavior also be demonstrated for persons who are not schizophrenic? Studies of three groups of stutterers, all of whom were out-
patients in a speech rehabilitation clinic, provide an affirmative
answer to this question. For these individuals, almost all of whose
pathology would be classified within the neurotic range, a link was
found between the kind of disruption in communicative behavior to
which they are vulnerable (their stutter) and another type of unconscious fantasy. In their case, in keeping with what the psychoanalytic clinical literature has most often viewed as pathogenic in
stuttering, the activation of a fantasy with anal content proved capable of exacerbating their speech disturbance. In each of the three
groups (total N=84), utilizing the same experimental paradigm that
has been described, the subliminal exposure of anal content led to
intensified stuttering that was not in evidence after subliminal neutral stimulation (Silverman, Klinger et al,,1972; Silverman, Bronstein & Mendelsohn, 1976).

The specificity of relationship between symptoms and unconscious fantasy was studied for the stutterers just as it had been for the schizophrenics. With one of the stutterer groups (Silverman, Bronstein & Mendelsohn, 1976), a third condition was introduced in addition to the anality and control conditions. This involved the same incest stimulus referred to earlier as having intensified homoerotic orientation in homosexuals. While the anality condition again intensified stuttering, the incest condition had no such effect. However, the latter condition did exacerbate other symptoms in the stutterers, i.e., certain forms of pathological nonverbal behavior, and for these the anality condition had no effect. Thus, it can be maintained that for nonschizophrenics as well as schizophrenics there has been an experimental demonstration of the proposition that different kinds of communicative disturbances are pathogenically linked with different unconscious fantasies.

VI

Let me now turn to the studies that have demonstrated that the activation of unconscious fantasy also has the power to ameliorate symptoms and thus enhance communicative behavior. The fantasy which has proven capable of having this effect is one that we term a "symbiotic-gratification fantasy." The stimulus used to activate this fantasy consisted of the verbal message MOMMY AND I ARE ONE. The initiation of work in this area owed itself, in part, to the writings of a few psychoanalytic clinicians (e.g. Limentani, 1952; Searles, 1960) who have reported observing an abatement of symptoms in schizophrenics when they seemed to be experiencing a "symbiotic relationship" with their therapist. Assuming that such a relationship stimulates unconscious fantasies of symbiotic gratification with mother, we introduced the stimulus mentioned above with the expectation that its subliminal presentation would have an ameliorative effect on their symptomatology.

The procedure followed along the lines of our earlier work on symptom intensification. Schizophrenic subjects were seen for two sessions, experimental and control, in each of which "baseline" and "critical" assessments were made of the two kinds of communicative disturbances described earlier: pathological verbalizations and pathological nonverbal behavior. Between the baseline and critical assessments, they were given four subliminal exposures of a verbal stimulus, either MOMMY AND I ARE ONE, or a neutral-control stimulus such as PEOPLE ARE WALKING or MEN THINKING. To date, eight studies have been carried out with the above described design, four by us in our own laboratory (Silverman et al. 1969; Silverman & Candell, 1970; Silverman et al. 1971; Bronstein, 1976), and four by others (Leiter, 1972; Kaplan, 1976; Kaye, 1975; Spiro, 1975). In all eight investigations, which involved 10 groups of schizophrenic patients (total N of almost 200), there was an identical outcome. The subliminal exposure of the symbiotic-gratification message led to a

reduction in symptomatology that was not in evidence in the control
session.[3]

Three of the investigations that have been cited addressed the
issue of specificity. In each of these, the question was asked if
a fantasy that had certain elements in common with MOMMY AND I ARE
ONE, yet in other respects was different, also would have an ameliorative effect on the communicative disturbances of schizophrenics. One
of these investigations Bronstein, (1976) addressed the question of
the cruciality of the nature of the internalization involved in the
symbiotic fantasy. Utilizing the categorization and definitions of
internalization suggested by Schafer (1968), he compared the effects
on different schizophrenics of the messages MOMMY IS INSIDE ME
(viewed as involving an introjection), MOMMY AND I ARE THE SAME
(sameness identification), and MOMMY AND I ARE ALIKE (likeness identification), as well as MOMMY AND I ARE ONE (conceptualized as a oneness identification). He found that while the oneness stimulus produced the same reduction in pathological communication that it had
in the other studies, none of the other internalization messages had
this effect. That is, the effects of these other stimuli on the
schizophrenics' symptoms was no different than that of the neutral-
control condition. Thus, it was concluded that the unconscious fantasy which, when activated, has an ameliorative effect on schizophrenics' communication, and must specifically involve a oneness internalization.

----

[3]This finding has been limited to "differentiated schizophrenics" defined as those who show a certain (predesignated) degree of the ability to maintain an image of themselves that is distinct from their
image of their mothers, as assessed by a testing procedure described
elsewhere (Silverman et al., 1969). We have found that such patients
comprise between 50% and 80% of the populations of hospitalized schizo
phrenics. For schizophrenics who are assessed as "undifferentiated"
on this procedure, the symbiotic-gratification is not therapeutic.

It should also be mentioned that in one of the experiments in
which a symbiosis stimulus was used (Silverman & Candell, 1970), there
was a third condition in which it was presented to the subjects supraliminally. This led to no symptom-reduction, thus further supporting
the contention that the subliminal presentation of fantasy-related
stimuli is the method of choice for the laboratory study of the effects of unconscious fantasies on psychopathology.

Finally, let me note that in some of the studies cited above,
the verbal message comprising the symbiotic stimulus was accompanied
by a congruent picture of a male and female merged at the shoulders
like siamese twins. In the recent study of Kaplan (1976), it was
found that this mode of presentation led to even more symptom reduction than when the symbiotic stimulus consisted of the verbal message
alone.

In a second investigation (Kaye, 1975), the investigator's interest was in the cruciality of the representation of "mother" as an element in the fantasy. Thus, the experiment involved a comparison of the effects of the stimuli MOMMY AND I ARE ONE, DADDY AND I ARE ONE, and MY GIRL AND I ARE ONE, in each case comparing the oneness message with a control message. For the MOMMY stimulus, there was a reduction of symptomatology; for the DADDY stimulus there was no change; and for the MY GIRL stimulus, there was significant symptom reduction, and moreover, to a degree that was substantially greater than that produced by the MOMMY stimulus. These results were interpreted in the following way. The fantasy of oneness, in order to be symptom ameliorating for schizophrenics, cannot involve just any significant figure in the schizophrenic's life (the DADDY stimulus had no effect), but must involve a maternal representation (the MOMMY and MY GIRL stimuli did have an effect). The fact that the MY GIRL stimulus was more effective, was taken to mean that the representation MY GIRL refers to an unequivocally positive mother substitute with whom fantasized merging is more desirable than with one's actual mother. Or, to state this conversely as it has been suggested occasionally in the clinical literature (e.g., Burnham, 1969), symbiotic fantasies can have threatening as well as gratifying connotations for schizophrenics; and the mother-substitute representation MY GIRL can lessen these.[4]

Finally, Kaplan (1976) addressed herself to the question of what is satisfied in a oneness fantasy that allows it to have its ameliorative effects. In addition to including a MOMMY AND I ARE ONE and neutral-control condition, she added conditions that involved the following messages, each of which she conceived of as referring to a need satisfaction that is mentioned in the clinical literature

---

[4]Bronstein's (1976) study, while replicating the finding of pathology reduction in schizophrenics after the MOMMY AND I ARE ONE stimulus, did not replicate Kaye's finding for the MY GIRL AND I ARE ONE stimulus. This, Bronstein ascribed, to an (inadvertent) omission of an aspect of Kaye's procedures that served to activate in the subjects, before subliminal stimulation was introduced, thoughts about their wives and girlfriends. This external activation, referred to in the subliminal literature as "priming" is sometimes necessary for a particular thought content to be in a sufficient state of readiness so that it can be "contacted" by a relevant subliminal stimulus (cf. Silverman, 1972, pp. 322-323). Apparently, in schizophrenics, while oneness fantasies about MOMMY are generally in a state of sufficient activation so that a congruent stimulus can trigger them off without prior priming, oneness fantasies about MY GIRL are in a more latent state and thus do require priming. This issue deserves (and is receiving) further attention in our laboratory.

as motivationally important in schizophrenia, and which thus might be
crucial in explaining the pathology-reducing power of the symbiotic
fantasy: MOMMY IS ALWAYS WITH ME intended to stimulate a fantasy
providing protection against object loss; MOMMY FEEDS ME WELL, a
fantasy that should counter a sense of oral deprivation; and I CANNOT
HURT MOMMY, a fantasy intended to counter the threat of unacceptable
destructive impulses. What she found was that while the MOMMY AND I
ARE ONE stimulus, once again, led to a significant reduction in the
schizophrenic's communication difficulties, none of the other experimental stimuli had this effect; i.e., they all acted no differently
on disturbance than the control condition. Thus, whatever the reasons may be why a oneness fantasy has its ameliorative effects (and
these are discussed in detail elsewhere, cf. Silverman, 1976), it
is not because such a fantasy implies a simple satisfaction of one of
the needs addressed by the messages Kaplan introduced.

In toto, the three studies that have just been cited offer compelling evidence for the degree to which the effects of unconscious
fantasy on behavior is a highly specific one. The fantasy MOMMY AND
I ARE ONE has an ameliorative effect on the communication disturbances
of schizophrenics, but a host of other fantasies that are identical
with elements of the MOMMY AND I ARE ONE fantasy but different in
terms of other elements do not have the same effect. This, I believe,
demonstrates the necessity of conceptualizing psychopathology not only
in terms of unconscious wishes, anxieties, and defenses, but unconscious fantasies as well. Only this latter concept defined as "an
organized constellation of ideas and images" allows for the kind of
specificity that has been demonstrated in these experiments.

VII

Can the activation of unconscious symbiotic-gratification fantasies also enhance the adaptation of nonschizophrenics? The recent
writing of a few psychoanalytic clinicians (Eckstein, 1972; Giovacchini, 1972; Rose, 1972) suggest an affirmative answer to this questio
These writers have made reference to the adaptation-enhancing function
that can be served by symbiotic gratifications for many different kind
of individuals at various times in their lives and in a variety of li
situations. Rose has detailed this quite explicitly.

"Mastering something by 'fusing' with it, temporarily obscur-
ing the boundaries between the self and object representations re-
calls the primary narcissism of the infant and the psychotic. But
to merge in order to reemerge, may be part of the fundamental process
of psychological growth on all developmental levels. Although fusion
may dominate the most primitive levels, it contributes a richness of
texture and quality to the others. Such operations may result in
nothing more remarkable than normally creative adaptation to circumstance. At the least, it affords what (William) James called the

'return from the solitude of individuation' refreshed to meet the moment. At the most, it may result in transcending the limitations of
earlier stages of narcissism to simplify, unify anew, and recreate
an expanded reality" (p. 56).

Experimental support for this view had emerged from five experiments carried out in our laboratory (Martin, 1975; Silverman,
et al. 1973; Silverman, Frank & Dachinger, 1974; Silverman, Ungaro
& Mendelsohn, in preparation; Silverman & Wolitzky, in preparation).
In each of these, the subliminal stimulation of a oneness fantasy improved adaptation in nonschizophrenic individuals; and in two of
these studies, it was specifically communicative behavior that was
positively affected. In one study (Silverman & Wolitzky, in preparation), we investigated whether the subliminal stimulation of the same
MOMMY AND I ARE ONE fantasy that has been under discussion would diminish defensiveness of nonschizophrenic subjects when they were asked
to be verbally expressive. Following the experimental paradigm that
has been described, a group of 10 research volunteers (hospital em-
ployees and medical patients) were seen for an experimental and control session in which they were asked to "make up stories" to TAT
cards. The stories were scored for two variables: openness of expression, and acceptance of responsibility for the plight of the
characters. On one of the two variables, "accepting responsibility"
there was a significant reduction in defensiveness after the symbiotic condition.

The above result brings to mind Shaffi's (1973) discussion of
how gratification of the wish for symbiosis with mother can be experienced in the psychoanalytic situation through the person of the
analyst, and result in a strengthening of the working alliance.
Drawing heavily from considerations advanced by Nacht (1964), Shaffi
writes:

"If the analyst is aware of (the importance of symbiotic gratification)
and allows it to temporarily blossom, it will enhance and deepen the
therapeutic bond and will help the patient to explore further the
depth of his unconscious for further growth and liberation" (p. 441).

In the laboratory study just cited, a microcosm of the process
Shaffi describes can be said to have been demonstrated. After the
activation of the fantasy of symbiotic gratification, the subjects
changed in a way that would be characterized in the psychoanalytic
situation as reflecting an enhanced working alliance, i.e., they
showed an increased ability to accept rather than externalize responsibility.

The relationship between symbiotic-gratification fantasies and
adaptation-enhancing communication in the treatment situation was
more directly demonstrated in another study, a discussion of which
will close this presentation. This investigation was different from

all those already described in that more than "laboratory effects"
were sought. It is part of a recently developed phase of our research in which we are asking whether the symptom-ameliorating effects of stimulating symbiotic-gratification fantasies can be utilized
for therapeutic purposes. In this aspect of our work, there were
three studies carried out, prior to the investigation to be described,
which yielded an affirmative answer to this question. In each of
these studies, a group of subjects with a particular psychiatric
disability was seen: male schizophrenics in one investigation (Silverman et al. 1975), women with insect phobias in a second (Silverman, Frank & Dachinger, 1974), and overweight women in a third (Martin
1975). In each investigation, all subjects received, over several
weeks, a therapeutic intervention designed to help them cope better
with their particular disability. For the schizophrenics, the intervention consisted of a specially designed procedure to help strengthen
reality testing; for the insect phobics, a variant of systematic desen
sitization; and for the overweight women, behavior modification treatment for overeating. In addition, embedded in the interventions for
each group, there was subliminal stimulation. During the sessions,
at specified times, the subjects were asked to look into a tachistoscope and were told that they would be shown flickers of light which
might help them to relax. For half of the subjects in each of the
groups, the subliminal stimulus was MOMMY AND I ARE ONE, while the
other half received a control message such as PEOPLE ARE WALKING.
In each of the three investigations, there was significantly more
symptom amelioration for subjects who had received the sumbiotic subliminal stimulation.

     With this as background, let me now describe the study that
bears on the effect of symbiotic-gratifications on adaptation-enhancing communication in the treatment situation. This investigation
(Silverman et al., in preparation) also involved overwieght women and
was intended as a follow-up to the study of Martin already described.
Our interest was, in part, to determine if we could replicate her fin
ing (that subliminal symbiotic stimulation can act as an aid in weigh
control), and, in part, to break new ground in a number of respects,
including the introduction of a new symbiotic stimulus for one subgroup of subjects. This contained the name of the therapist in the
place of MOMMY (e.g., ROSEANN AND I ARE ONE). Our rationale here was
the following. It is our hypothesis that an important if not crucial
therapeutic agent in nonanalytic forms of therapy is the inadvertent
activation of symbiotic-gratification fantasies (c.f. Silverman, 1976
While at their root, these fantasies are assumed to involve symbiosis
with mother, more immediately they involve a fantasy of symbiosis wit
the therapist. Thus, we were interested in comparing the results obtained with the "oneness with mother" stimulus and a "oneness with
the therapist" stimulus.

     The subjects were divided into three groups, matched for rele-
vant independent variables, with four therapists seeing equal numbers

of subjects in each of the groups. For one of the groups, the stimulus MOMMY AND I ARE ONE accompanied the weight control program; for
a second, ROSEANN AND I ARE ONE (or ERIC AND I ARE ONE, etc.); and
for a third, the control group, PEOPLE ARE WALKING. As far as the
replication part of the experiment was concerned, the behavior modification program, again, was enhanced by the MOMMY AND I ARE ONE
condition. However, here, my interest is not in the effect of symbiotic stimulation on weight loss, but on communication in the treatment situation. While we originally had not planned to investigate
this variable, something unexpected happened that indicated that the
symbiotic stimulation had an effect on this behavior as well as on
degree of overeating. At the study's completion, three out of four
therapists spontaneously commented that although they had carried
out the procedures blindly, they thought they knew which subject
group was receiving the oneness-with-therapist condition, and in
each instance the therapist's postdiction was correct. In giving
the basis for their judgments, each of the therapists referred to
something special about the way a number of the subjects in this group
communicated during the sessions. They described behavior characterized by: (a) unusual freedom of expression (in the words of one
of the therapists "as if they were in psychotherapy rather than in
behavior therapy"); (b) intense involvement with the therapist; and,
(c) indications of having internalized characteristics of the therapist. Since this special kind of communicative behavior distinguished
the subjects in the oneness-with-therapist condition not only from
the control subjects, but also from those receiving the MOMMY AND I
ARE ONE stimulus, further support is available for a hypothesis that
has been addressed throughout this paper: communicative behavior is
reactive in a very differentially sensitive manner to rather finely
distinguishable unconscious fantasies.[5]

SUMMARY AND CONCLUSIONS

     In this paper, a series of laboratory studies have been described
bearing on the role of unconscious fantasy on communicative behavior.

---

[5]The support for the conclusion that the subjects who received the
oneness-with-therapist stimulus were different in their relationships
with their therapists than the subjects in the other two groups is
admittedly "soft" and in need of systematically collected and controlled data. Such data are actually available for one of the behavioral qualities mentioned above: "indications of having internalized
characteristics of the therapist." Both at the beginning and at the
end of the (12 week) treatment period, measures were obtained of the
degree to which the subject maintained an image of herself that was
distinct from her therapist, assessed by the same testing procedure
referred to in Footnote 3. The subjects in the oneness-with-therapist
condition, in comparison with the subjects in both of the other groups
showed, from pre-to-post-testing, significantly greater similarity between their perceptions of themselves and their perceptions of their
therapists.

The data that have emerged from these investigations allow for conclusions to be drawn that are related to our dual aims: (1)   to
provide appropriate experimental tests of various clinically based
psychoanalytic propositions; (2)   to provide laboratory data that
can further the development of the psychodynamic aspects of psychoanalytic theory.

With regard to the first aim, it can be concluded that abundant
experimental support now exists for both general and specific psychoanalytic propositions implicating unconscious fantasies in behavior,
particularly pathological behavior.   Here, it should be noted, that
the method that has yielded these data--"subliminal psychodynamic
activation"--allows for the most stringent controls against extraneous variables influencing results.   It is, as far as I know, the only
experimental method that has been utilized to test aspects of psychoanalytic theory that is carried out in "double-blind" fashion, therefore allowing for the ruling out of demand characteristics and experimental bias as contaminating variables.   Thus, the findings that
have been reported pose a substantive challenge to those within the
fields of psychology and psychiatry who have ignored or disputed the
proposition that psychopathology is motivated by the kinds of "id-
related" unconscious fantasies that always have been at the heart of
psychoanalytic theory.   This conclusion seems particularly warranted
in light of the fact that in our studies of symptom exacerbation, we
have been able to demonstrate not only that symptoms intensify when
these kinds of unconscious fantasies are activated, but that there
are specific relationships between particular symptoms and particular
unconscious fantasies.

Concerning the contribution of our laboratory method to the
further development of psychoanalytic theory, the following conclusions seem warranted.   First, the replicated and clear-cut results
bearing on the motivational role of both oral-aggressive and symbiotic fantasies in schizophrenia are consonant with the views of some
psychoanalytic clinicians, but discordant with the views of others
(cf. Silverman, 1975a); thus they can be viewed as contributing toward the resolution of an issue that clinical data have left ambiguous.   Second, the finding that the stimulation of unconscious symbiotic fantasies can lead to more adaptive behavior in nonschizophrenics
as well as schizophrenics provides experimental support for a postulate that only recently has been proposed in the clinical literature
(cf. Silverman, 1976); thus, it could contribute toward bringing this
view more into the mainstream of psychoanalytic thinking.   Finally,
the results bearing on the high degree of specificity that characterizes fantasies related to symptom amelioration have not been inferrable, as far as I know, from clinical data; thus they allow for refinements of psychoanalytic theory.   I am referring here to such findings as: schizophrenics show symptom amelioration when there is activated a fantasy involving "oneness" with mother but not "likeness"
or "sameness" with mother; and nonschizophrenics relate differently

in a treatment situation when there is an activation of a fantasy of oneness-with-therapist than when the fantasy of oneness-with-mother is activated.

One final point. My enthusiastic advocacy of experimental methods in general, and the subliminal psychodynamic activation method in particular, for further developing psychoanalytic theory makes necessary a restatement of the following caution and qualifier. All experimental methods, including our own, have built-in limitations and thus should not be utilized in isolation for theory development. Rather, they should be viewed as providing data that are complementary and supplementary to that obtained both in the clinical situation and through the use of nonexperimental research paradigms. It is only when utilized in conjunction with other investigatory approaches that the experimental approach can optimally serve its unique functions.

REFERENCES

Arlow, J. Unconscious fantasy and disturbances of conscious experience. The Psychoanalytic Quarterly, 1969, 38, 1-27.

Beres, D. The unconscious fantasy. The Psychoanalytic Quarterly, 1962, 31, 309-328.

Bronstein, A. An experimental study of internalization processes in schizophrenic men. Unpublished doctoral dissertation, Yeshiva University, 1976.

Buchholz, E. S. A study in the management of aggression by schizophrenics and normals. Unpublished doctoral dissertation, New York University, 1968.

Burnham, D. L., Gladstone, A. I. & Gibson, R. W. Schizophrenia and the need-fear dilemma. New York: International Universities Press, 1969.

Eckstein, R. On telling secrets. In P. L. Giovacchini (Ed.), Tactics and techniques in psychoanalytic therapy. New York: Science House, 1972.

Freedman, N. & Steingart, I. Kinesic internalization and language construction. Psychoanalysis & Contemporary Science, Vol. 4. New York: Macmillan, 1975.

Giovacchini, P. L. On symbiosis. In P. S. Giovacchini (Ed.), Tactics and techniques in psychoanalytic therapy. New York: Science House, 1972.

Kaplan, R. The symbiotic fantasy as a therapeutic agent: An experimental comparison of the effects of three symbiotic elements on manifest pathology in schizophrenics. Unpublished doctoral dissertation, New York University, 1976.

Kaye, M. The therapeutic value of three merging stimuli for male schizophrenics. Unpublished doctoral dissertation, Yeshiva University, 1975.

Leiter, E. A study of the effects of subliminal activation of merging fantasies in differentiated and nondifferentiated schizophrenics. Unpublished doctoral dissertation, New York University, 1973.

Lewin, B. D. Claustrophobia. The Psychoanalytic Quarterly, 1935, 4, 227-233.

Limentani, D. Symbiotic identification in schizophrenia. Psychiatry, 1956, 19, 231-236.

Litwack, T. A study of certain issues concerning the dynamics of thinking and behavioral pathology in schizophrenics through the use of subliminal stimulation. Unpublished doctoral dissertation, New York University, 1972.

Lomangino, L. The depiction of subliminally and supraliminally presented aggressive stimuli and its effect on the cognitive functioning of schizophrenics. Unpublished doctoral dissertation, Fordham University, 1969.

Martin, A. The effect of subliminal stimulation of symbiotic fantasies on weight loss in obese women receiving behavioral treatment. Unpublished doctoral dissertation, New York University, 1975.

Nacht, S. Silence as an integrative factor. International Journal of Psychoanalysis, 1964, 45, 299-300.

Pine, F. The bearing of psychoanalytic theory on selected issues in research on marginal stimuli. Journal of Nervous and Mental Disease, 1964, 138, 205-222.

Rose, G. Fusion states. In P. L. Giovacchini (Ed.), Tactics and techniques in psychoanalytic therapy. New York: Science House, 1972.

Sandler, J. & Nagera, H. Aspects of the metapsychology of fantasy. Psychoanalytic Study of the Child, 1963, 18, 159-194.

Schafer, R. Aspects of internalization. New York: International Universities Press, 1968.

Searles, H. F. Integration and differentiation in schizophrenia. Journal of Nervous and Mental Disease, 1959, 129, 542-550.

Shaffi, M. Silence in the service of the ego: Psychoanalytic study of meditation. International Journal of Psychoanalysis, 1973, 54, 431-443.

Silverman, L. H. An experimental approach to the study of dynamic propositions in psychoanalysis: The relationship between the aggressive drive and ego regression - initial studies. Journal of the American Psychoanalytic Association, 1967, 15, 376-403.

Silverman, L. H. Further experimental studies on dynamic propositions in psychoanalysis: On the function and meaning of regressive thinking. Journal of the American Psychoanalytic Association 1970, 18, 102-124.

Silverman, L. H. An experimental technique for the study of unconscious conflict. British Journal of Medical Psychology, 1971, 44, 17-25.

Silverman, L. H. Drive stimulation and psychopathology: On the conditions under which drive-related external events evoke pathological reactions. In R. R. Holt & E. Peterfreund (Eds.), Psychoanalysis and Contemporary Science, Vol. 1. New York: Macmillan, 1972.

Silverman, L. H. An experimental method for the study of unconscious conflict: A progress report. British Journal of Medical Psychology, 1975a, 48, 291-298.

Silverman, L. H. On the role of laboratory experiments in the development of the clinical theory of psychoanalysis: Data on the subliminal activation of aggressive and merging wishes in schizophrenics. International Review of Psychoanalysis, 1975b, 2, 43-64.

Silverman, L. H. The unconscious symbiotic fantasy as a ubiquitous therapeutic agent. Paper presented at the annual meeting of the American Psychoanalytic Assoc., Baltimore, Maryland, May 8, 1976.

Silverman, L. H., Bronstein, A., & Mendelsohn, E. The further use of the subliminal psychodynamic activation method for the experimental study of the clinical theory of psychoanalysis: On the specificity of relationships between manifest psychopathology and unconscious conflict. Psychotherapy: Theory, Research and Practice, 1976, 13, 2-16.

Silverman, L. H. & Candell, P. On the relationship between aggressive activation, symbiotic merging, intactness of body boundaries and manifest pathology in schizophrenics. Journal of Nervous and Mental Disease, 1970, 150, 387-399.

Silverman, L. H., Candell, P., Pettit, T. F., & Blum, F. A. Further data on effects of aggressive activation and symbiotic merging on ego functioning of schizophrenics. Perceptual and Motor Skills, 1971, 32, 93-94.

Silverman, L. H., Franks, S., & Dachinger, P. A psychoanalytic re-interpretation of the effectiveness of systematic desensitization: Experimental data bearing on the role of merging fantasies. Journal of Abnormal Psychology, 1974, 83, 313-318.

Silverman, L. H., Klinger, H., Lustbader, L., Farrell, J., & Martin, A.D. The effect of subliminal drive stimulation on the speech of stutterers. Journal of Nervous and Mental Disease, 1972, 155, 14-21.

Silverman, L. H., Kwawer, J. S., Wolitzky, C., & Coron, M. An experimental study of aspects of the psychoanalytic theory of male homosexuality. Journal of Abnormal Psychology, 1973, 82, 178-188.

Silverman, L. H., Levinson, P., Mendelsohn, E., Ungaro, R., & Bronstein, A. A clinical application of subliminal psychodynamic activation: On the stimulation of symbiotic fantasies as an adjunct in the treatment of hospitalized schizophrenics. Journal of Nervous and Mental Disease, 1975, 161, 379-392.

Silverman, L. H. & Silverman, S. E. The effects of subliminally presented drive stimuli on the cognitive functioning of schizophrenics. Journal of Projective Techniques, 1967, 31, 78-85.

Silverman, L. H., Spiro, R. H., Weisberg, J. S., & Candell, P. The effects of aggressive activation and the need to merge on pathological thinking in schizophrenia. Journal of Nervous and Mental Disease, 1969, 148, 39-51.

Silverman, L. H. & Wolitzky, C. The effects of the subliminal stimulation of symbiotic fantasies on the defensiveness of "normal" subjects in telling TAT stories. In preparation.

Silverman, L. H., Ungaro, R., & Mendelsohn, E. A further study of the effects of subliminal stimulation on weight loss. In preparation.

Spiro, T. The effects of laboratory stimulation of symbiotic fantasies and bodily self-awareness on relatively differentiated and nondifferentiated schizophrenics. Unpublished doctoral dissertation, New York Univesity, 1975.

SOME ASSUMPTIONS OF PSYCHOANALYTIC COMMUNICATION: IMPLICATIONS

OF SUBLIMINAL RESEARCH FOR PSYCHOANALYTIC METHOD AND TECHNIQUE

Howard Shevrin

University of Michigan Medical Center

Ann Arbor, Michigan

Communication in psychoanalysis is of a very special nature.
Although two people talk to each other, it is not merely conversation. Although words are spoken, it does not altogether depend on
language. Although the main intent of both parties is to be understood, it is the difficulties in communication which are at the heart
of the matter. Finally, although much is said, it is mainly what remains unspoken that is important. Communication meeting these requirements is not ordinary; it is constrained by a method, requiring
that one person reveal his thoughts unsparingly to the other person
who is listening carefully enough to identify gaps, confusions, inconsistencies, and contradictions in the communication, as well as
the tenor of expressed and intimated feelings. The psychoanalyst's
third ear is glued to a psychic stethoscope which magnifies the otherwise unheard stirrings in the unconscious that point to underlying
disorder. Further, a special relationship quickly develops between
the people involved in this enterprise. Once we recognize that psychoanalytic communication is not ordinary conversation, nor simply
one person giving an account of himself to another, but constitutes
a highly specialized and uniquely constrained form of dialogue, then
we can appreciate how important it is to arrive at some clear idea
as to what this method is and what its assumptions are. Further,
it is important to know how this method is related to: (1) a body
of confirmatory or supportive evidence, and (2) particular applications in a given case (technique).

In a recent paper, Ramzy and I (1975) have reviewed and evaluated
the sparse literature dealing with psychoanalytic method as distinct
from psychoanalytic technique. By method, we meant the rational basis
on which the psychoanalyst arrives at his understanding of the patient;

by technique, we meant the wording and timing of interventions. Much attention has been paid to technique, but very little to method. And yet, our appreciation of the communication between patient and analyst must suffer if we do not increase our understanding of the logic in our listening. In this paper, I will explore some implications of my own research on subliminal perception for the assumptions basic to the psychoanalytic technique. I will start with a clinical illustration.

CLINICAL ILLUSTRATION[1]

In the 227th treatment hour, the patient, a young man who had entered psychotherapy because of a persistent conviction that he was small and inadequate, was struggling with the fantasy of taking away his therapist's girl. Typically for him, he was trying to convince the therapist that the fantasy was too frightening for him to explore. The therapist interpreted the patient's resistance as a defensive regression to the position of a weak, frightened little boy--the very condition for which he originally entered treatment. He had recently come into an inheritance following his father's death; he was convinced that his fee would be raised and, in fact, this had been discussed in a previous hour. His defensive regression was then also intended to ward off the therapist's expected attack on him for being like his father, a rich, "flashy womanizer" who must pay for his expensive habits. He admitted that he often fantasied being rich and powerful and potent sexually, but he also considered that way of life to be shallow, empty, and lonely. He recalled being proud of his father's greater affluence as compared to his friends' fathers. When he was about 10, he recalled really wanting to be like his father; but then he had the disconcerting thought that to grow up to be like his father would involve being his mother's lover. The therapist pointed out that there was a difference between being like his father and replacing him. He was affected by this interpretation. The therapist then related this to the patient's often expressed feeling that only one of them--patient or therapist--will come out on top. Although he recognized this understanding to represent a "synthesis" of many seemingly divergent feelings, he reported feeling inexplicably angry--wanting to scream, having images of his father the therapist, and a high-school teacher he idolized. All during this latter part of the hour, the patient seemed studiously to be avoiding looking at a picture in front of him, depicting a man and woman embracing. Instead he was staring at a plant placed beneath this picture.

In the very next hour, he announced with considerable reluctance, that he went to an art auction and bought a painting for $75.00. His

---

[1] I am indebted to Mr. James Staebler for his permission to use this psychotherapy excerpt based on his process notes.

interest in painting was totally new. He admitted it was an impulsive action, and that he was at a loss to account for it. Although
he confessed that he was anxious in discussing this, at the same time
he described his main attitude as being, "Why all the fuss?" He described how, at the auction, he was acting the part of the "rich womanizer" and related it to an image of his father. When he was questioned about why he had suddenly bought a picture, he reported feeling
anxious, but had no further thoughts. Of interest is the fact that,
during the hour, he talked about hanging the picture he had bought on
his wall; he also referred to his interest in Indian art. The picture
he had bought was a Western scene. The picture in the therapist's office was East Indian. Occasionally his eyes moved toward the picture
then quickly focused on the plants again.

The patient missed the next hour because he forgot about a change
in his starting time and came at the old time. In the next hour, he
revealed that he planned to seduce a girl he had recently met, and to
sleep with her while his girlfriend was away. However, he cancelled
the date when he realized that he was "acting out" again and had not
given himself a chance to talk about it. When the therapist pointed
out that he had "acted out" by forgetting the changed therapy time,
the patient returned to the fantasy of taking the therapist's woman
away, which was the most pleasurable part of his planned seduction,
for he imagined that the girl in question was the therapist's girl.
He added that he was so engrossed in planning the seduction that he
forgot about the change in time. The therapist suggested that the
last time he was mainly anxious about buying a picture; this time he
was upset about his taking the therapist's woman away. Perhaps buying the picture was a more disguised version of the latter. The patient then recalled a picture in a previous office the therapist had
used, which he thought was "very appropriate" for a psychologist's
office. He described the poster as showing a large spiral with a long,
thin rod-like object sticking up the middle of it.

The hour ended at this point. Unfortunately the therapist did
not return to the picture on his office wall. The therapist ended
his note for this last hour by saying, "Suffice it to say this is a
striking example of selective repression in the visual sphere. Although I too have stared at the poster in my previous office for well
over four years, I had never before noted its obvious 'appropriateness' in the patient's sense. His association was to a symbolic
representation of intercourse, when the most recent stimulus for his
jealousy and anxiety was a far more graphic painting of a woman and
a man embracing."

In this illustration we have reasonably clear, but not conclusive,
clinical evidence of a stimulus of which the patient is unaware playing
a key role in his thinking, feeling and--most important--his actions.
Suddenly he became interested in art, and purchases a picture for the
first time in his life. As far as we can tell, he remained totally

oblivious to the connection between his new artistic interest and its
origin. At the same time, it fit in well with the immediate status
of the transference; finally, there was a remarkable symbolic transformation of the picture, involving a displacement from the picture
in the therapist's current office to an earlier one; its symbolic
and abstract character is in contrast to the concrete erotic portraya
in the picture staring him in the face. Further, we see the use of
avoidance in looking at the plant rather than directly at the pictures. We may wonder at the therapist's unwillingness, or his possible oversight, in not calling the patient's attention to the picture. As an intervention this would have been a confrontation. Or
would it? Generally a confrontation calls the patient's attention
to some implication of his behavior, thought, or feeling of which
he was unaware or attempting to ignore. But in this instance, it
would be calling his attention to an apparently unconscious perception.

     Thus far I have dealt with the clinical material in customary
psychodynamic clinical fashion. Other clinicians might place a
somewhat different emphasis on this or that factor, or their interpretation might differ substantially from mine. Nonetheless, they
would be relying on the same assumptions. What I would like to
describe next is the contribution of research on subliminal perception in supporting and clarifying the underlying assumptions of a
psychodynamically based treatment method. Without these assumptions,
the patient's communications would be understood in an entirely different way. Moreover, the analyst's communications would also be
understood in a very different manner. Following this discussion,
I will conclude by dealing with further implications for technique,
although this area is more problematic than the first.

IMPLICATIONS OF SUBLIMINAL RESEARCH FOR PSYCHODYNAMIC TREATMENT AS-
SUMPTIONS

     There are three assumptions I would like to explore: (1) Under-
lying all apparent discontinuities of behavior, there is a continuity
determined by psychological unconscious processes (Rapaport, 1944).
(2) Every conscious process goes through a previous unconscious
phase.   (3) At any given time, the whole weight of the individual's
personality is brought to bear during this unconscious phase.

     Assumption 1: Underlying all apparent discontinuities of be-
havior, there is continuity determined by psychological unconscious
processes. In the clinical illustration, the therapist was using the
assumption of a psychological unconscious at every turn. Thus, the
therapist's view of the patient's fear of exploring his rivalrous
fantasy, as caused by a defensive regression to being a little boy,
is itself based on the assumption that such unconscious forces are
at work, that there is, in fact, a wish to be small, and thus to escape attack, as well as the wish to be rid of oppressive father figures, and to take their place in the scheme of things. Others need

not make this assumption. A behaviorist would simply say that there
was a learned association between anxiety and "little boy" behavior.
No more is psychologically involved than in thinking of <u>table</u> after
<u>chair</u>. There is no need to invoke any unconscious processes involv-
ing motives, fantasies, feelings, etc. All this is superfluous. One
might well counter this argument by saying that this oversimplified
explanation does not account for a good deal, e.g., why did the patient ignore the picture? Why the sudden love of art? Why the fantasied seduction, etc.? The reply would be that all that is very
complex, and we would need to know a good deal more about the patient's repertory of learned responses. In any case, we could likely
"extinguish" his "little boy" response with a very simple behavioral
modification regimen which, for the behaviorist, would represent
"proof" that no psychological unconscious is involved and no complex
interpretations are necessary. Of course, the success of his method
is not more proof of his propositions than the success of our therapist's interpretations (and I might add the eventual successful treatment of the patient). Usefulness and predictability are no guarantee
of validity. It is instructive to have an antagonist who can fall
into the same logical pitfalls, although he stumbles into them from
a completely different direction.

No clinical science can progress without a productive relationship with related basic sciences. We are more fortunate than many
of us realize in this particular area. Subliminal research has
clearly demonstrated that complex unconscious cognitive processes
do indeed exist. Several literature reviews (Fisher, 1957; Bevan,
1964; Dixon, 1971) have amply demonstrated that there is substantial
convergent evidence for the assumption of a psychological unconscious.
To those who would assert, "But we already knew there was an unconscious," I would simply reply, "No, we did not know there was an unconscious. We <u>assumed</u> that there was, and found it useful. Others
are not bound to make this assumption. But as the weight of evidence
from a variety of sources begins to accumulate, they may be forced to
do so."

I would like in particular to describe those subliminal studies
and their findings that do not depend on complex psychological or
clinical judgments, for only in these studies do we have clearcut
convergent evidence based on totally different operations from those
relied on in our clinical work. In my own work, I have demonstrated
that subliminal stimuli can elicit a discriminatory brain process in
the form of an average evoked response (Shevrin & Fritzler, 1968a,
1968b; Shevrin, Smith & Fritzler, 1969, 1970, 1971; Shevrin, 1973).
Although the subject is clearly unaware of having seen anything,
there is nevertheless reason to believe that a complex brain discrimination is being made without any awareness of it. Further, association data reveal, on the basis of an objective scoring system, that
associational processes have been set in motion. Lastly, these associations are related to the stimulus and are also correlated with the

discriminating brain wave component. The experimental procedure involves presenting the subject with repeated exposures of either an experimental or control stimulus. The stimuli are matched for such variables as size, orientation, total inner and outer contour, color, etc., so that only the fact that the experimental stimulus is composed of meaningful objects (a pen and a knee), and the control stimulus of nonsense forms, differentiates the two (see Figure 1). Electrodes are placed on the left occipital region and the frontal region just below the hairline. In most of our studies, the bipolar occipital-frontal leads provided the main findings: a larger positive going peak amplitude in the 40 to 260 msec. post stimulus interval for the experimental stimulus as compared to the control stimulus. This difference was found both for the 1 msec. subliminal condition and a 30 msec. supraliminal condition (see Figure 2). It was this amplitude which we found to be correlated with associations to the experimental stimulus. These findings have been replicated by my co-workers and myself. Recently Schwartz and Rem (1975) reported a related finding showing that in the absence of better than chance discrimination between pairs of the same stimuli we used, brain wave cross correlations demonstrate a discrimination between the two subliminal stimuli. In other words, although subjects could not make a conscious discrimination between the pairs, a brain discrimination was present (Shevrin, 1975).

There is also other convergent evidence derived from cortical studies of stopped retinal images and neurophysiological studies of the cortical conditions for consciousness. In brief, it has been found that when an image is stabilized on the retina so that no matter how the eyes move the image remains in the same place, the subject reports an intermittent fading of the image from consciousness. Originally it was thought that this was a peripheral satiation effect, but Riggs and Whittle (1967) found that even when the image fades, retinal potentials and, more important, cortical evoked potentials remain and are identical to those found when the image is in consciousness. What better evidence for the separation of consciousness from cognition! This finding is further supported by the work of Libet, et al. (1967, 1971) who found that a unique condition is necessary for consciousness--a 500 msec. cortically activated pulse train. In its absence, the existence of evoked critically activated levels indicate that cognitive activity is present but without benefit of consciousness.

A behaviorist would have difficulty maintaining his position in the face of these findings. Yet these findings provide critical support for a fundamental psychoanalytic assumption. Complex cognitive activity of the kind involved in our patient's thoughts, fantasies, and wishes can indeed go on without benefit of consciousness, and yet many influence conscious processes. There is a significant convergence between clinical necessity and research findings.

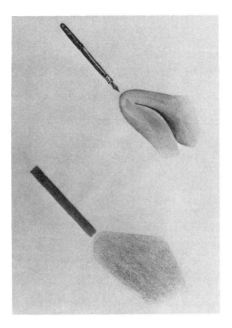

Figure 1.

Assumption 2:   Every conscious process goes through a previous
unconscious phase.   In an interesting paper, Basch (1975) has pointed
out that Freud expressed two different viewpoints with respect to the
pathway traversed by perception.   In the Project (1895), he insisted
that all perceptions must first be unconscious, but later in The Ego
and the Id (1923), he argued that perceptions and consciousness are
identical.   Why is this important clinically, and how does this effect communication in the therapeutic process?   The full import of
this assumption will become clearer when we turn our attention to
the third assumption.   Suffice it to say at this point that the model
proposed by Fisher (1957) in which he posited on the basis of considerable subliminal research, that all percepts must first go through
an unconscious phase is not only consistent with subliminal findings
but also clears up difficulties in Freud's "picket fence" model designed to explain the cognitive regression to perception necessary
to understand dreaming.   As Libet's work has shown, consciousness
is a final and optional step, dependent on the activation of a special process.   The activation of this process may depend on internal
factors (defensive needs) as well as external factors (weak stimulation).   It would follow from this evidence that all communication between patient and analyst goes through an unconscious phase before
becoming conscious.   Conversely, no communication is conscious first.
By unconscious, I mean the presence of complex cognitive and effective processes going on without benefit of consciousness.   In communication we do not first become aware and then repress, even though

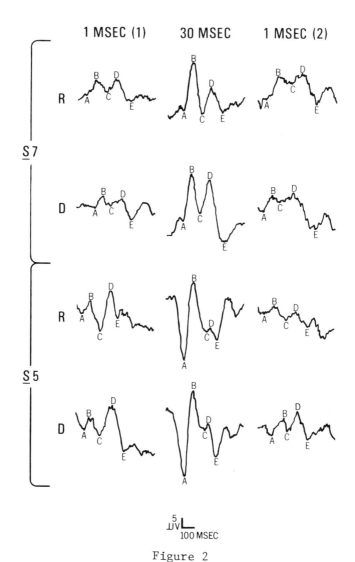

Figure 2

introspection tells us that this is what appears to happen. The
initial awareness of an unacceptable content would already speak
to the failure of a defensive process. The best example of this is
a slip of the tongue in which we communicate more than we consciously
wish.

Assumption 3: At any given time the whole weight of the individual's personality is brought to bear during this unconscious phase.
The tabula rose concept in psychology dies hard. Even G. Klein, for
all of his emphasis on the person in perception, found a place for a
neutral registration process preceding perception (1959). Clearly,

there must be some correspondence between our preceptions and its objects, but how this comes about is another matter. No process, no matter how veridical, is uninfluenced by the individual's unique characteristics. It is a question of how much, not whether. Therefore, all communications have already been put through the sieve, not only of unconscious processes, but of the communicator's unique personality. First I would like to cite some evidence in support of this proposition, and then it will be of interest to pursue some of its implications for communication in psychoanalysis.

In several studies, we have found that Rorschach based ratings of repressiveness were negatively correlated with the AER amplitude differentiating between the two subliminally presented stimuli. This differential amplitude occurred at approximately 160 msec. post stimulus. High repressive subjects had significantly smaller AER subliminal amplitudes than low repressive subjects. In other words, in less than a sixth of a second, a complex cognitive discrimination and dynamic process had taken place involving attention, perception, judgment, and motivation. We also found that repressive subjects free associated _fewer_ stimulus related words, thus demonstrating that associative processes were also affected. It could be argued that Klein's neutral registration could have taken place before personality factors entered the picture. This may indeed be true, although future research may prove otherwise. We can only say that work done to date reveals that dynamic personality factors are effectively present surprisingly early; and perhaps more important, that these events go on without any apparent reflection in conscious experience. One could not infer from what the subject was aware of in our experiments that the events described were occurring. The subject's conscious communication was a simple statement that he was seeing nothing other than a black dot, the fixation point. When he was giving his free associations, he was equally unaware that there was some change in certain categories of association. Subliminal perception works silently; dynamic personality factors operate with equal silence. Conscious communication can be remarkably opaque. There is an entire realm of subliminal experience entirely psychological in nature and subject to the dynamic laws of the unconscious which exist without any trace appearing in consciousness. One is reminded of the ocean depths far below the surface where an entirely different world exists, unpenetrated by sunlight, in which the animals and plants are entirely different from those found up above.

IMPLICATIONS FOR PSYCHOANALYTIC COMMUNICATION

As a point of departure, I would like to propose that communication in psychoanalysis is based on what I will call a _model of mild decompensation_. Analytically, we have referred to this as the patient's necessary capacity for controlled regression. The classical example is a slip of the tongue, in which a sudden lapse in repression

results in a minor symptomatic process, self-limited, spontaneous,
and revealing. From this transient symptom, we learn a good deal
about the individual's unconscious attitudes and motives. The therapist in my example was alerted to the significance of the picture by
the patient's studious efforts to avoid looking at it. Luborsky's
work on momentary forgetting is another example of a parapraxes which
can be significantly revealing (1973). In the most general sense,
the psychoanalyst is alert to any discontinuities that may appear
in the course of communication. Often these discontinuities are
instances, as with slips, of momentary defensive lapses or of structured and persistent symptoms. Symptoms are especially valuable because they are a permanent record of an unconscious influence on conscious processes. It is because a symptom provides this entre into
the unconscious that makes them so useful in treatment. Much good
and speedy work becomes possible when, in Freud's phrase, the symptom
enters into the therapeutic conversation, for then its relationship
to the transference can be explored, and the way open to discovering
its dynamic and genetic origins. On the other hand, our task is difficult, time consuming, and not always successful when we are confronted by well-entrenched character patterns which appear to be
self-contained and unassailable. We resort to confrontations in which
we point out unacceptable consequences, the deleterious impact of
certain actions on others, wasted opportunities, and, in particular,
the patient's difficulties in using the treatment for which he came.
We are thus reduced to treating the patient from "outside" the unconscious with no purchase available as with slips or symptoms. I
recall a 50-year old patient with a well organized compulsive character structure, a man totally incapable of experiencing anger or
any strong feeling, whose marriage was disintegrating as he stood
helplessly by. The treatment went on unproductively until, one day,
the patient locked his briefcase and airline ticket in his car in
the airport parking lot as he was on his way to an important busi-
ness meeting. He was utterly flabbergasted by this totally unchar-
acteristic action. He was always too thorough and organized to permit any such "accidents." This event made possible the first significant advance in the treatment. With many more narcissistically
organized people than my patient, few such "accidents" occur, or if
they do, they are not reported. Yet, we assume that an unconscious
is active in these people as well. Subliminal stimuli of all kinds
are also affecting them. How might we be in a better position to
take advantage of this knowledge we possess?

Before proceeding with some thoughts on that score, there has
been one significant omission from the repertory of psychoanalytic
communications which has a special place in this context. I refer
to dreams. It is of some interest to note that the dream begins,
quite often, with an indifferent perception of the dream day, and
proceeds to weave it into a texture of unconscious wishes and memories. Free associations unravel this fabric, separating the indifferent from the significant, the present from the past. We sometimes fail to discover what the indifferent dream instigator was.

Certainly the patient may have forgotten. But subliminal research tells us that he may have never been aware of it. A dream may appear to lack an anchor in conscious experience. It may prove to be an intriguing question as to what difference it makes clinically, that for certain dreams the residue is available and for others not. Generally we anticipate that the link to the present is vital for it gives us the most recent displacement. The transference is the best example of this. (Some interesting research might be done on the clinical value of dreams with day residues and those without, that is, those without consciously retrievable residues.) The question I am posing is this: could our work with some forms of character pathology be accelerated if we had some better idea, in advance, as to how these patients deal with subliminal inputs of various kinds? Would we be better prepared to pick up the slightest trace of unconscious influence on conscious thought and behavior? Or would it be best to continue to rely on the slow, careful patient clinical approach which awaits its opportunities with forebearance?

And yet one is tempted to wonder if one may perhaps increase the likelihood of therapeutically useful mild decompensations through the use of judicious subliminal exposures prior to, or coordinate with, therapy sessions. Silverman (1975) has described a series of experiments in which subliminal stimuli apparently activate mild, reversible pathological effects. One draws back before this undertaking because it would appear to violate a tacit assumption shared by patient and analyst--that the psychoanalyst will only undertake to influence the patient through the logic of his understanding, which he will share with the patient when deemed appropriate. Were we to use subliminal adjuncts, we would be returning to the earlier hypnotic and suggestion models which were intended to circumvent resistances and to penetrate to hidden unconscious conflicts and memories. In its place, Freud developed the model based on the transference neurosis brought about mainly by interpreting resistances. However, this model depends on the presence of mild decompensation, and runs into difficulties when opposed by deeply rooted character pathology. How do we transpose an ego, equal to developing a neurotic symptom, into an ego capable of the mild decompensations necessary for psychoanalytic work? The usual answer to this question has been to propose various parameters in treating these people, including a recommendation that analysis not be the treatment of choice. Is there some way of increasing the likelihood that analytic treatment, considering its greater thoroughness, might be made more applicable to such difficult cases? We have learned from subliminal research that it is likely that much dynamic processing of inputs goes on without any show of it in consciousness. How can this processing be made available without compromising the treatment method itself? Certainly the value of subliminal studies for diagnostic purposes has not been fully exploited. To some degree a thorough exploration of the way in which conflict related and unrelated subliminal stimuli are managed may assist the therapist's task.

SUMMARY AND CONCLUSIONS

Let me return to the clinical illustration and, using what we know of subliminal processes and psychodynamic theory, try to reconstruct what took place. I will also indicate at what points the three assumptions enter in. Clearly, at the start of the hour, the patient is already at a certain point in the transference. He has a fantasy about depriving the therapist of his girl. This is by now conscious, although in previous hours it was gradually working its way toward consciousness with the therapist's help. The resistance now is evidenced by assuming the position of a frightened little boy. The therapist understands this to be another instance of the patient's use of regression as a defense against hostile oedipal wishes to triumph over the therapist. We can see how the first assumption was already used in order to understand the "little boy" behavior as a defense, which is itself unconscious, as well as the reason for it. (As already indicated, a behavior modifier, or for that matter an intelligent layman, might understand it differently and perhaps from their point of view, in a simpler fashion. They would not be making the same assumption, however, as the psychoanalyst.) Much work has already been done on this defense but, as often happens, it needs further work. When the therapist interprets the defended against wish to triumph over the therapist, the patient, although recognizing the value of the interpretation, becomes angry and experiences images of his father, the therapist, and the revered high school teacher. The hostile affect, held in check by the "little boy" defense, now emerged toward the various transference figures and toward the original figure, the father, although significantly, not <u>directly</u> toward the therapist (recall that it was toward an image of the therapist). Again we rely on the first assumption to arrive at the understanding that this affect, or at least its disposition, was unconscious.

As this was going on, the patient was trying not to look at the picture of the couple embracing. Here, experimental research comes to our assistance in understanding what was now taking place. We know from the work of Luborsky and Blinder (1964, 1965) that repressive people, of whom this patient is a striking example, will tend to limit their number of eye fixations as compared to nonrepressive people, and will cluster their fixations on the nonthreatening parts of a TAT picture. We know from my own work that, nevertheless, there is a subliminal perception of the picture and therefore an unconsciously guided avoidance of it: he looks at the plant instead of the picture. (One is reminded of the New Yorker cartoon depicting a prim elderly lady standing before this immense portrayal of The Rape of the Sabine Woman and looking fixedly at a lower corner where the painter's signature appeared.) According to the second assumption, the erotic painting was blocked from achieving consciousness by an act of repression which was sustained by avoidance in the face of the continued presence of the painting. We would surmise that he

could say nothing about the painting because it was not in consciousness.

Nevertheless, the repressed painting influenced a decisive action he took prior to the next hour. Uncharacteristically, he attended an art auction and purchased a painting. Note that he did
so in the fantasied role of the rich flashy womanizer in which he
resembled his father. Here we draw on our third assumption: the
entire personality was responding to the subliminal pictorial input.
It was not simply a picture, but it entered significantly into the
patient's conflict, typical defenses, object relations, etc. I believe this is what we mean when we say that some content, for example, has become an instinctual derivative. The painting has not been
perceived as an object in the impersonal "outer" world, but from
the start, it became part of the individual's inner world. The
second assumption makes it possible for us to take this into account:
the therapist's painting would ordinarily have been "seen," that is,
it would immediately have been delivered into consciousness with
only a residue of personal flavor. But because it was drawn into a
whirlpool of conflictual feelings, its movement toward consciousness
was blocked, repressed and, instead, it became part of a complex unconscious system resulting in symptomatic behavior, the impulsive
purchase of the painting. As the therapist later pointed out, the
painting as the therapist's possession became the displaced representation of the therapist's woman. Buying a painting at the auction was thus a displaced achievement of the same goal without directly challenging the therapist. Again we invoke the first assumption, and are thus enabled to explain his resistance to discussing
the purchase and his effort at minimizing its significance. In this
hour, he again must avoid looking at the painting in order to preserve the necessary repression.

However, the conflict is moving closer to consciousness. Again,
on the verge of acting out, he almost follows through on a plan to
seduce a girl who he fantasied was the therapist's woman. He "for-
gets" the changed time. In the next hour when the therapist interpreted the reason for his buying the picture as related to his wish
to take the therapist's woman away, the patient recalled--not the
painting in the office in front of him--but a picture in a previous
office which actually was a symbolic version of that painting! The
interpretation could not lift the repression of the painting right in
front of his nose. The disguise was still necessary. From this,
using all three assumptions, we arrive at the hypothesis that much
work will be necessary on the patient's oedipal rivalry revealed in
the transference. He must remain unconscious of a reality literally
staring him in the face; he must do so because of his particular neurotic character organization and the conflicts now coming to the fore
in the transference; and all this is going on unconsciously with respect to an immediate stimulus.

Subliminal research provides us with significant convergent evidence which serves to validate our basic treatment assumptions, but which cannot be independently validated in the course of treatment. If our behavior modifier or a less biased intelligent layman were to listen to the clinical material I shared with you, he too might have some question about the nature of the therapeutic interpretations. Other explanations would appear plausible. However, if we were to tell him about the experimental findings based on completely different operations, he might be more impressed by the psychodynamic approach to understanding the patient's communications and behavior. The contributions of a basic science of psychoanalytic psychology should strengthen the foundation of clinical psychoanalysis, and should in time lead to an enhanced understanding of psychoanalytic communication.

REFERENCES

Basch, M. Perception consciousness in Freud's 'Project'. Annual Psychoanalysis, 1975, in press.

Bevan, W. Subliminal stimulation: A pervasive problem for psychology. Psychological Bulletin, 1964, 61:81-99.

Dixon, N. F. Subliminal perception: Nature of a controversy. London: McGraw-Hill, 1971.

Fisher, C. A study of the preliminary stages of the construction of dreams and images. Journal of the American Psychoanalytic Association, 1957, Vol. 5, No. 1, 5-60.

Freud, S. (1895). Project for a scientific psychology. Standard Edition, 1:283-344. London: Hogarth Press, 1966.

Freud, S. (1923). The ego and the id. Standard Edition, 19:3-63. London: Hogarth Press.

Klein, G. S. Consciousness in psychoanalytic theory: Some implications for current research in perception. Journal of the American Psychoanalytic Association, 1959, 7:5-34.

Libet, B., Alberts, W. W., Wright, E. W., & Feinstein, B. Responses of human somatosensory cortex to stimuli below threshold for conscious sensation. Science, 1967, 158:1597-1600.

Libet, B., Alberts, W. W., Wright, E. W., & Feinstein, B. Cortical and thalamic activation in conscious sensory experience. Neurophysiology Studied in Man. Proceedings of a symposium held in Paris at the Faculte des Sciences, July 20-22, 1971.

Luborsky, L.   Forgetting and remembering (momentary forgetting) during psychotherapy: A new sample. Psychological Issues, 1973, Monograph 30:29-55. New York: International Universities Press.

Luborsky, L. & Blinder, B.   Eye fixation and the contents of recall and images as a function of heart rate. Perceptual and Motor Skills, 1964, 18:421-436.

Luborsky, L. & Blinder, B.   Looking, recalling, and GSR as a function of defense. Journal of Abnormal Psychology, 1965, 70, 4: 270-280.

Ramzy, I. & Shevrin, H.   The nature of the inference process in psychoanalytic interpretations: A critical review of the literature. Journal of Psychoanalysis, 1975.

Rapaport, D.   The scientific methodology of psychoanalysis.   In Collected papers of David Rapaport. New York: McGill, 1944.

Riggs, L. & Whittle, P.   Human occipital and retinal potentials evoked by subjectively faded visual stimuli. Vision Research, 1967, 7:441-451.

Schwartz, M. & Rem, M. A.   Does the averaged evoked response encode subliminal perception? Psychophysiology, 1975, 12:390-394.

Shevrin, H.   Brain wave correlates of subliminal stimulation, unconscious attention, primary- and secondary-process thinking, and repressiveness. Psychological Issues, 1973, 8:2, Monograph 30, 56-87.

Shevrin, H.   Does the averaged evoked response encode subliminal perception? Yes. A reply to Schwartz and Rem. Psychophysiology, 1975, 12:4, 395-398.

Shevrin, H. & Fritzler, D.   Visual evoked response correlates of unconscious mental processes. Science, 1968, 161:295-298. (a)

Shevrin, H. & Fritzler, D.   Brain response correlates of repressiveness. Psychological Reports, 1968, 23:887-892. (b)

Shevrin, H., Smith, W. H., & Fritzler, D.   Repressiveness as a factor in the subliminal activation of brain and verbal responses. Journal of Nervous & Mental Disease, 1969, 149:261-269.

Shevrin, H., Smith, W. H., & Fritzler, D.   Subliminally stimulated brain and verbal responses of twins differing in repressiveness. Journal of Abnormal Psychology, 1970, 76:39-46.

Shevrin, H., Smith, W. H., & Fritzler, D. Average evoked response
and verbal correlates of unconscious mental processes. Psychophysiology, 1971, 8,2:149–162.

Silverman, L. H. On the role of laboratory experiments in the development of the clinical theory of psychoanalysis: Data on the
subliminal activation of aggressive and merging wishes in schizophrenics. International Review of Psychoanalysis, 1975, 2:43–64.

ISSUES POSED BY SECTION 4

Peter H. Knapp

Boston University School of Medicine

Boston, Massachusetts

The two papers under discussion deal with one kind of research--experiment. It is not the only kind, although assigned an ascendant position in the current hierarchy of scientific values. Experiment strives for the greatest possible control over phenomena under investigation. This means defining, and in most cases measuring. The reward is power, epitomized by the null hypothesis. Experiment aims to show that a finding is not the effect of chance, but the answer, selected out of nature by virtue of the precision with which a question has been asked. Questions, as well as answers, almost always involve simplification. The result may be loss of relevance or outright distortion. A case in point was the early work reviewed by Sears (1943), purporting to test psychoanalytic propositions.

Over the years such disadvantages have led to a disappointing distance between psychoanalysis and experimentation. Leaving aside efforts to test theory by inappropriate data, a number of analytically interested and sophisticated investigators remain; yet their efforts to extend the clinical insights of psychoanalysis by way of experiment have proved extraordinarily difficult.

Studies in primitive ideation and symbol formation, such as the early work of Silberer (1912), despite exciting leads, never reached fruition possibly because of unsolved problems in dealing with ipsative data and with quasi-aesthetic questions lurking in the whole area of symbolism. Memory, suggested as a crucial area by Rapaport

From the Division of Psychiatry, Boston University School of Medicine. Supported in part by Grant MH 11299-6 and Grant MH26183-03, National Institute of Mental Health.

(1942), proved complex and elusive. Simplification in experiments
of retention and recall seemed remote from interesting psychoanalytic considerations.

Hypnosis and suggestion had more potential. Theoretical difficulties in defining the parameters of the hypnotic state and in
bringing it into relationship with psychoanalytic constructs were
partially solved by Hilgard (1970), Gill and Brenman (1959), and
others. Perhaps a more serious obstacle was the largely latent
clash in ideology between the meticulously careful breed of analysts
who had abandoned hypnosis and the charismatic, active persona of
the mesmerist. In the case of suggestion, Fisher's pioneer experiments (1953) held extraordinary promise though this again remained
largely unfulfilled. Studies of dreaming ended up having more to do
with the psychophysiology of dreaming than with unanswered questions
about its psychology. Again, Fisher's work (1954) which began with a
replication of Poetzl's experiment (1960) was a major exception. It
led, in turn, to some of the work discussed here.

Investigations of stress made brilliant use of psychoanalytic
concepts, as in the early experiments of Reiser (1955), Sachar
(1963, 1968), and Wolf (1964), and their colleagues. However,
psychoanalytic formulations proved complex and difficult to corre-
late with biochemical and endocrine measures. Another exception
here was the work of Horowitz (1975), using language and perceptual
measures following stressful stimulation.

Indeed, the general areas of perceptual and cognitive psychology
prove more viable for experiment than the equally important problems
connected with free association, which Colby (1960, 1961) opened,
but which have never been pursued. In particular, George Klein and
his associates (1970) provided perhaps the most successful examples
of laboratory experiments bearing upon psychoanalysis. These formed
a major part of the stream from which came the work we are considering here.

Broadly speaking, we see: (a) conceptual difficulties in building bridges between psychoanalytic propositions and observations from
other, particularly biological perspectives; (b) practical difficulties in reproducing experimentally the powerful motives and emotions with which psychoanalysis is concerned, and finally (c) ideo-
logical and temperamental difficulties, which made most psychoanalysts, emulating the early Freudians, predominantly clinical practitioners, or at best naturalists rather than experimenters.

Despite these conceptual, practical, and temperamental problems,
necessary tools have gradually become available, and the power of
curiosity has begun to prevail over embattled adherence to schools.
The experimental approach has steadily gained momentum in psycho-

analytic investigation, as evidenced by the two preceding contributions. I shall discuss each of these, giving a slightly wider view of the author, based on parts of his work which could not be presented here; and I will try to comment on some of the central issues raised by the methods and findings of each. In closing, I will touch on the question of how research findings such as these are related to clinical practice, an issue that both authors address to varying degrees.

Shevrin's work, insofar as it has dealt with subliminal perception, has resulted in a number of findings:

(1) Presentation of a perceptual stimulus at a rate too rapid for conscious recognition has been shown to leave psychological "traces," namely an increase in words associated to the presented stimulus by rational links ("pen," leading to "ink," "paper," etc.) and words associated to the stimulus by "primary process" links ("pen" leading to "pennant"; "pen and knee" leading to "penny").

(2) Such subliminal presentation also leads to neurophysiological traces, namely an alteration in the amplitude of components of the Averaged Evoked Potential (AEP) (cf. Shevrin et al., 1968, 1971).

(3) These components are the same ones which in other studies have correlated with attention, both in Shevrin's work and in the extensive studies of others, such as Mirsky (1969) and Tecce (1976).

(4) Using identical twins, presumed to have a considerable congruence of neurologic substrate, Shevrin et al. (1968, 1970) found pairs who differed on psychological measures of "repressiveness." Such pairs also differed in the degree to which they showed these two parallel sets of "trace" phenomena. High repressors showed diminished psychological traces and lower deflections of the attention-related AEP component.

(5) This trend was reversed when supraliminal exposure was used. Then high repressors showed greater amplitude of the "attentional" component.

Shevrin's data are an outstanding demonstration that psychological processes outside of conscious awareness are accompanied by lawful and meaningful electro-physiological activity. Such an interrelation is exciting, and suggests a number of further lines of investigation. Let me comment on four of these.

The first concerns the "continuity" of psychological processes. Shevrin points out elsewhere (1970) that the very notion of unconscious processes assumes a continuum from obvious, macroscopic, conscious events to those that are entirely beyond awareness. Demonstra-

tion of such a continuum requires careful observation and inference.
I cannot entirely agree that it demands correlation with some external criterion, such as a physiologic measurement, for the correlation itself poses problems of reconciling frames of reference that
are easily confused. Nevertheless, such correlations are a convincing and dramatic way of approaching validation. In Shevrin's case
we are left with further questions: Exactly what does AEP "measure?" Presumably something to do with attention, but what sort of
processes are involved? Do they refer to the exclusion of some
peripheral stimuli or heightened focusing by some sort of feedback
activity on certain other stimuli? Some of the most interesting
questions that Shevrin raises have to do with the nature of repression—not as a mysterious mechanical or hydraulic barrier, but as
deployment of attention, directing it away from sources of danger or
distress. Yet for this to happen, some preliminary fleeting recognition of "danger" must have taken place.

We need to know more about the traits and states which maximize
and minimize repression, so viewed. This takes us to a second set of
implications which Shevrin discusses; namely his statement that "the
whole weight of an individual's personality is brought to bear during
the unconscious phase of perceptual organization." To distinguish
trait from state, we need further exploration, using a variety of
stimuli somewhat along the lines that Silverman has followed, working
them up gradually to the threshold of conscious recognition in order
to observe the changes that take place as consciousness manifests
itself. Detailed step-wise explorations of this type are made difficult by the particular technology of AEP, which requires repeated
exposure to a single stimulus.

Both on an immediate and a long term basis, we need to know more
about the links between electrographic potentials, such as AEP, and
other processes, conceptualized both psychologically and physiolog-
ically. Alerting and affective "interest" seems involved; this
probably involves some kind of generalized central "arousal." It may
be similar to more macroscopic, and peripheral, alterations in heart
rate which Spence (1972) found in psychodynamically skilled listeners
as they detected meaningful cues in speech.

At the neurophysiological level, expanding knowledge continually
raises further questions and changes our tentative formulations.
Shevrin has made sensitive use of a neurophysiologic measure, timed
to coincide with a precise psychological stimulus, thus solving one
of the major difficulties of psychosomatic investigation, that of
synchronous timing. We do not actually know where the AEP deflections originate, what other neurophysiologic activities they represent, nor the sites of these. We are still some distance removed
from identifying, far less localizing, most of the complex patterns
associated with mental states or traits. Shevrin gives us a tanta-
lizing look at virtually simultaneous processes identified within two

different frames of reference, but he hasn't quite closed the brain-
mind gap. Put otherwise, the research for precise coincidence in
time does not solve problems of structure, dynamic mechanism, causal-
ity in the widest sense.

Along with Luborsky (1975), we have tried to approach some of
these problems by looking at petit mal attacks. The "absence" is a
neurological phenomenon that can be identified accurately, coming on
while the individual is in the midst of speech. Yet even when we can
identify the syllable coinciding precisely with a deflection in a concomitant electrographic tracing, we are left with uncertainties. Was
the conscious mental event, culminating in speech, a trigger setting
off the brain dysrhythmia? Was there an antecedent state--containing
both "thoughts" and "feelings" and including dysfunctional brain processes? Indeed, could actual disturbances of both communication and
EEG be found prior to the full blown burst, as some of our observations have suggested? If so, the etiologic question is pushed further back: What was the main initiating event--electro-cerebral instability or instability in the surrounding social sphere? If the
latter, was the dysrhythmia a reflection of strong primitive instinctual processes, or did it reflect some mechanism for warding off
such processes?

These are some of the questions which can be raised, and which
can be answered only piecemeal over time by this type of coincident
observation of brain events and psychological activity, made possible
by Shevrin's kind of expanded neurophysiological technology. In such
studies we should recall the slightly outdated and overstated, but
none the less pertinent maxim of Fournié (1887, quoted by Lashley,
1951): "Speech is the only window through which the physiologist can
view the cerebral life."

Let me comment on a third theoretical assertion of Shevrin, that
every conscious thought goes through a prior unconscious phase. Common sense immediately questions such a view. We can understand how
manipulation with a tachistoscope might lead to fleeting perceptions
which then might undergo distortion, rotations, fragmentations, re-
combinations, and finally appear as part of a stable end product.
But surely, we feel, at other times we have some perceptions and
thoughts which are stable from their onset. Exactly at this point, we
must remind ourselves of the basic scientific contributions of perceptual research. It has shown that thoughts are continuously constructed, as Schilder originally put it (1922, 1935), out of a moving
flux of images. Our representations of self and others, our life
space, our more detailed image of reality, the sentences we utter, all
have a permanence that is only apparent, and a clarity which results
from the organization we bring to bear on this fluid matrix.

In an earlier paper, Shevrin suggested that the "pen-knee" stimulus may stir up repetitive "ringing" neurological activation, charac-

terized by rhythmic burst of alpha waves. He wonders whether the
latter may originate in nondominant hemispheric activity associated
with focused attention. Such a notion is congruent with considerable
current neurophysiologic speculation; it points the way toward examination of primitive roots observable within both psychological and
brain frames of references.

Finally we come to the clinical illustration that forms a central part of Shevrin's present paper. Here I am less happy. Essentially he deals with a common phenomenon--the elimination from consciousness of an unpleasant stimulus and, hence, of the disturbing
trains of thought and feeling which it might evoke. These find their
way back into the material by devious disguised routes. Observing
the sequence, we make constructions about motivational operations
being carried out beyond awareness.

However, in this illustration, there is really no evidence of
"unconscious perception." The patient was looking directly at the
stimulus in question, a picture in the therapist's office. He seemed
to avert his gaze; certainly he diverted his thoughts. But this is a
commonplace sequence. Shevrin's analysis of it is informed by his
work in the area of subliminal activities, but nothing in the fragment really demonstrates their existence. Knowledge of their activity will (he believes, and so do I) give us a better understanding
of crucial processes such as perception and repression. But this
clinical fragment does not really illustrate them. To use an analogy,
it can be explained by classical rather than quantum physics.

Such an analogy highlights the difficulties of going from experimental to clinical data. In our clinical encounters, we see
numerous examples that come close, as does this one, to genuine subliminal perceptual activity. I recall one sequence in which an asth-
matic patient passed me, while I was standing in line at a theater
with my wife who was pregnant in her eighth month carrying twins. The
patient completely repressed what must have been fleeting perception;
but during the next hours he brought in an enormous amount of material directly related to pregnancy. He almost managed to get his girl
friend pregnant, and finally in a culmination, complete with an asth-
matic attack, he reported a dream of strangling a bully, who represented an unwanted younger sibling. Here, too, a case could be made for
truly subliminal activation of conflict; but without the accuracy of
the tachistoscope, we are hard put to argue that he did not have more
than ample time for supra-liminal registration, followed by appropriate defensive manipulation of what had been perceived.

What is exciting to me about Shevrin's experimental work is the
exquisite timing, which allows us to link perceptual processes with
simultaneous brain processes. Further extension of this work into
the clinical area, for instance, by the use of subliminal priming before or during free associative sessions, which Shevrin hints at, is

an interesting terrain that remains to be explored.

Silverman, for more than a decade, has gathered an impressive and coherent body of data using subliminal stimulation in a different way. Again, let me try to place the present paper in a wider context of his published work.

(1) Methodologically, he has used tachistoscopic exposure at speeds well below discriminatory capacity (four msec.), and has checked his subjects to determine whether or not any conscious discrimination or perception took place. Moreover, as outlined in his paper, he has used a double blind technique.

(2) Subliminal exposure of pictures depicting aggressive impulses, either of a charging lion or a man in an aggressive act, when compared with neutral and bland stimuli, have been shown to disrupt thought in schizophrenic subjects. Disruption was judged by use of Rorschach or TAT cards. These original measures have been supplemented by other indices, such as word associations, story recall, overt behavior in the testing situation, and in some later, more long range studies, by observation of ward behavior.

(3) Supraliminal exposure of the same stimuli has not led to that type of disruption.

(4) Vocalization of aggression by the schizophrenics, however, has tended to restore the disruptive effect, presumably as they have struggled with awareness, implications and extension by further stimulation of the original aggressive schemata that have been activated.

(5) Similar changes have been observed in a normal population, provided that they are primed with an aggressive stimulus (reading them a story with blatant aggression in it). Such normal subjects have responded with paradoxical increases in libidinal responses (possibly as some type of defensive counter-mobilization or reaction formation to aggressive stimulation).

(6) Libidinal stimulation has not produced thought disturbance, although it has led to some minor evidences of behavioral disturbance, such as inappropriate laughter or tic-like movements.

(7) However, one particular libidinal stimulus, directed toward "merging" fantasies, has had a specific effect in diminishing schizophrenic thought disturbance. As indicated in the present paper, the author has been exploring whether this merging stimulus can be most simply conveyed by words referring to a mother or mother representative, and how narrowly such stimuli serve that purpose.

(8) The beneficial effects of this "merging" subliminal stimulus,

tend to appear at "cost" of faulty self-other differentiation. Silverman has attempted to counteract this tendency by specific instructions on self-differentiation--the technique of Des Lauriers. This
maneuver seems to have transient beneficial effect, which may become
more enduring when coupled with ministrations by a concerned person.

(9) Most interesting, from a scientific point of view, are the
explorations which Silverman and his collaborators have begun with
different stimuli in different disorders. They have obtained some
evidence that anal subliminal stimuli may enhance pathology in stutterers (1972), although, as originally reported, this effect was not
entirely clear-cut and was confused by a similar effect in some subjects following oral-aggressive subliminal stimuli. As mentioned in
his paper today, Silverman has found some effects in male homosexual
subjects, induced by an "oedipal" stimulus. He is also exploring the
effects of "merging" stimuli on obese subjects, thus extending his
work into the psychosomatic area.

These investigations raise some questions. How exactly was disruption of thought gauged after subliminal stimulation? Were the
same Rorschach and TAT test cards used as before; if not, what means
were taken to insure comparability of the demand characteristics of
the different TAT and Rorschach cards used?

Secondly, in the more long range studies, what measures have
been used to insure a continued double blind status? R. Rosenthal
(1966) has taught us how easy it is for cues to leak out, either by
covert communication between technician and tester, or, in studies of
repeated exposure during therapy, by information conveyed on one test
and its reflection in the assessment of a subsequent test.

A different question has to do with interpretation of the though
disturbance. In his original work, Silverman interpreted the effect
in terms of energy. Aggressive energy is aroused, and somehow "in-
filtrates" ego functions. It seems to me an advance that he is now
talking about unconscious fantasy, a term that can more readily be
made precise and operational. I still am not clear about his view of
the thought disturbance. In some of his writing, he speaks about
merging of ideas, as is encountered in typical "looseness of association," and sees it as somehow paralleling the merging of subject and
object, postulated to be part of the schizophrenic behavioral disorder. We run into dangers of mixing levels of discourse. Other explanations need to be systematically spelled out and explored. For
example, after subliminal stimulation, aggressive fantasy, mobilized
in latent form, might lead to partial abandonment of some kind of
mature psychological activity, a "surrender" in some regressive way to
less organized primitive imagery. The explanation would be a defensive adaptive view, which at times Silverman seems to favor. On the
other hand, there might be a direct heightening of primitive imagery,
a quasi-mechanical contamination and spread. This, in turn, might be

related to a particular heightened physiologic arousal, which has been postulated as part of the schizophrenic process, either as cause or effect, or in reverberating feedback fashion.

Silverman is aware of the different models, and is working on ways of defining them carefully in his continued explorations. It is conceivable that these explorations may even make contact with the AEP, which Buchsbaum and others are exploring as part of the theory of hyper-arousal in schizophrenia. Certainly it is important to test the effects in different subjects, selected according to careful diagnostic criteria pertaining to chronicity, prognosis, etc., a consideration that Silverman has himself drawn attention to in some of his studies. Differential reactions of different groups in successive experiments may have been due to the fact that they are drawn from differing schizophrenic populations. The more these can be specified in advance, the stronger the subsequent findings.

Clearly, the step to clinical applications is going to be difficult. Silverman's recent results, suggesting an adjunct role for subliminal stimulation in therapy, require controls against observer bias, and call for assessment over a long time span. One wonders if it might be useful to follow the vicissitudes of self and other both as external alliance and as internal representation, by multiple methods along with Silverman's technique, somewhat along the lines suggested by Horowitz earlier in this meeting. The phenomenon of merging as part of the schizophrenic process is real and important. Evidence for it has come from a number of sources. In terms of therapy, one might suspect that a good alliance leads to both some degree of fusion at one level, and to some degree of differentiation at another. Thus the patient, like the lover, may ultimately have the best of both worlds.

The most fascinating aspect of Silverman's work, in some ways, is the use of different stimuli in different conditions. This appears mostly in unpublished doctoral dissertations. One hopes that as these become more widely available, and replicated, they will offer a promising avenue for the investigation of specificity, not only in psychological but in psychosomatic disorders. I think of one stutterer, who had entered analysis with an almost incapacitating stutter. After brilliantly successful treatment, he was able to talk about his symptom with rare insight. He was an "S" stutterer. He said that four words had been particular nodal blocks: "shame," "sex," "shit,"--and finally "stuttering." Such conceptual feedback is similar to what we have seen in one petit mal patient, whose seizures occurred prominently in early interviews in relationship to the word "epilepsy."

A puzzling feature remains: Silverman asserts that words, as well as images, can be discriminated at extraordinarily rapid subliminal exposure times, and can then go to produce lasting effects.

I would be interested in his explanation of this phenomenon. It
bears on crucial theoretical implications of his work, namely the
contrast between subliminal and supraliminal stimulation. The way
the effects of subliminal stimulation appear to "spread" and "make
contact with other elements"--as Silverman puts it--suggest a potential tool for investigating and exerting some influence on mental
processes. In the latter regard, it is (perhaps fortunately) limited: attempts at subliminal influence on television viewers, like
similar attempts to influence sleeping subjects, have failed. Perhaps a special kind of readiness, occasioned by sitting in front of
a tachistoscope, is necessary, as Fisher postulated in his early extension of the Poetzl phenomenon (1954). A particular set, in other
words, shaped by instructions, may be necessary.

Conscious awareness certainly cannot be replaced or even overwhelmed. It may be supplemented in systematic fashion by certain
specific inputs to a prepared or open system. One of these may be
ESP. In the Journal of Nervous and Mental Disease, next to Silverman's most recent article, is one by Ehrenwald (1975) showing drawings of brain injured patients and of subjects doing ESP card recall
tasks. Both are strikingly similar to the drawings Fisher elicited
after subliminal stimulation (1954). Leaving aside such uncertainties, we should remain open ourselves to the possibilities of subliminal activation. It may belong in a total armamentarium of con-
sciousness-altering-activity, as we explore new modes of therapeutic
intervention.

In conclusion, the central focus, which I have selected from the
studies presented here, is that of imagery, as one type of nondiscur-
sive psychological process. Elsewhere I have argued that it forms a
universal substrate underlying clear, verbalizable (secondary process)
mental activity. The present studies point to the efficacy of this
stratum in mental life, the rapidity with which its impressions can
be registered, the way processes can ramify in it without reaching
conscious awareness and--by inference--the way in which such awareness itself must be a hierarchically organized level of psychological
activity.

Both authors have raised important questions about the structural
organization of these levels. Let me close by summarizing some of the
various models which have been suggested to describe their relationship. These are depicted in Figure 1. Freud's topographical and
structural models, each with different explanatory properties, constitute one set of overlapping zones. MacLean (1973) has suggested a
model from phylogony and ontongony to account for certain characteristics of cognitive activity, affective elaboration, and primitive
drive. Contemporary linguistics, I suggest, has within it the seeds
of still a further model: this goes from "surface" structures to
"deep" structures. Such terminology must make allowance for the fact
that Chomsky's original use of these terms (1965) was more precise and

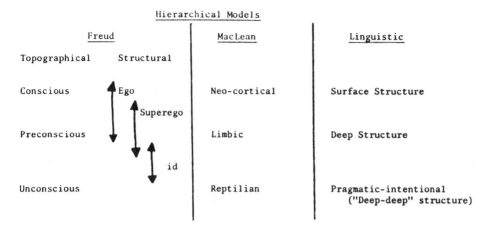

Figure 1

restricted. I propose to extend his terminology considerably by
suggesting under the "deep" structural layer there is even "deeper"
stratum, which I have designated pragmatic-intentional. This layer
may be seen as generating "deep" structures, much as the latter generate "surface" ones.

My point is that a number of workers, using various frameworks
have arrived at a tripartite view of psychological organization.
Such views postulated an intermediate stratum populated by imagery:
this serves to organize more primitive, "lower" organ-bound systems
that mediate drives; yet at the same time it remains ambiguous; in
turn it is organized, made precise, by higher cognitive and linguistic processes. These "higher" processes have great adaptive value.
During the course of development they become shared and socially acknowledged, unlike the layer of image-related activities which are in
some ways "richer"--that is, highly textured and evocative--but
private.

The major theoretical contribution of subliminal stimulation experiments, I suggest, is to demonstrate and explore the continuous
activity of this "image stratum." We ignore it under the illusory
sense of fully controlling our every thought and action. Bert Lewin
used to comment on this habitual illusion by saying: "Here we are
talking together while we are dreaming about each other." Mental
life undergoes a constant ebb and flow of imagery; we visualize, form
vague plans, and even, as Freedman has shown so elegantly in this
volume, picture them with gestures. The "image stratum," I might add,
has direct access to endocrine and autonomic systems that mobilize us
for action. It is with this stratum as equipment that the child first
meets the social world of his mother and other crucial individuals.
We have seen how early he begins to circumscribe and ward off his open

interchange with this world.

I suspect that the lasting clinical implications of the studies
on imagery and subliminal perception will not be to introduce a new
therapeutic technique, but to sharpen our thinking about how processes of perception and defense work, as Shevrin in particular has
done. They may also expand our awareness of what goes on in the
therapeutic encounter. Felix Deutsch in some of his early studies
(1953) was a pioneer in emphasizing the communicative significance
of gesture and posture within the psychoanalytic situation. Birdwhistell (1952), among others, has documented the ubiquity of communication, much of it micro-kinesic, virtually invisible except as
captured by a slow motion film projector. The individual is constantly sending messages to the outside world, and subliminal studies
help to establish that this kind of communication is a two way street.

Let me close by discussing, in slightly more detail, three clinical implications. First, Helene Deutsch, another gifted pupil of
Freud, used to remark: there can be no secrets in analysis. She
meant it as a moral maxim, urging scrupulous honesty with patients.
I suggest that it is true in a wider sense. The analyst is not a
blank screen. His relative silence and the paucity of his feedback,
puts him in a unique communicative position. But he is also a real
person and is constantly transmitting information about himself, his
character, his traits, and his state from moment-to-moment. His marginal, subliminal cues--possibly also, as I hinted earlier, cues
transmitted by as yet unknown, nontraditional communicative path-
ways--are inevitably transmitted to the patient. Possibly the more
disturbed and primitive the patient, the more surely he or she is
likely to pick up such cues. Thus, technically, we must be open ourselves as far as possible to our own unconscious processes. My own
belief, moreover, is that we had best acknowledge these when, as increasingly is the case, we are challenged by our patients' awareness
of them.

Secondly, we must pay particular attention to the manifestation
of the inner stratum of imagery. Horowitz remarked earlier in this
volume that we are on the verge of rediscovering the hypnoid state.
It, and variants thereof, appear in many current "schools" of neo-
analytic therapy. Furthermore, if we do not interfere with them, the
manifestations of imagery, the dreaming self, will appear as part of
a well-conducted psychoanalytic therapy, given an open and sensitive
therapist.

Thirdly, I am suggesting some theoretical modifications from the
old model of the detached analyst, who intervenes only by his scrupu-
lously worded and timed interpretations. Actually these modifications
have taken place slowly, at an almost imperceptible rate of growth
within the most orthodox bastions of psychoanalysis. They imply a
degree of reapproachment with Sullivan and the transactional analysts

Without fully acknowledging or often knowing the extent of such predominantly Sullivanian influence, psychoanalysis has gradually been
shifting toward a much more open model, one which acknowledges the
paramount role of social and communicational influences. The attention of Zetzel (1970), Stone (1966), and others to the therapeutic
alliance or nonneurotic transference, the emphasis by Greenson
(1967) on the real relationship to the analyst, the recognition by
Winnicott (1958) and many others of the fact that the core relationship to the analyst repeats aspects of the early relationship to the
mother, and the theoretical awareness especially enunciated in his
recent Presidential Address by Wallerstein (1973) of the fact that
outer social reality plays a crucial continuing role in the lives of
our patients--all of these developments suggest that we are moving
from an older closed model to a newer open model of the psychoanalytic relationship.

Figure 2 depicts progression from the concept of a detached
"analytic" observer focusing on drive versus defense in order to pro-
mote mastery by insight, to a newer model, which includes this overall conceptualization, but which adds that the analyst is inevitably
involved. He is necessarily a participant observer; in addition to
his long range aim of focusing on insight, he must also be providing

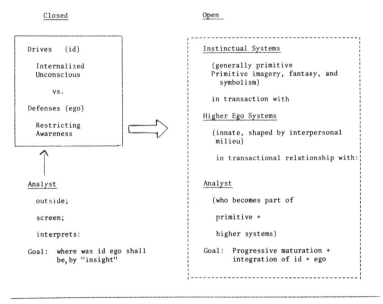

Figure 2   Changing Models

a nutrient medium for growth.

An eventual psychoanalytic psychology, still recognizing its inevitable relationship to biology, and studying how biological forces are shaped by learning, must include the discoveries from Sullivan, the expressive schools and, I would add, the existentialist view of the therapeutic encounter. Such an eventual psychology will gain from the work presented here by these pioneering investigators of subliminal perception.

REFERENCES

Birdwhistell, R. L. Introduction to kinesics. Louisville, Ky.: University of Kentucky Press, 1952.

Chomsky, K. M. Aspects of theory of syntax. Cambridge, Mass.: MIT Press, 1965.

Colby, K. M. Experiment on the effects of an observer's presence on the imago system. Behavioral Science, 1960, 5:216.

Colby, K. M. On the greater amplifying power of causal-correlative over interrogative inputs on free association in an experimental psychoanalytic situation. Journal of Nervous & Mental Disease, 1961, 133:233.

Deutsch, F. Instinctual drives and intersensory perceptions during the analytic procedure. In R. Loewenstein (Ed.), Drives, affects and behavior. New York: International Universities Press, 1953.

Ehrenwald, J. Cerebral localization and the Psi syndrome. Journal of Nervous & Mental Disease, 1975, 161(6).

Fisher, C. Studies on the nature of suggestion I and II. Journal of the American Psychoanalytic Association, 1953, 1:222-255, 406-437.

Fisher, C. Dreams and perceptions: The role of preconscious and primary modes of perception in dream formation. Journal of the American Psychoanalytic Association, 1954, 2:389-445.

Gill, M. & Brenman, M. Hypnosis and related states. New York: International Universities Press, 1959.

Greenson, R. R. The technique and practice of psychoanalysis. New York: International Universities Press, 1967.

Hilgard, J. Personality and hypnosis. Chicago: University of Chicago Press, 1970.

Horowitz, M. Intrusive and repetitive thoughts after experimental
stress: A summary. Archives of General Psychiatry, 1975, 32:11,
1457-1463.

Klein, G. Perceptions, motives and personality. New York: A. Knopf,
1970.

Lashley, K. S. The problem of serial order in behavior. In L. A.
Jeffries (Ed.), Cerebral mechanisms in behavior. New York: John
Wiley, 1951.

Luborsky, L., Doherty, J. P., Todd, T. C., Knapp, P. H., Mirsky,
A. F., & Gottschalk, L. A. A context analysis of psychological
states prior to petit mal EEG paroxysms. Journal of Nervous &
Mental Disease, 1975, 160:4, 282-297.

MacLean, P. D. A triune concept of brain and behavior. In Boag, T.
& Campbell, D. (Eds.), The Hincks Memorial Lectures. Toronto:
University of Toronto Press, 1973.

Mirsky, A. F. Neuropsychological bases of schizophrenia. In D. L.
Farnsworth (Ed.), Annual Review of Psychology, 20. Palo Alto:
Stanford University Press, 1969.

Poetzl, O. The relationship between experimentally induced dream
images and indirect vision. Psychological Issues, 1960, 2:7.

Rapaport, D. Emotions and memory. Baltimore: Williams & Wilkins,
1942.

Reiser, M. F., Reeves, R. B., & Armington, J. Effects of variations
in laboratory procedure and experimenter upon the ballistocardio-
gram, blood pressure, and heart rate in healthy young men. Psychosomatic Medicine, 1955, 17:183.

Rosenthal, R. Experimenter effects in behavioral research. New
York: Appleton-Century-Crofts, 1966.

Sachar, E. J., Mackenzie, J. M., Binstock, W. A., et al. Cortico
steroid responses to psychotherapy of depressions. II. Further
clinical and physiological implications. Psychosomatic Medicine,
1968, 30:23.

Sachar, E. J., Mason, J. W., Kolmer, H. S., & Artiss, K. L. Psycho-
endocrine aspects of acute schizophrenic reactions. Psychosomatic
Medicine, 1963, 25:510.

Schilder, P. The image and appearance of the human body: Studies in
the constructive energies of the psyche. London: Kegan, Paul,
French, Trubner & Co., 1935.

Schilder, P. Medical psychology (English trans.). D. Rapaport, Translator & Editor. New York: International Universities Press, 1952.

Sears, R. Survey of objective studies of psychoanalytic concepts. New York: Social Science Research Council Bulletin, 1943.

Shevrin, H. The physical reality of the unconscious. Presented at Annual Meeting, American Psychoanalytic Association, New York City, December 19, 1970.

Shevrin, H. & Fritzler, D. Visual evoked response correlates of unconscious mental processes. Science, 1968, 161:295-298.

Shevrin, H. & Fritzler, D. E. Brain response correlates of repressiveness. Psychological Reports, 1968, 23:887-892.

Shevrin, H., Smith, W. H., & Fritzler, D. E. Repressiveness as a factor in the subliminal activation of brain and verbal responses. Journal of Nervous & Mental Disease, 1969, 149:261-269.

Shevrin, H., Smith, W. H., & Hoobler, R. Direct measurement of unconscious mental processes: Average evoked response and free associative correlates of subliminal stimulation. Proceedings of the 78th Annual Convention APA, 1970.

Shevrin, H., Smith, W. H., & Fritzler, D. E. Subliminally stimulated brain and verbal responses of twins differing in repressiveness. Journal of Abnormal Psychology, 1970, 76:39-46.

Shevrin, H., Smith, W. H., & Fritzler, D. Average evoked response and verbal correlates of unconscious mental processes. Psychophysiology, 1971, 8:2, 149-162.

Silberer, H. On symbol formation. Jhb. Psa. Psychopath Forsch, 1912, 4:661-723.

Silverman, L. H. Further data on the relationship between aggressive drive activation and the impairment in thinking: The effects of blocking of aggressive discharge on the thought processes. Journal of Nervous & Mental Disease, 1965, 141:1, 61-67.

Silverman, L. H. A study of the effects of subliminally presented aggressive stimuli on the production of pathologic thinking in a nonpsychotic population. Journal of Nervous & Mental Disease, 1966, 141:4, 443-455.

Silverman, L. H. An experimental approach to the study of dynamic proposition in psychoanalysis: The relationship between aggressive drives and ego repression--Initial studies. Journal of the American Psychoanalytic Association, 1967, 15:2, 376-403.

Silverman, L. H. Further experimental studies of dynamic propositions in psychoanalysis: On the function and meaning of regressive
thinking. J. of Amer. Psychoanal. Assoc., 1970, 18:1, 103-124.

Silverman, L. H. Drive stimulation and psychopathology: On the conditions under which drive-related external events evoke pathological reactions. In R. R. Holt & E. Peterfreund (Eds.), Psychoanalysis & Contemporary Science, Vol. 1. New York: International Universities Press, 1972.

Silverman, L. H., Klinger, H., Lustbader, L., Farrel, J., & Martin,
A. D. The effects of subliminal drive stimulation on the speech of
stutterers. J. of Nervous & Mental Disease, 1972, 155:1, 14-21.

Silverman, L. H., Levinson, P., Mendelsohn, E., Ungarro, R., & Bronstein, M. A clinical application of subliminal psychodynamic activation on the stimulation of symbiotic fantasies as an adjunct in
the treatment of hospitalized schizophrenics. Journal of Nervous &
Mental Disease, 1975, 161:6, 379-392.

Silverman, L. H. & Spiro, R. H. The effects of subliminal and supraliminal and verbalized aggression on the ego functioning of schizophrenics. Journal of Nervous & Mental Disease, 1968, 146:1, 50-61.

Spence, D. P. et al. Cardiac change as a function of attention to
and awareness of continuous verbal text. Science, 1962, 176:1344.

Stone, L. The psychoanalytic situation. New York: International
Universities Press, 1961.

Tecce, J. J. & Cole, J. O. The distraction arousal hypnosis, CNV and
schizophrenia. In D. I. Mostofsky (Ed.), Behavior control and
modification of physiologic activity. Englewood, N. H.: Prentice
Hall, 1976.

Wallerstein, R. S. Psychoanalytic perspectives on the problem of
reality. J. of Amer. Psychoanal. Assoc., 1973, 21:1, 5-33.

Winnicott, D. W. Metapsychological and clinical aspects of regression
within the psychoanalytic setup. Collected papers. London: Tavistock Publications, 1958.

Wolff, C. T., Friedman, J. B., & Hofer, M. A. Relationship between
psychological defenses and mean urinary 17-hydroxy corticosteroid
excretion rates, Parts I and II. Psychosomatic Medicine, 1964,
26, 576-609.

Zetzel, E. The capacity for emotional growth. New York: International Universities Press, 1970.

SECTION 5
COMMUNICATIVE BEHAVIOR IN
THE PSYCHOANALYTIC SITUATION:
THE ROLE OF MOTOR PHENOMENA

INTRODUCTION

A fundamental issue in psychoanalytic theory is the understanding of the various transitions in thought which emerge during associative discourse: the transition from primary to secondary process
thought; the transition from preconscious to conscious ideation; or,
leaving aside theoretical models, the transition from the previously
unverbalized to the verbalized. The central problem highlighted by
these transitions is how images or ideas are transformed into verbalized speech. The psychoanalytic exploration of this problem has
focused upon the impact of the analytic dyadic, i.e., the impact of
object relationships in the transference, analytic interventions, or
interpretations. However, we have already seen in Sections 2 and 3,
that auto-regulations are also powerful regulators of the communicative process. Motor factors which accompany or precede speech
appear to reflect important processes which aid the transition from
the unverbalized to the verbalized.

The three contributions to this section explore the relationship between motor phenomena and verbal communication in the analytic situation. They are unique in their theoretical formulations.
They are also unique on methodological grounds, in that each author
combines formal experimental observations with naturalistic yet
systematic observations of the clinical process.

Gottschalk's work seeks to establish a causal chain consisting
of a kinesic-semantic (verbal) connection. His methodology entails
the use of a basic clinical study to generate hypotheses which are
then tested by formal experiment. The initial clinical observations
were straightforward. In the presence of continuous hand-to-snout
approximations, oral sexual themes emerged in speech. When the hands
rested quietly at the side, such content was absent. The clinical
observations provided a paradigm for the experimental study reported
in this volume. The experimental findings, however, were more complex than the clinical ones. They indicated large individual differences in the relationship between body movement and specific
semantic content. Such differences do not, however, negate a ki-
nesic-verbal connection. As Gottschalk points out, the significance
of body movements may be in their influence upon psychological states

broader than encompassed by a specific semantic category. The papers by Santostephano and Mahl offer two kinds of models which might
account for such a relationship.

Santostaphano views motor manifestations in an explicit developmental context. His model corresponds to the classical psychoanalytic theory which postulates a developmental progression of various
modes of representation from action, to fantasy, to verbal expression.
Within such a model, the appearance of motor behavior in communication constitutes an alternative, albeit regressive, discharge mode
which is reactivated in preparing the ground for verbal representation, the highest form of symbolic expression. Santostephano's work
on this kinesic verbal interaction is first described through the
presentation of experimentally derived normative data on children in
successive age groups. The conceptions arising from these studies
are then applied to findings in the developmental progression emerging in the process of the psychoanalytic treatment of a single child.
In his case presentation, the importance of the regressive reactiva-
tion of earlier action modes in the repetition and working through
of the analytic process is given much weight.

Mahl's contribution (based upon earlier experimental studies)
presents a unique phenomenon which he terms the A--B sequence: A, a
motor manifestation indicative of an as yet unverbalized message:
B, the verbal representation of that message after the motor act
drops out. His theoretical treatment of this A--B sequence views
motor phenomena as core components in the process of something
emerging in conscious experience. This view differs quite fundamentally from that of Santostephano's in that here the motor act is considered central to the representational process itself rather than
simply one of several alternative modes of representation. For Mahl,
motor phenomena serve to prime conscious experience. That is, Mahl
postulates that feedback from the sensory-motor bodily innervations
of symptomatic behavior constitute an essential transitional stage in
the process of something becoming conscious. In this view, conscious
communicative behavior is, at every moment, a distant derivative of
such core schemata.

In all, the studies reported in this section provide an interesting continuity with the issues of motor regulation raised in the
work on kinesics reported in earlier chapters by Freedman, Dittmann,
and Grand, and early sensory-motor regulations described in the reports of Sander and Beebe & Stern. Within the present context of
the psychoanalytic situation, these papers raise a host of new issues
concerning the role of motor phenomena in relation to both theoretical and clinical aspects of psychoanalytic technique.

BODY MOVEMENT, IDEATION, AND VERBALIZATION DURING PSYCHOANALYSIS[1]

George F. Mahl

Yale University

New Haven, Connecticut

INTRODUCTION

I will focus on one role of actions in the process of verbalization in psychoanalysis. The kind of actions I will discuss is familiar to every analyst, who usually regards them as expressions of the repressed. In his case reports, and technique papers, Freud cited such actions and saw them in that light. (Freud, 1893-95, 1905, 1909a, 1909b, 1913, 1914, 1918). To mention but one example, he noticed that Dora repeatedly opened her handbag and put her finger in it during one of her analytic hours. Only a few days earlier, she had claimed she had no memories of masturbating in childhood. Freud concluded that Dora betrayed her secret in these actions (Freud, 1905).

In Remembering, repeating, and working through, Freud (1914) proposed that such actions were instances in which the analysand "does not remember anything of what he has forgotten and repressed, but acts it out. He reproduces it not as a memory but as an action; he repeats it, without, of course, knowing that he is repeating it" (p. 150. Italics original). And he said, "...in the end we understand that this is his way of remembering " (p. 150). Freud added that this repetition was a function of the resistance.

Our findings suggest that many such actions are not simply alternative ways of remembering. Instead many of them appear to be integral to recollection and verbalization. The following observation,

---

[1] A version of this paper was presented to the Western New England Psychoanalytic Society, June 20, 1970.

made over 15 years ago during a study of initial interviews at an outpatient clinic (Mahl, Danet, & Norton,1959;Mahl, 1968) suggested this alternative view.

When Mrs. B. was discussing her inferiority feelings as a wife and homemaker, she once placed her fingers over her mouth for a moment. Three minutes later she was saying, spontaneously, that her feelings of inferiority dated from her childhood. Then she had felt she was homely and not as pretty as her sister, because she then had two ugly protruding front teeth. We inferred that the slight action of putting her fingers to her mouth anticipated, and perhaps facilitated, this recollection and verbalization about her childhood buckteeth.

The remainder of this paper is concerned with the phenomenon illustrated by this observation. For convenience, I call it the A-->B phenomenon. The initial interview study provided several other instances of it. Then I began to notice it occurring during the analytic hours of three analysands. Eventually I started to keep daily records of portions of two additional analyses, so as to establish a systematic body of clinical data pertaining to the phenomenon.

These records consist of process notes, supplemented by detailed records of the analysand's nonverbal behavior. I recorded the behavioral observations immediately following the hour, annotating them with mnemonic keys to the verbal content of the hour. The more complete reconstruction of the hour was nearly always completed later the same day, and always before the analysand's next analytic hour. The global postures were recorded in stick figure drawings comparable to Felix Deutsch's posturograms (F. Deutsch, 1952). Smaller unusual, or repetitive, idiosyncratic actions, as with the hands, for example, were indicated in improvised sketches, or with appropriate labels. Such systematic, daily records are the raw data for nearly all that follows in this paper.

At no time did I comment to my analysands about their A-->B phenomena. I tried not to vary my interaction with them because of this research. I continued to mostly listen...and watch.

The presentation is organized as follows: First, I will summarize and sometimes illustrate what I believe to be certain attributes of the A-->B phenomenon. Then I will present excerpts from the first few weeks of a single analysis. Finally, I will discuss theoretical ideas prompted by all the clinical observations.

SOME ATTRIBUTES OF THE A-->B PHENOMENON

1. The empirical paradigm covering most of the clinically observed A-->B's is shown in Figure 1. While the person is talking

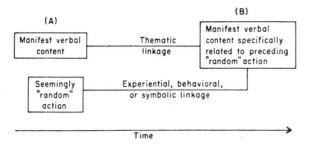

Figure 1 First Empirical Paradigm

about one thing at Point A, he performs a certain action, which is usually not obviously related to what he is saying. Then later, at Point B, the person spontaneously mentions something else which is thematically linked to the first topic and very clearly related to the former action. The pattern of events is such that the action has anticipated the subsequent verbalization. This paradigm schematizes what is observed in most clinical instances. It will become apparent in this paper, however, as it did in my research, that this is an incomplete paradigm.

2. The frequency of A-->B's. It is my impression that for most patients a minimum of one clear-cut A-- B occurs every three or four analytic hours, but I have not rigorously documented the frequency. The important point is that they are not rare events.

3. The A-->B time interval. This may range from seconds to several weeks. Impressionistically, most clear-cut sequences seem to be completed within one to three analytic hours. Long term A-->B's may span several weeks, during the course of which many relevant short-term A-->B's may occur as though in the service of the long-term process. Resistance does seem to prolong the time interval.

4. Specific muscular tensions and preparations for actions may substitute for overt acts in the A-->B sequence.

5. All components of the personality may be expressed in the A-actions: Id -- impulses, Ego -- defenses, and central Super-ego attitudes or developmental experiences.

The preceding five points about the A-- B phenomenon have been stated in summary fashion. I will illustrate the next three points, using material that will also illustrate some of the preceding points.

6. A-->B phenomena stem from most important aspects of the person's life. And they may occur during very significant phases of the analytic process. One day, near the end of his third year of analysis,

Alec, a young, recently married man, was discussing a prospective
visit he and his wife might make to his parents. It would be the
first real visit they would have had since his marriage. While he
was saying that he didn't want to go because he knew his mother
would be full of critical comments about how he and his wife were
leading their lives, he removed the pillow from under his head and
placed it against the wall beside the couch. He lay his head back,
flat down on the couch, and continued speaking dysphorically about
the visit. In about a minute, he replaced the pillow under his head
and, without making reference to this singular action, he continued
along the path of his conscious thinking. This was the only occasion
in his nearly four years of analysis that he did this with his pillow.
I have never seen another patient do this.

Two hours later Alec recalled something new concerning his mother and his adolescent masturbation: (a) His mother and father
went out one evening, saying they would return about eleven o'clock.
About nine, he was in bed masturbating against his pillow. Suddenly
his mother's voice filled the room. They had returned early and she
was standing in the doorway to his bedroom. (b) His mother punished
him by taking away his pillow for four years. As he said now, while
he used to tell his curious adolescent friends that there was never
a pillow on his bed because he preferred to sleep without one, the
absence of his pillow was always a private symbol of his guilt over
masturbating. Here is a clear-cut A-->B phenomenon. While speaking
dysphorically about what he anticipated would be his mother's disapproval of his current marital (sexual) life, he removed his pillow
on the couch. A short time later, crucial, relevant memories emerge
for the first time. This example also illustrates how the Superego,
and passivity-activity shifts, may contribute to the actions in the
A-->B sequences. He felt guilty about his marriage, and he now pun-
nished himself as his mother had punished him; he took his pillow
away from himself.

This A-->B was one step in an extended phase of his analysis
dealing with his masturbatory complex, and during which he and his
wife were attempting to achieve conception. There were visits to
the fertility clinic, and then his adolescent phantasies that he was
using up his sperm each time he masturbated emerged. Soon after, his
wife was pregnant. Thus, this man's pillow A--»B involved a very
significant dimension of his life. It was also an important feature
in an on-going phase of his analysis.

7. The sensory feed-back from the transitory actions may be
consciously perceived and become part of the associative drift leading to the verbalizations. (a) This feed-back may be kinaesthetic.
A pregnant woman, Mrs. C., felt the tensing of her abdominal muscles
while she imagined her analyst's penis was erect. This awareness of
the tension led to her telling that recently she had been contracting

her abdominal muscles to make her baby-filled belly stick out in a
hard protruding ball. In a moment we will follow this episode further. (b) The feedback may be an indirect consequence of the action rather than kinaesthetic. Another time, Mrs. C. noticed the
tingling she had produced in the back of her hand by rubbing it
against the roughly plastered wall by the couch as she spoke of
her affectionate transference feelings. She then recalled "bear-
hugs" with her father in her childhood. When he came home in the
evening he would hold her in his lap and they would hug and rub
cheeks vigorously. The stubble of his five-o'clock shadow would
leave her cheeks tingling. Most A--⟩B sequences include no report
about such sensory feedback.

8. Dreams containing imagery highly relevant to the A action
may occur in the midst of an A--⟩B sequence that extends over two or
more days. The pregnant woman just mentioned had a dream the night
after her abdominal muscles contracted in the analytic hour. In the
dream, she is lying down, and can see her large abdomen looming up.
The baby inside is moving about, causing the wall of her abdomen to
be pushed out in places as though the baby is pushing out with a leg
here, a leg there, an arm here, and then there. Then, either her
navel or a spot near is pushed out, making a protuberance about the
size of a thumb. Her associations to the dream included the thought
that the baby might have had an erection which caused this protrusion near her navel. Then she recalled that as a little girl she
had thought her navel was her penis.

This woman's unconscious, childhood wish to have a penis was
first expressed in the abdominal tensing, then in the abdominal
imagery of her dream, and then it was recalled and verbalized.

I have completed listing attributes of the A--⟩B phenomenon and
I turn now to some excerpts from the first 35 hours of the analysis
of Edward.

THE INTRICATE INVOLVEMENT OF A--⟩B PHENOMENA IN THE ANALYTIC PROCESS

Edward is a youngish married man who sought analytic therapy because he was experiencing certain heterosexual inhibitions and he
feared his reaction to the possibly pending death of his mother. She
had undergone surgery for a serious illness a few months earlier.
The material I will present is one-sided, coming primarily from the
more ego-alien trends in his personality. In contrast to the impression one might form solely on the basis of what follows, Edward was
quite effective in his occupation and showed much 'masculine' strength.
Table 1 summarizes the events I will describe more fully; reference
to it may make it easier to follow the narrative description.

Edward removed his wallet from his hip pocket and placed it on
the side table as he got onto the couch at the outset of the second

Table 1

Summary of Edward's A-->B Sequences

Time Span of Sequence	A Bodily Action (Theme of Verbal Content)	Primitive Ideation	B Subsequent Verbalization
Within 2nd hour	Places wallet on table		Hopes analyst will be tough but kind: honest and warm. "No bullshit." "Ass on table."
4th-5th hours	Wiggles and settles buttocks onto couch		Father's wiping him after bowel movement, and shaming him, age 7-8.
	Slams calendar on table (analyst's absence)		Mother's delay causes him to soil pants, age 6-7-8.
Within 5th hour	Two-handed bosom. (Mother doesn't take care of his needs)		Mother's mastectomy. Anger at her indifference to loss of femininity.
6th-18th hours	Left hand breast, 6th-11th hours. (women, needs for nurturance)		
	Buttock wiggling onto couch, chest expansion, pelvic thrust; two-handed bosom, 12th hour. (My evaluation of his work competence)	Image of self as naked woman on couch, facing me, 12th hour.	Wish to be woman on couch, 13th hour.
	Urge to sit up and look at me, to walk about room, 12th hour.		
			Adolescent fixation on girl's breasts, loss of love objects, identification with them.
			Mother's illness--feminine identification.
			Father substitute mother. (14th-18th hours)
Within 33rd hour	2-hand bosom. (Phantasy that analyst more interested in women, than him.)		Wish he were female. Father's desire for little girl.
			Playing "girl" with brother as child.
			Envy of woman's passive role in intercourse.
33rd-35th hours	"Finger-inside," 33rd hour (his phallic penetration in intercourse). Sensation of having to move bowels, 33rd hour (Forgotten dream of woman)	Image: Woman lying on floor, exposed thighs and buttocks, ready for intercourse. (33rd hour)	
	Breasts and bosoms; pectoral spasms, 34th hour (Anger at analyst's absence, making-up.)	Dream: Anal intercourse between man and woman. (after 34th hour)	Discovery of anal-erotism; passive homosexual phantasies in reaction to mother's serious illness; wish for analyst's penis in rectum. 35th hour "Loss" of wallet, after 35th hour.

hour. He moved his buttocks about slightly on the couch as he settled into it. Later in the hour, he said he wanted me to be tough,
kind, honest, and warm. He thinks I will be. In the screening
period, I had seemed tough, like I would stand for no "bull-shit."
The expression, "Ass on the table" came to mind when he thought of
the impression I made on him. Placing his wallet on the table preceded these spontaneous verbalizations. It is also the beginning
of other A-->B sequences in which the less prominent buttock wiggl-
ing-in is important.

At the beginning of the fourth hour, Edward checked his trouser
pockets carefully and spent what seemed to be quite a long time wiggling and settling his buttocks into the couch. Then he started to
talk.

At the beginning of the next hour (the fifth), only a trace of
this buttock wiggling was apparent, but he slammed his calendar onto
the table. He used the calendar partly to verify the dates of three
sessions I would be missing the following week. Towards the end of
the hour, two significant childhood anal memories emerged. Until
he was seven or eight, he would always call for his mother or father
to wipe him after a bowel movement. One time, his father asked, "Am
I going to have to wipe you until you are 10?" Edward felt shamed.
He then recalled another experience from about the same period of
time. Suffering from diarrhea, he had rushed straight home from
school to go to the toilet. But when he arrived, the door was locked.
While his mother took her time unlocking the door, he lost control
and soiled his pants. He was furious at her for keeping him waiting
so long. His excessive buttock wriggling on the couch and his slamming his calendar onto the table preceded the emergence of these two
memories. The wiggling onto the couch seems most relevant to being
wiped by his father; the slamming of his calendar, to his infuriat-
ing, maybe infuriated, loss of control because of his mother's momentary absence.

His thoughts drifted on to his mother's current health. He worried that she will die. He also complained about the lack of affection by his parents. His mother, particularly, didn't take care of
his needs, like in the episode just described. As he was voicing
these complaints, his two hands appeared over his pectorals in the
position shown in Figure 2. He had made on himself, for the first
time, what I will be calling a two-handed bosom. He then spoke
bitterly about her "sick" joking about her left mastectomy. She
had recently said the left side of her chest was like a boy's now;
and, her remaining breast was like a penis. He cursed in the hour
at her lack of concern for her femininity. Here, Edward had first
made breasts nonverbally, and had then immediately spontaneously verbalized highly relevant thoughts and feelings. Had he also made himself into a woman? A woman on the couch? And if so, would he be
speaking of this?

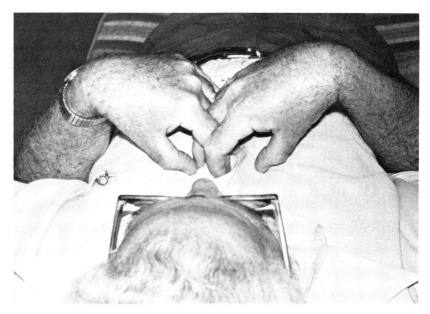

Figure 2   Two-handed bosom.

From the sixth through the eleventh hours he made a left-hand breast for brief periods of time.   Typically he did this when his thoughts touched on women and on his needs for nurturance.   His buttock-wiggling onto the couch became unnoticeable in these hours.

When he was settling himself on the couch at the outset of the twelfth hour, however, his buttock-wiggling was again noticeable, and was followed by several deep sighs or chest expansions and thrusting of his pelvis.   In a few minutes he was making a very prominent two-handed bosom, while speaking, incidentally, of how I might respond to any inquiries about him from his employer.   Soon he reported an urge to sit up and look at me, to walk about the room. Later he was telling of an article he had once read about Susan Strassberg's experience in Reichian therapy.   She had sat naked, facing the therapist.   Then an image formed in his mind's eye--he was a woman on the couch and was facing me.   In the next hour his associations drifted to his explicitly saying that he wishes he were a female here; if he were, I would be warmer to him.

He had made himself into a woman with his two-handed bosoms and breasts.   In this hour, this act was joined by other consonant ones, including a motor urge.   There followed an image containing a pictorial rendition of his motoric state earlier in the hour.   The next hour he verbalized the wish.

In the next four hours, material emerged that began to fill-out
the background of his feminine actions. Object-loss, grieving, and
identification formed the nexus of this material. He told of how,
in adolescence, the girl he first loved suddenly broke-off with
him. He had worshipped her. He never had enough of "suckling" her
breasts. He mourned losing her for over a year. He also recounted
his grieving the assassination of one of the Kennedys. While listening to the news reports, with his family, he went alone into another room, closed the door, and fell to the floor where he lay weep-
ing and sobbing. Thus he identified with his adored hero who was
now mortally wounded. He mourned Kennedy's death for a long time.
Once, telling me of a television documentary about the life of Kennedy, moved him to uncontrollable, convulsive crying.

His thoughts also touched upon the loss of his mother's breast,
and the anticipated loss of her whole self. Associations to a dream,
in which he succeeded in sucking on his own penis, led him to recall
that he became troubled by thoughts about fellatio and of semen re-
sembling milk after he had heard of the necessity for his mother's
operation. At the same time, he had started to feminize his appearance. His thoughts drifted on to memories of some prepubertal homosexual play involving the boys' buttocks. Then he fell silent and
covered his brow. Struggling against a sense of shame, he said,
"I may want something from you... a bill... a rich analysis... maybe
something homosexual." I replied, "If you do, it would seem to be
substitute mothering, a replacement for your mother." He answered,
"My father replaced my mother for me in many ways. He was more gen-
erous, and more giving, and more emotional." When I handed him the
bill at the end of the next hour, incidentally, he stuck it in his
mouth, between his teeth, while he put on his coat.

A picture of Edward emerges: object loss grieves and angers
him deeply. He copes with it by powerful identification. The immediate basis for his current feminine transformation -- which was
first and so clearly manifested in his nonverbal behavior -- was
the loss of his mother's breast, the real or phantasied loss of her
motherliness, and the threatened loss of her totally. Thus identified with her, he has turned to his father for the masculine versions
or equivalents of mothering. His A-->B's, starting from his first
hours, and the material of the last four hours, bring us to this
point, (and the end of his 18th hour).

The theme of femininity now largely disappeared from his verbalizations for approximately two weeks. But in nearly every hour
of the dormant phase, breasts and bosoms appeared briefly, and on
occasion were followed by relevant brief verbal references -- to
embraces, soft-breasts, and cravings for oral stimulants. Thus,
nonverbally, he was continuing to partly make himself into a woman
in the analytic situation. But consciously he was attempting to
strengthen his sense of masculine strength -- to build his "ego
muscles," he said.

In the 33rd hour, he spent a great deal of time talking about a woman acquaintance who was in psychotherapy. Finally, he said that he felt like his hour was being devoted to her, not to him; that he was a messenger between her and me. I replied that he seemed concerned that I would be more interested in her than in him. Thereupon, he made a two-handed bosom which he held as he told the following. What I had said was true. And he has often had the phantasy of being a girl on the couch. He has wished he were a girl. If he were a female patient, I would be more interested. "I really believe that I believe this about myself," he said. He then made brief, but new, references to his childhood. His father wanted a girl after he was born. His brother used to dress him up in girls' clothes when he was a youngster. His mother let his hair grow long when he was little. Finally, his father became enraged and had it cut.

He also spoke of his envy of the woman's passive role in intercourse: they don't have to work, and they don't have to get an erection. His hands were still in the two-handed bosom position. He went on to say that usually his penis only became fully erect when he had "penetrated" and was "inside." In the course of this associative drift to "penetration" and being "inside," the bosom was transformed into the form shown in Figure 3. This "finger inside" position had never appeared before. He held the "finger inside" and went on to think about the way his penis recently emerged from his wife covered with blood. He also became aware that he had dreamt about women last night. While he tried unsuccessfully to recall the dream, he felt as though he had to move his bowels. He then thought about a woman co-worker. His hands now separated. An image formed in his mind: she was lying on the floor of his office ready for intercourse, with her skirt pulled up exposing her large thighs and buttocks. This sight was unattractive to him, and her genitals would be unattractive looking. I only want to point out about this material that the sensations in his bowels joined the "finger inside," and that a highly relevant image followed. We saw this kind of sequence in an earlier episode. But one cannot help but also hypothesize that in this hour he had bodily made himself into a girl with an erection inside her, all done on the couch -- ie. on me?

A four day separation now occurred, occasioned by one of the long week-end holidays. He had forgotten my having told him earlier of this break. When we resumed work in the 34th hour, he spent a great deal of time being angry about my taking a holiday and then making-up with me. While doing these things, he also made breasts and bosoms with his hands almost continually throughout the hour. He was apparently also doing so within his body, for he felt spasms in his left pectoral muscle group and massaged it.

We hypothesized that before the break, Edward had pantomimed a girl with a penis inside her and had felt bowel activity. After the

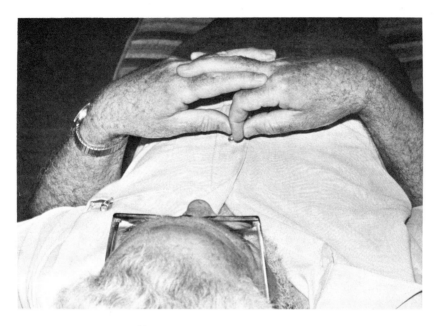

Figure 3 "Finger-inside" hand position.

break, he was making breasts strenuously. In the next hour, he reported a dream which had occurred during the break. Thus, it had
actually followed the complex of "finger-inside," bowel activity,
and image of the large thighs and buttocks of his woman colleague.
The dream report was as follows: A man and woman are naked. Their
faces aren't in focus. The man is sitting down in a chair and the
woman is straddling him, but with her back to him. [cf. analytic
situation]. They are having intercourse. His penis is very large,
and she is going way up, down, way up. The man is white, but his
penis is a brownish-red color, as though the skin had been pulled
off. He then said the color of the man's penis reminded him of a
"piece of shit." I commented, "and the scene is as though his penis
were in her rectum." He then made the "finger-inside" gesture, and
except for one brief right breast, he held the "finger-inside" position as he spoke about the following anal-erotic material for the
first time.

He has often thought of having anal intercourse with his wife.
Shortly before his mother's operation, but after he had heard it
might be necessary, he learned about his own rectum. He felt it,
put his finger in it, and then did this while masturbating. His
wife occasionally does it to him during intercourse. After discovering his rectum, he started having passive homosexual phantasies,
both of fellatio and of anal intercourse. His thoughts drifted to

his relationship to me. He mentioned, again, seeing me as tough and successful. His wanting to have my penis in him is a wish to absorb my power.

The emergence of these anal trends completes the immediate short-term sequence that started three hours earlier with the "finger-inside" and the bowel urge, progressed to the image of the anal woman, then to the dream, and finally to explicit verbalization. This emergence was also part of a long-term sequence that started with that little A-->B in the second hour when he placed his wallet on the table and later said I reminded him of the expression "Ass on the table." In a phone call following this 35th hour, Edward furnished evidence that this might be so. He called to ask if he had left his wallet in my office that morning. "It's gone. It's probably stolen," he said, "but I wanted to check with you before reporting it."

DISCUSSION

Freud repeatedly raised the questions: What is the difference between something that is unconscious and that which is conscious? How does the unconscious become conscious? Perhaps the data about the A-->B phenomenon can make a contribution to the solution of these questions, for the sequences we have described included events that we refer to as the "emergence of the repressed," or as "the unconscious becoming conscious."

REPETITION INSTEAD OF RECOLLECTION; OR MOTORIC EXPRESSION OF THE REPRESSED

If we treat the first empirical paradigm with the concepts Freud presented in his paper on repetition and recollection, we have the theoretical paradigm presented in Figure 4. This contains the usual psychoanalytic explanation of what is observed. It assumes that the later conscious content with unconscious at point A, that it was dynamically operative then, that it either produced the A-content or was, in some way, associatively connected with it, that it found sidewise expression in the action, and that it later became conscious when the defenses were mitigated. Thus, there is first repetition instead of recollection. Later there is recollection.

THE INTERVENING OCCURRENCE OF BODY-PERCEPTIONS, IMAGES, AND DREAMS

Our investigation showed that such primitive cognitions often followed relevant motor acts and that, in turn, relevant verbalization occurred. This calls for a modification of the first observational paradigm which will recognize the intervening occurrence of body-perceptions and primitive ideation. Figure 5 contains this second empirical paradigm.

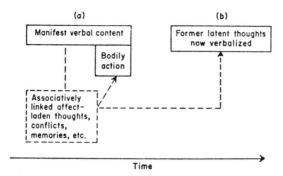

Figure 4   First Theoretical Paradigm   (From Mahl, 1968)

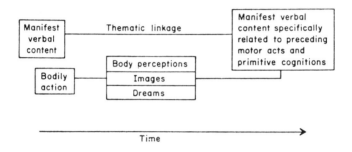

Figure 5   Second Empirical Paradigm

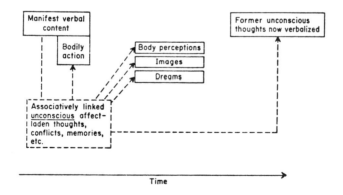

Figure 6   Second Theoretical Paradigm

The comparable theoretical paradigm is presented below in Figure 6. It is essentially the same as the one presented in Figure 4, the only difference being that the primitive cognitions, as well as the motor acts, are viewed as being produced by the unconscious processes. This is the usual view of the primitive cognitions and, of course, of dreams. According to this paradigm, the new elements in it are simply alternative side-effects of the unconscious.

But are the motor acts merely alternative side-effects to the process of something becoming conscious and verbalized, or are they integral to that very process? We will turn to this question now, considering two alternatives to the theoretical formulation we have followed so far.

FACILITATION OF THE UNCONSCIOUS BECOMING CONSCIOUS

The first alternative, schematized in Figure 7, is the proposition that in some instances nonverbal expression facilitates the spontaneous process of something becoming conscious. This hypothesis speaks of repetition in the service of recollection, in addition to repetition instead of recollection. This is a modest proposal, for it only suggests that some, not all, nonverbal expression may have this facilitative effect. It does not propose any other changes in customary view of unconsciousness or the process of becoming conscious. Some of the observations suggest one possible way in which facilitation might come about--namely, by way of sensory feedback that becomes part of the conscious associative process.

There is good reason to suppose that essentially the same facilitative process may occur spontaneously without consciousness of the sensory feedback from the body action. As with stimuli in experiments on subliminal perception, it is possible that the feedback may be registered though not consciously perceived. One effect of such registration might be the direct emergence of the repressed into consciousness and verbalization. Another effect of such an unconscious registration might be the instigation of primary process ideation such as images or dreams, and then the emergence and verbalization of the repressed.

Neither we, nor the speaker, may have direct evidence that the feedback entered into the flow of events. But both psychoanalysis and cybernetic studies have shown that feedback is an integral factor in behavior. We know now that feedback operates silently and ubiquitously in such complex behavior as language and secondary process functioning just as in simple motor skills (Lee, 1950a, 1950b; Klein, 1965; Mahl, 1961, 1972).

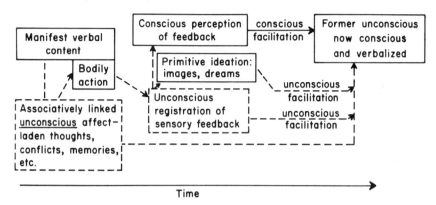

Figure 7   Third Theoretical Paradigm - The Facilitation Hypothesis

The role of "unconscious perception" of body feedback and the hypothesized progression from it to primitive imagery and to eventual consciousness that we are suggesting here is envisaged as analogous to the common nighttime experience in which a bodily need arises in the middle of our sleep, is first manifested in our consciousness by a "dream of convenience" -- after having been necessarily registered mentally but unconsciously -- and is eventually consciously appreciated when we wake up to satisfy the need.

TRANSITIONAL STAGES IN BECOMING CONSCIOUS

The second alternative to the usual theoretical formulation is more speculative and differs more radically from it than does the facilitation hypothesis. In the earlier paradigms we assumed that the thoughts, memories, etc. verbalized at point B were present but repressed at point A, and were being expressed in the actions and associated verbalizations at that time. Just as Freud did in his repetition and recollection paper, we were explaining the observable events by means of the early paradigms he developed to account for hysterical symptoms and later extended to dreams. In both cases, Freud assumed that the unconscious memories and wishes existed in cathected ideational form. Hysterical symptoms were the result of the "discharge" of the charge of affect on the memory trace (Freud, 1894); dreams were thoughts (wishes, purposive ideas) transformed into sensory images by regression and the dream work (Freud, 1900). In Repression (1915a), Freud wrote in the same vein. What was repressed was:

"...an instinctual representative, and by the latter we have understood an idea, or group of ideas which is cathected with a definite quota of psychical energy (libido or interest) coming from an instinct" (p. 152).

The idea or derivatives of it could become conscious, and the quota of energy could be discharged over body pathways, resulting in affect. In the paper The Unconscious (1915b), when discussing the same theoretical idea, he spoke of "...the development of affect and the setting-off of muscular activity" (p. 179). These statements comprise the theoretical framework for Remembering, repeating, and working through (1914) which was published a year earlier.

At the same time, however, Freud began to discard this theoretical framework. In the paper, The Unconscious, he also spoke of the theoretically "enigmatic Ucs" (p. 196), and of many transitional stages in the process of something becoming conscious. In hypothesizing the unconscious "thing-cathexes" and the preconscious "word-cathexes," and translation of the former into the latter as the essence of something becoming conscious, Freud was clearly introducing a new theoretical paradigm. He no longer believed that the dynamic unconscious contents were of the same form or substance as when they were conscious.

But what were "thing-cathexes"? In the case of objects, he said only, "...[thing-cathexis] consists in the cathexis, if not of the direct memory-images of the thing, at least of remoter memory-traces derived from these" (p. 201). In the case of thoughts and wishes, his discussion of "organ-speech" in the schizophrenic and of hysterical symptoms seems to clearly imply that he considered the thing-cathexis to consist of bodily innervation. Beginning with a reference to Tausk's patient, who experienced a jerk in her body and a sense of having her body position being forcibly changed by somebody, Freud wrote as follows:

"The physical movement of 'changing her position', Tausk remarks, depicted the words 'putting her in a false position' and her identification with her lover. I would call attention once more to the fact that the whole train of thought is dominated by the element which has for its content a bodily innervation (or, rather, the sensation of it). Furthermore, a hysterical woman would, in the first example, have in fact convulsively twisted her eyes, and, in the second, have given actual jerks, instead of having the impulse to do so or the sensation of doing so: and in neither example would she have any accompanying conscious thoughts, nor would she have been able to express any such thoughts afterwards" (pp. 198-199, Italics original).

These remarks imply that Freud would include bodily innervation as part of the thing-cathexis, but he never came out and explicitly said that a potential for bodily innervation was part of the thing-cathexis, a step he never hesitated to take in discussing the nature of an unconscious emotion.

I believe Freud's indefiniteness about the nature of the thing-cathexis was scientific uncertainty, not stylistic vagueness. He made this scientific uncertainty quite explicit when he again discussed these issues in The Ego and the Id (1923). There he wrote,

"...an idea that is conscious now is no longer so a moment later, although it can become so again.... In the interval the idea was -- we do not know what" (p. 14), and, ..."I have already, in another place, suggested that the real difference between a Ucs. and a Pcs. idea (thought) consists in this: that the former is carried out on some material which remains unknown, whereas the latter (the Pcs.) is in addition brought into connection with word-presentation" (p.20).

It is at this point that the observations we have made might make a contribution. (1) The frequency with which one can observe that relevant bodily events precede conscious experiences suggests that at bottom the essence of an unconscious wish or memory, of a thing-cathexis, may be a potential for bodily innervation, or perhaps covert innervations and their sensory feedback. (2) The frequency with which one can observe the regular progression from a bodily expression, to primitive ideation, to eventual verbalization suggests that these are some of the usual transitional stages in the process of something becoming conscious. (3) The considerations we presented in discussing the facilitation hypothesis suggest that sensory-feedback plays an important role in the progression from one stage to the other.

If we combine these three assumptions we arrive at the theoretical paradigm contained in Figure 8. This paradigm comes from our observations taken together with Freud's distinction between thing-cathexes and word-cathexes and his remarks linking bodily innervations to thing-cathexes.

The hypothesis outlined in Figure 8 assumes that the nucleus of the unconscious content at point A is a potential for body innervation. The core of the "thing-cathexis" becomes, for us, nearly identical with Freud's idea of the essence of an unconscious affect: a potential for bodily innervation. What we have in mind here is the assumption that the nucleus of unconscious wishes and memories consists of excitatory potentials for very concrete bodily excitations which are specific instances of the abstract categories termed "wish," or memory. The core of the unconscious wish of the woman who rubbed her hand on the rough wall until it tingled, for example, is assumed to be the excitatory potential tending to reproduce the actual experiences of the bear-hugs with her father. Similarly, the core of Edward's unconscious wishes to be a woman is assumed to consist of the corresponding concrete bodily strivings for excitation of his anus and for female breasts on his chest.

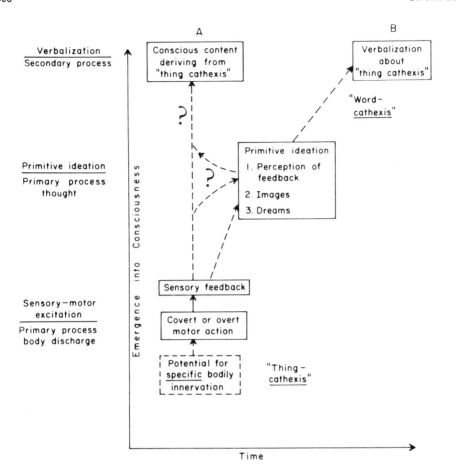

Figure 8   Fourth Theoretical Paradigm - Transitional Stages
            in Something Becoming Conscious

The scheme of Figure 8 raises the possibility that the verbal content at point A derives from the unconscious potential assumed to be operative then. Perhaps the A-->B sequence operates at every moment -- nearly simultaneously, as well as being perceptibly spread out over longer time intervals. But this is so speculative as to deserve the question marks shown.

REFERENCES

Deutsch, F. Analytic posturology. Psychoanalytic Quarterly, 1952, 21, 196-214.

Freud, S. (1893-95) Studies on hysteria. Standard Edition, Vol. 2. London: Hogarth Press, 1955.

Freud, S. (1894) The neuropsychoses of defence. Standard Edition, Vol. 3. London: Hogarth Press, 1962.

Freud, S. (1900) The interpretation of dreams. Standard Edition, Vols. 4 and 5. London: Hogarth Press, 1953.

Freud, S. (1905) Fragment of an analysis of a case of hysteria. Standard Edition, Vol. 7. London: Hogarth Press, 1953.

Freud, S. (1909a) Analysis of a phobia in a five-year-old boy. Standard Edition, Vol. 10. London: Hogarth Press, 1955.

Freud, S. (1909b) Notes upon a case of obsessional neurosis. Standard Edition, Vol. 10. London: Hogarth Press, 1955.

Freud, S. (1913) On beginning the treatment. Standard Edition, Vol. 12, London: Hogarth Press, 1958.

Freud, S. (1914) Remembering, repeating, and working through. Further recommendations on the technique of psychoanalysis, 2. Standard Edition, Vol. 12. London: Hogarth Press, 1958.

Freud, S. (1915a) Repression. Standard Edition, Vol. 14. London: Hogarth Press, 1957.

Freud, S. (1915b) The unconscious. Standard Edition, Vol. 14. London: Hogarth Press, 1957.

Freud, S. (1918) From the history of an infantile neurosis. Standard Edition, Vol. 17. London: Hogarth Press, 1955.

Freud, S. (1923) The ego and the id. Standard Edition, Vol. 19. London: Hogarth Press, 1961.

Klein, G. S. On hearing one's own voice. In M. Schur (Ed.), Drives, affects, behavior. Vol. 2. New York: International Universities Press, 1965.

Lee, B. S. Some effects of side-tone delay. Journal of the Acoustic Society of America, 1950, 22, 639-640. (a)

Lee, B. S. Effects of delayed speech feedback. Journal of the Acoustic Society of America, 1950, 22, 823-826. (b)

Mahl, G. F. Sensory factors in the control of expressive behavior. Acta Psychologica, 1961, 19, 497-98.

Mahl, G. F. Gestures and body movements in interviews. In J. M.
  Shlien (Ed.), Research in psychotherapy, 3. Washington, D. C.:
  American Psychological Association, 1968.

Mahl, G. F. People talking when they can't hear their voices. In
  A. W. Siegman & B. Pope (Eds.), Studies in Dyadic Communication.
  New York: Pergamon Press, 1972.

Mahl, G. F., Danet, B., & Norton, N. Reflection of major personality
  characteristics in gestures and body movements. American Psychology
  1959, 14, 357. Abstract.

FURTHER STUDIES ON THE RELATIONSHIP OF NON-VERBAL TO VERBAL BEHAVIOR:

EFFECT OF LIP CARESSING ON SHAME, HOSTILITY, AND OTHER VARIABLES AS

EXPRESSED IN THE CONTENT OF SPEECH

Louis A. Gottschalk and Regina L. Uliana[1]

University of California, Irvine

Irvine, California   92664

INTRODUCTION

This study grew out of a long therapeutic psychoanalysis in which a patient's speech was tape-recorded before and after he periodically touched different parts of his body. Two types of observations were made during this psychoanalysis on these psychokinesic sequences; (1) impressionistic evaluations of the relationships between hand movements and the content of free-associations, and (2) independent and objective scoring of the content of speech and its statistical relationship to hand movements and placements. These two types of assessment of the data of observation gave results which supplemented one another, the former method allowing more broad generalizations but less certainty, and the latter method enabling more specific evaluations and greater potential for statistical assessment of probabilities.

Some of the main observations noted by the impressionistic method were as follows:

1. If the analysand moved his hands, he generally touched a part of his anatomy related to a psychological or biological function he was experiencing or describing. The relationship of the hand activity and position to the content of his speech could be very concrete or symbolic.

_____

[1]From the Department of Psychiatry and Human Behavior, College of Medicine, University of California at Irvine, Irvine, California 92664. Herman Birch, Ph.D., provided statistical consultation.

2. Hand movements around his mouth or lips tended to be associated with talking about women, a longing for the breast or for the
whole body or to be part of a woman, in a sexual or nonsexual context. These associations tended to be affectionate or positive
rather than negative.

3. Touching his eyelids was often related to talking about
seeing or understanding.

4. Touching his abdomen was often associated with thoughts
about the vagina and sexual intercourse.

5. Touching his nose was associated with sexual interest in
forbidden women, diarrhea, or disliked women.

6. These psychokinesic relationships remained fairly stable
and unchanging without specific analytic intervention. They could
be altered, however, by interpretive comments or, sometimes, by
simply calling the patient's attention to specific hand movements
and thought contents.

The more objective method of content analysis provided statistically significant evidence that the analysand spoke more frequently
of women and expressed positive feelings toward all objects (animate
and inanimate) when he was touching his oronasal area as compared to
when his hands were at his side (Gottschalk, 1974).

In this natural history study, where the hand-mouth activity
appeared spontaneously during the psychoanalytic situation and where
the hand movements around the oronasal area served a soothing function leading to a temporary feeling of security and the capacity to
feel separate and autonomous from the analyst, there was, of course,
no information enabling one to generalize how commonly such hand-
mouth activity might evoke such specific speech content in others.
Also, except for the inferences one might make on the basis of temporal relationships, it could not be determined whether the hand-
mouth contact did, indeed, evoke certain memories and thoughts and,
hence, such speech content, or whether this directly observable and
recordable speech content and its underlying unrecordable associated
mental content caused the hand-mouth activity.

One approach to exploring the cause and effect aspects of such
kinesic-semantic relationships was considered to be an experimental
study with a group of individuals, in which the hand-mouth activity
would be systematically alternated with a hand position away from
the face. On a broader basis, such an experimental method, in contrast to the natural history method, was seen as a means of exploring the ways in which such kinesic activity might affect speech content and of contributing to our understanding of the interplay of
early life experiences and object relations on mental content. Another purpose of this study was a heuristic one; namely, to apply

hypotheses generated from the psychoanalytic situation to measurement theory and practice outside psychoanalysis to determine how
kinesic activities, such as lip touching, can influence the measurement of psychological states, not only by content analysis but, by
extension, through other means, such as self-report and rating scale
procedures (Gottschalk, 1975).

METHODS AND PROCEDURES

    Subjects. Twenty college students, 10 males and 10 females,
with a mean age of 21.45, were paid volunteers for this study. Only
those subjects who reported, during an initial interview, that they
were in good general health and that they had not taken any drugs,
for example, depressants or psychoactive drugs, during the preceding
month were allowed to participate in the study. Furthermore, because the use of birth control pills has been demonstrated to influence speech content (Silbergeld et al., 1971), although the phases
of the menstrual cycle can also do so (Gottschalk et al., 1962; Ivey
& Bardwick, 1968), only women who were not taking such hormones were
offered the possibility of participating in the study.

    Procedure. Each subject gave four five-minute speech samples
in the presence of one of the authors (RU). Each five-minute period
of speech was accompanied by either hand-position "A" (hands at one's
side) or hand-position "B" (one hand caressing one's lips), balanced
for both men and women in either the sequence ABBA or BAAB to control
for possible order effects. The speech was elicited by asking each
subject to talk for five minutes about any interesting or dramatic
life experiences, following standardized instructions used previously
in many investigations of content analysis of speech (Gottschalk &
Hambidge, 1955; Gottschalk & Gleser, 1969). Speech samples were
tape-recorded in full view of the subjects, and these tapes were
later transcribed.

    After giving the four five-minute speech samples, each subject
completed the following measures:

    1. The Luborsky et al. (1973) Social Assets Scale, which is a
self-report procedure constructed of 33 weighted items relating to
an individual's psychosocial background, including details of parent-
child relations, parent loss, sibship, educational level and so forth.
The composite score from this measure is called a "social assets"
scale score, and this measure has been found valuable in predicting
improvement from brief psychiatric hospitalization and the frequency
of episodes and severity of certain specific illnesses (herpes simplex, arthritis). This social assets scale score, in 25 acute
schizophrenic patients, was significantly negatively correlated
($r = -0.46, p < .01$), before treatment with a major tranquilizer, with
social alienation-personal disorganization content analysis scores

Table 1

Correlations of Social Assets Scale Scores (Luborsky) and Various Behavioral and Psychological Measures Before (days 1, 3, and 6) and After (day 8) Thioridazine (4mg/kg) by Mouth in Acute Schizophrenic Patients (N = 25)

Behavioral or Psychological Measure	Social Assets Scale (Luborsky)			
	Day 1	Day 3	Day 6	Day 8
BPRS				
1. Depression				-0.45*
2. Thinking Disorder				
3. Anergia	-0.54**	-0.64****	-0.59***	-0.37
4. Excitement-Disorientation				-.56***
Hamilton Depression Scale				
1. Sleep Disturbance				
2. Somatization	-0.37	-0.47*	-0.31	-0.44*
3. Anxiety Depression				
4. Apathy	-0.28	-0.37	-0.45*	-0.23
Wittenborn Scale				
1. Anxiety				
2. Somatic-Hysterical	-0.36	-0.36	-0.16	-0.42*
3. Compulsive-Phobic				-0.37
4. Retardation	-0.40*	-0.33	-0.37	-0.45*
5. Excitement				-0.45*
6. Paranoia				
Social Alienation-Personal Disorganization Scale			-0.46*	-.53**

*p   .05
**p   .01
***p   .005
****p   .001

(a measure of the relative severity of the schizophrenic syndrome derived from the content analysis of speech (Gottschalk & Gleser, 1969), with the Anergia Factor (r= -0.59,p<.005) of the Overall Gorham Brief Psychiatric Rating Scale (1962), and the Apathy Factor (r= -0.46, p<.05) of the Hamilton Depression Scale (Guy & Bonato, 1970). The predrug social assets scores were also significantly correlated with various other measures from these patients two days after a single oral dose of thioridazine (4mg/Kg) (Gottschalk et al., 1974, 1975). (See Table 1.)

2. A questionnaire designed by the authors, composed of 22 questions about various aspects of the subjects' history of oral activities (See Schedule 1).

The typescripts of the speech samples were then content analyzed, without the content analysis technician knowing the hand position with which the speech sample was associated, for the dependent variables of this study:

(a) Hope scale scores (Gottschalk & Gleser, 1969; Gottschalk, 1974a), which are derived from a verbal content analysis scale composed of seven content categories (4 weighted positively and 3 weighted negatively) counted for their frequency of occurrence within each grammatical clause of verbal communication. This scale was devised to measure the intensity of the optimism that a favorable outcome is likely to occur, not only in one's personal earthly activities, but also in cosmic phenomena and even in spiritual or imaginary events. The total hope scale score is arrived at by summating the weights of all relevant hope content categories used per speech sample, and expressing this raw score in terms of a corrected score per 100 words spoken, so that these scores can be compared within an individual over different occasions and between individuals, regardless of the total number of words spoken during the five minutes of speech.

(b) Hostility scale scores (Gottschalk et al., 1963; Gottschalk & Gleser, 1969). These are validated content analysis scales covering three types of conscious and preconscious hostility: hostility outward (overt and covert), hostility inward, and ambivalent hostility.

(c) Anxiety scale scores (Gottschalk et al., 1961; Gleser et al., 1961; Gottschalk & Gleser, 1969). These are validated content analysis scales covering conscious and preconscious total anxiety with six anxiety subscales: death anxiety, mutilation anxiety, separation anxiety, guilt anxiety, shame anxiety, and diffuse anxiety.

(d) Object Relations Scale (Gottschalk, 1974b, pg. 282-283) which classifies each reference to "objects" for references to

females, males, sexually unspecified humans, inanimate objects, and
for the expression of positive and negative feelings toward any object.

(e) Oral references occuring in the speech samples (See
Schedule 2 for the classification of Oral References).

In a previous report (Gottschalk & Uliana, 1976), we described
and discussed our initial findings in this psychokinesic study, and
we will summarize them here.

(i) Subjects, on the average, spoke significantly
fewer words (t=2.14, p<.05) during the five minute period when
they caressed their lips than when they kept their hands at their
sides.

(ii) There were more verbal references per 100 words
during lip caressing (t= -1.84, N=20, p<.08, two-tail test) to "not
being or not wanting to be or not seeking to be the recipient of
good fortune, good luck, or God's favor or blessing" (Hope Scale
content category #5).

(iii) In line with a prestudy hypothesis, the group
of subjects with lower social assets scale scores (lower 1/3) tended
to have greater increases in hope scores (B-A) while touching their
lips (t= -1.84, N=12, p<.05, one tail) than the group with the higher
(higher 1/3) social assets scale scores. Likewise, the subjects who
had the greater increases in total hope scores during hand-mouth
approximation, as compared to when their hands were at their sides,
tended to be those subjects who had the lower social assets scale
scores (t= -2.21, N=12, p<.05, one tail).

(iv) When the subjects had their hands at their
sides (position A), significant negative correlations of their hope
scale scores occurred with total anxiety (r= -0.64, p<.002), guilt anx
iety (r= -0.67, p<.001), diffuse anxiety (r= -0.62, p<.003) total
hostility outward (r= -0.55, p<.01), and overt hostility outward
scores (r= -0.51, p<.02). Significant positive correlations occurred
between their hope scale scores and object relations scores (r=0.86,
p<.001) while their hands were at their sides.[2] Studies of intercorrelations between these scores of psychological states among
other samples of subjects, including both adults (Gottschalk & Gleser,
1969; Gottschalk, 1974) and children (Gottschalk, 1974; Gottschalk,
1976) also reveal similar significant correlations when subjects are

---

[2] Intercorrelations between these various psychological dimensions were
calculated for each of the two conditions A and B. Since two verbal
samples were elicited from each subject per condition, these intercorrelations were based on the sum of the scale scores or the sum of each
of the subscale scores for the two verbal samples per condition.

not caressing their lips. When subjects in the present study changed
their hand position and caressed their lips with a finger (position
B), all these significant correlations disappeared, that is, became
nonsignificant, except for the negative correlation between hope
scores and overt hostility outward (r=-0.45, p< .05).

(v) When the subjects held their hands at their
sides (position A), their object relations scale scores correlated
significantly negatively with total anxiety scores (r=-0.51, p <.02)
and guilt anxiety scores (r= -0.51, p<.02). When these same subjects
fingered their lips (position B), no correlations occurred between
object relation and total anxiety scores (r=-0.06) or guilt anxiety
scores (r=-0.06).

(vi) Four of the subjects consistently made a pre-
ponderance of references to objects of all kinds (animate and inanimate) associated with positive affects while fingering their lips
(0.91 $\pm$ 0.33), and four other subjects consistently voiced more
negative feelings (0.37 $\pm$ 0.18; t=5.14, p <.02) associated with
verbal reference to objects while lip stroking. Three out of the
four subjects with increased object relations scores during lip
stroking (hand position B) also had more references to women during
hand position B than during hand position A. These three subjects,
one male and two females, had similar quantitative changes in their
references to objects while lip stroking as did the psychoanalytic
patient studied by Gottschalk (1974). Three (all males) of the four
subjects who had decreased object relations scores during lip stroking had fewer references to women during this hand position (B).

(vii) Male-female differences. Women made significantly more verbal references than men (t= -2.42, N=20, p<.05, two-
tail) to the self or others getting or receiving help, advice,
support, sustenance, confidence, esteem (Hope Scale content category H-1) when their hands were at their sides. Females had significantly more references than males to food when their hands were
at their sides (t=2.26, N=20, p <.05). Males had more references
to food than females while they were lightly rubbing their lips
(t= -2.40, N=20, p<.05, two-tail). Finally, there were significantly
more oral anatomical references by both sexes during hand-mouth approximation than with hands at sides (t=-2.20, N=20, p <.05, two-tail).

(viii) There was more likely to be an increase in
hope scale scores when subjects fingered their lips if the subjects
had lower Social Assets scale scores; they had been breast fed; they
did not chew their fingernails; they rarely got cold or canker sores
around the mouth.

Additional Results. Further analysis of data obtained in our
study of 20 subjects, 10 males and 10 females, had revealed the following additional, heretofore unpublished, findings.

RELATIONSHIP BETWEEN HOSTILITY OUTWARD SCORES AND HAND ACTIVITY

Freedman et al. (1972, 1973), doing natural and nonexperimental studies, noted that hand movements involving the body (body-focused hand movements) were associated with increased covert hostility outward content analysis scores and, moreover, that hand movements involving objects external to the speaker (object-focused hand movements) were associated with increased overt hostility outward scores derived from their speech. These findings prompted our examining whether, in an experimental situation, there was an increase in covert hostility outward scores in the speech of our subjects while they caressed their lips as compared to when they positioned their hands at their sides.

There were no significant differences between average overt hostility outward or covert hostility outward scores and hand activity when the subjects' hands were at sides or fingering their lips.

SHAME AND GUILT ANXIETY (SUPER EGO OR EGO IDEAL CONSTRAINTS) AND LIP FINGERING

The previous natural history study of Gottschalk with a psycho-analytic patient (1974) and the experimental study with 20 subjects in which hand movements were alternated systematically as part of a research design (Gottschalk & Uliana, 1976) indicated that in some individuals caressing one's own lips enhanced an individual's sense of security and evoked positive feelings, possibly by mobilizing pleasant memories of supportive, nurturing women. But some individuals in the experimental study, judging from the content of their speech, apparently were reminded of unpleasant feelings and tended to have fewer thoughts of women when fingering their lips. In these and other subjects who were not soothed and supported by lip fingering, did such activity in an experimental situation arouse super-ego and ego-ideal constraints and inhibitions against openly and publicly indulging in oral pleasures? Some support for this conclusion seems to be available in the finding of an average increase in the number of references in the speech of the 20 subjects, when fingering their lips, to not wanting to be favored, blessed, or rewarded (Hope Scale category item H-5, $0.08 \pm .09$ with hand position A versus 0.17 ± 0.2 with hand position B; $p < .08$, two-tail). Accordingly, several analyses were carried out examining various relationships occurring between shame and guilt anxiety and lip fingering.

There was a nonsignificant interaction effect between sex and hand position ($p < .10$ by analysis of variance) such that lip fingering was associated with an increase in shame anxiety scores in males as predicted ($t=-1.59$, $N=10$, $p < .10$) and with a decrease in shame anxiety scores in females (See Table 2).

Table 2

Effect of Hand Position and
Sex on Shame Anxiety Scores

Hand Position	Males (N=10)	Females (N=10)
A	0.65 $\pm$0.33	0.79 0.41
B	0.85 $\pm$0.39	0.70 $\pm$0.30

Average shame anxiety scores of both sexes showed no significant difference under the two hand positions, namely, hands at sides (0.72 $\pm$ 0.37) and at lips (0.77 $\pm$ 0.35). The same is true of average guilt anxiety scores under the two hand conditions.

An attempt was made to test the psychodynamic hypothesis that the subjects who had the least amount of increased hopefulness during lip fingering were individuals who had higher amounts of guilt or shame. The 20 subjects were divided into a subgroup of the six subjects whose hope scores increased the most during lip fingering, as compared to when they had their hands at their side, and a subgroup of six subjects whose hope scores increased the least during lip fingering. Neither guilt anxiety scores nor shame anxiety scores showed any significant differences in these two subgroups.

The six subjects with the highest average shame anxiety scores and the six subjects with the lowest average shame anxiety scores derived from speech samples given during lip fingering (hand position B) were identified. The six subjects with the highest shame anxiety scores showed an average increase in negative valences associated with references to objects during lip fingering as compared to the position when hands were at the sides (B-A= -0.05 $\pm$ 0.48), whereas the six subjects with the lowest shame anxiety scores showed, on the average, a decrease in negative valences associated with references to objects with lip fingering (B-A=0.38 $\pm$ 0.73). The difference in these mean change scores for negative valences associated with object references was statistically significant (t=2.47; p <.05, two-tail, see Table 3). No significant differences in change scores occurred in other components of the Object Relations scale scores (positive valences and references to males or females) or Hope scale scores in these high and low shame anxiety groups of subjects.

Table 3

Differences of Responses in Speech Content to
Lip Fingering in High and Low Shame Anxiety Subjects

Subject #	Shame Anxiety Scores	Changes (B-A) in Negative Valences (Feelings) Associated with Object References During Lip Fingering (B) as Compared to Hands at Side (A)
11	1.49	-0.31
12	1.30	-0.58
4	1.25	0.16
3	0.99	-0.99
5	0.99	-0.18
1	0.98	-1.09
13	0.51	-0.36
14	0.49	1.67
10	0.45	0.10
18	0.38	0.17
17	0.27	0.75
19	0.22	-0.04

EVIDENCES OF SEXUAL DIFFERENCES IN THE PSYCHODYNAMIC EFFECTS OF
LIP FINGERING

Previous data analysis revealed that lip fingering eliminated
significant negative correlations between various affect scores
(anxiety and hostility) and hope scale and positive object relations
scores. We wondered whether these intercorrelations as well as the
dynamic effect of lip fingering were uniform across the sexes. Hence
possible sexual differences in these intercorrelations were analyzed
with the following results:

Males, while they had their hands at their sides, had significant positive correlations between separation anxiety scores and
verbal references to inanimate objects with neutral valence (r=0.69,
p<.03), to all inanimate objects regardless of valence (r=0.69,
p<.03) and to total negative valences, but no significant correlations occurred between any components of the Object Relations scale
and guilt or shame anxiety scores, whereas, when fingering their
lips, males lost all significant correlations between separation
anxiety and any kinds of verbal references to inanimate objects or
negative valences. But they developed significant negative correlations between guilt anxiety scores and references to males with

positive valence (r=-0.69, p<.03), references to females with neutral valence (r=-0.67, p<.03), to females with all valences (r=-0.66,
p<.041), and references to inanimate objects with negative valence
(r=0.69, p<.03). No correlations occurred between shame anxiety
scores and object relations.

     Females, while holding their hands at their sides, had a signi-
ficant negative correlation between separation anxiety scores and
references to males with positive valence (r=-0.63, p<.05); and a
significant negative correlation between guilt anxiety scores and
references to others with neutral valence, regardless of gender
(r=-0.64, p<.05); a significant positive correlation between guilt
anxiety scores and references to other females with negative feelings
(r=0.95, p<.001), and a significant positive correlation between
shame anxiety scores and references to females with negative feelings
(r=0.69, p<.03), whereas, while fingering their lips, females had
significant positive correlations between separation anxiety scores
and references to inanimate objects with negative feelings (r=0.68,
p<.03); and between guilt anxiety scores and references to positive
feelings towards males (r=0.70, p<.03). No significant correlations
occurred among the women while fingering their lips, between shame
anxiety scores and any components of the object relations scale
content categories.

     Significant correlations of males and females, taken separately,
between hostility scores and all components of the object relations
scale content categories during the two different hand positions,
showed numerous changes, including reversals. They will not be detailed here.

     There were no significant effects produced among either males or
females on the magnitude of positive affects or valences by lip
fingering as compared to the hands-at-side position.

DISCUSSION

     Our studies indicate that there are individual differences with
respect to the effects of hand-mouth activity on speech content and,
by extension, mental events, including perceptions and the evocation
of memories. Though lip fingering significantly reduced the average
rate of speech of 20 subjects, five subjects spoke an increased number of words over a five-minute period. Though lip fingering evoked
evidence of positive, optimistic, pleasurable feelings in a few
people, other individuals had negative and unpleasant feelings during
such motor activity. Some individuals were induced to speak more
hopefully during lip caressing, whereas, others were not so affected.

     What are the reasons for these individual differences and for the
capacity of some of us to be soothed and comforted by our touching a
part of our facial anatomy, and others to be unaffected or, even, to

to have negative responses?

Developmental psychology, learning theory, and clinical psychoanalytic theory would, in general, be in agreement that a person's
childhood experience and later past history could likely account for
these differences. There is supportive evidence from our studies
that past experience can account, in part, for the variety of responses to hand-mouth movements.

Individuals with a past history of relative childhood psychosocial deprivation (lower social assets Scale scores), including,
less satisfactory parenting, limited education, and so forth, were
among the group of subjects having significantly greater increases
in hope scores during lip fingering than subjects with higher social
assets scores. Likewise, subjects who had been breast fed and who
did not have the history of chewing their fingernails were more
likely than others to have an increase in hope scores when fingering
their lips.

There is always a possibility of constitutional or genetic factors playing a part in the kind of response of an individual to lip
fingering or any other kinesic activity. Our studies in this area
were not well designed to examine such a possibility. A few leads
can be derived from our findings that may be pertinent.

Subjects who rarely got cold or canker sores around the mouth
were more likely to have an increase in hope scale scores when fingering their lips. Since cold or canker sores are a result of a
localized infection with the herpes simplex virus, such a finding
would seem to point to the involvement of a genetic factor. However,
this virus is ubiquitous and it typically finds a nidus for localized
infection with localized trauma. The common cold, dental work, lip
biting, pipe smoking, and so forth can trigger the onset of cold or
canker sores around the mouth. While it is understandable by someone
with cold sores around the mouth may not enjoy or be soothed with lip
rubbing, it is not so clear why such a person would be predisposed
not to enjoy lip rubbing when no oral cold sores are present. Also,
if lip sucking, biting, or chewing-- which behavior can itself lead to
oral cold sores--were genetically determined (which is highly ques-
tionable), then perhaps we would have some evidence.

Male-female differences in response to lip fingering could be
seen as evidence of a biological factor accounting for varying responses to lip caressing. We found that males had significantly
($p < .05$) more references to food than females when lip fingering.
Also, males tended to have more shame anxiety than females ($p < .10$)
when fingering their lips. And females gave significantly more verbal references to getting or receiving help, advice, support, or
esteem than males when their hands were at their sides, and away from
their lips. But many aspects of sexual role are learned in our

society (Money, 1955; Stoller, 1968) and sex differences in behavioral responses cannot be automatically attributed to hereditary factors and/or hormonal differences.

Response differences, to kinesic activity, such as lip fingering, could result not only from unmet dependency needs in childhood, but also from adult inculcations and warnings that certain kinds of hand-body activity are taboo. We are much more familiar in the clinical literature with case histories of the sexual inhibitions and associated neuroses resulting presumably from parental disapproval of hand-genital stimulation. Lip and nose fingering and finger sucking are often subjected to parental ridicule and scolding. We could not establish, however, that average shame or guilt anxiety scores were significantly different in our subjects under the different hand conditions. But we did note that significant negative correlations between hope and object relations scores with anxiety and hostility scores derived from content analysis of speech when hands were at one's side tended to disappear completely with lip fingering. This suggests that our research design, permitting and requiring public lip fingering as it did, may have provided a partial sanction to dissociate old taboos and, hence, shame or guilt, from feelings of hopefulness and optimism.

Studies of psychokinesics should distinguish between natural science and experimental observations. Most research workers in the area of kinesics, that is, nonverbal behavior, choose the natural science method over the experimental method. Examples of the natural science method, stemming from a psychoanalytic orientation, are the studies of Deutsch (1966) and Scheflen (1966). Deutsch has been credited with catalyzing the awakening interest in body communication. He found, in the patient's gestures and postures, evidence for underlying drives and defenses. To a large extent, he perceived a one-to-one relationship between a gesture and underlying drive and/or defense. The evidence for Deutsch's system for interpreting kinesics consisted of its plausibility, internal coherence, and consistency with some aspects of psychoanalytic theory. For Scheflen, however, matters were more complicated. He held that only rarely was the meaning of a single gesture clear, and then only in the simplest instances, as in pointing out directions to a location. Scheflen noted complex patterns of communication in which the body language was one element, and to be understood, it must be considered in its complicated interaction with the patient's verbal behavior. Deutsch believed that nonverbal behavior frequently took the place of verbal behavior or customarily did so, for example, in expressing unconscious, unverbalized drives or defenses. How one might objectively validate that a gesture or posture represented a deeply unconscious mental event was never elaborated, except on the basis of plausibility and internal consistency. Scheflen was more likely to study a piece of nonverbal behavior and fit it into a larger pattern of communication extending over as

long as 15 minutes. Hence, he was more likely to see the nonverbal
behavior as mirroring, emphasizing, or otherwise modulating the
semantic or paralanguage facets of the communication process.

The work of Freedman and his co-workers (Freedman et al., 1972;
Grand et al., 1973) continues the line of inquiry of Deutsch and
Scheflen as sophisticated natural science research in psychokinesis.
The investigations of these workers adds scientific rigor and the
application of the mathematical assessment of data of observation to
the intuition and breadth of these earlier workers. The present conference on "Communicative Structures and Psychic Structures" organized by Norbert Freedman is a culmination of the stimulation and contributions of this group to the field.

While the natural science approach to this field of inquiry has
predominated, the experimental approach has been used occasionally.
Experimental studies, involving manipulation of independent variables
such as total body, face, or extremity movements, while dependent
variables such as speech content or other behavioral or physiological
variables are recorded, have been avoided. This avoidance has been
based on the notion that the experimental method would be "artificial"
and because the methodological and theoretical problems using the
experimental method are difficult and challenging.

The use of the experimental method in the present report to
supplement and pursue unanswerable questions arising from a natural
science study, specifically, a therapeutic psychoanalysis, is one way
in which the two methodological approaches may fruitfully interdigi-
tate to add scientific information in the area of psychokinesis. In
so doing, we must remind ourselves that one method is not a simple
substitute for the other. The findings that prevail under the conditions of a natural science approach may not obtain under the conditions of the experimental method and vice versa. And, unfortunately,
one cannot freely generalize that what scientific discoveries are established in one kind of situation, be it experimental or psychoanalytic, necessarily apply to another situation.

What advice or guidelines can basic research of the kind here in
psychokinesics offer the practicing psychotherapist? The surest advice, I am afraid, is almost banal but now carries the weight of new,
hard empirical data from the present study and others: do not ignore
but carefully watch what your patient is doing with gestures, postures
and other body movements while talking. When the question arises,
what do the body movements mean, we do not seem to have come much beyond the level of understanding of Deutsch and Scheflen. Some specific movements do, as Deutsch suggested, tend to signify specific
things. On the other hand, as Scheflen insisted, the message of any
specific body movement may change in varying communication contexts
and settings. Body movements may influence the psychodynamic interrelationships between speech content in such a way that the inter-

correlations between the magnitude of certain affects and other psychological states may be enhanced or diminished among a group of subjects. There is no simple formula that has been discovered for discerning the precise effects of such kinesic-psychological activities within one individual. Knowing what these interrelationships are for one individual will not necessarily help predict what they will be within another individual. The main solution to this problem is to keep an eye on your patient and try to learn his inner formula which he also needs to learn and understand. Remember that a significant correlation between some aspects of his verbal associations and body position can disappear when he moves, for example, his fingers to lips. In this connection, other studies examining various psychosomatic relationships have revealed that a diuretic drug used in the treatment of essential hypertension (hydrochlorothiazide) can eliminate the significant correlation between hostility outward (content analysis) scores and blood pressure (Gottschalk et al., 1964), and that marihuana smoking can cancel the usually significant relationship between certain affect (content analysis) scores and various hemodynamic variables (Gottschalk et al., 1976). That a non-drug event, lip fingering, can also terminate usually significant psychodynamic correlations in the speech of subjects, indicates the potency of some such body movements.

What are the implications of our findings as applied to the measurement of psychological states whether by self-report, rating scale, or content analysis procedures? Our findings raise the question whether kinesic activities, such as hand-body touching, modify the empirical phenomena on which assessments are made by these various measurement procedures. We believe it is likely that such kinesic activities add to the error variance occurring in such measurements.

REFERENCES

Deutsch, F. Some principles of correlating verbal and nonverbal communication. In L. A. Gottschalk & A. H. Auerbach (Eds.), Methods of research in psychotherapy. New York: Appleton-Century-Crofts, 1966.

Freedman, N., O'Hanlon, J., Oltman, P., & Witkin, H. A. The imprint of psychological differentiation on kinetic behavior in varying communicative contexts. Journal of Abnormal Psychology, 1972, 79:239-258.

Gleser, G. C., Gottschalk, L. A., & Springer, K. J. An anxiety scale applicable to verbal samples. Archives of General Psychiatry, 1961, 5:593-605.

Gottschalk, L. A. A hope scale applicable to verbal samples. Archives of General Psychiatry, 1974, 30:779-785. (a)

Gottschalk, L. A. The psychoanalytic study of hand–mouth approximations. In L. Goldberger & V. H. Rosen (Eds.), Vol. 3, Psychoanalysis and Contemporary Science. New York: International Universities
Press, 1974. (b)

Gottschalk, L. A. Drug effects and the assessment of affective states
in man. In W. B. Essman & L. Valzelli (Eds.), Current developments
in psychopharmacology. Chapter 8. New York: Spectrum Publications,
1975.

Gottschalk, L. A. Childrens speech as a source of data toward the
measurement of psychological states. Journal of Youth and Adolescence, 1976, 5:11–36.

Gottschalk, L. A., Aronow, W. S., & Prakash, R. Effects of marijuana
and placebo-marijuana smoking on psychological state and on psychophysiological cardiovascular functioning in anginal patients. (To
be published, 1976.)

Gottschalk, L. A., Biener, R., Bates, D., & Syben, M. Depression,
hope, and social assets. Unpublished study, 1974.

Gottschalk, L. A., Biener, R., Noble, E. P., Birch, H., Wilbert, D.
E., & Heiser, J. F. Thioridazine plasma levels and clinical response. Comprehensive Psychiatry, 1975, 16:323–337.

Gottschalk, L. A. & Gleser, G. C. The measurement of psychological
states through the content analysis of verbal behavior. Berkeley:
University of California Press, 1969.

Gottschalk, L. A., Gleser, G. C., D'Zmura, T., & Hanenson, I. B.
Some psychophysiological relationships in hypertensive women. The
effect of hydrochlorothiazide on the relation of affect to blood
pressure. Psychosomatic Medicine, 1964, 26:610–617.

Gottschalk, L. A., Gleser, G. C., & Springer, K. J. Three hostility
scales applicable to verbal samples. Archives of General Psychiatry
1963, 9:254–279.

Gottschalk, L. A. & Hambidge, G., Jr. Verbal behavior analysis: A
systematic approach to the problem of quantifying. Journal of
Projective Techniques, 1955, 19:387–409.

Gottschalk, L. A., Kaplan, S. M., Gleser, G. C., & Winget, C. N.
Variations in magnitude of emotion: A method applied to anxiety
and hostility during phases of the menstrual cycle. Psychosomatic
Medicine, 1962, 24:300–311.

Gottschalk, L. A., Springer, K. J., & Gleser, G. C. Experiments with a method of assessing the variations in intensity of certain psychological states occurring during two psychotherapeutic interviews. In L. A. Gottschalk (Ed.), Comparative psychoanalysis of two psychotherapeutic interviews. New York: International Universities Press, 1961.

Gottschalk, L. A. & Uliana, R. A study of the relationship of nonverbal to verbal behavior: Effect of lip caressing on hope and oral references as expressed in the content of speech. In P. H. Ornstein & S. M. Kaplan (Eds.), Memos to Maury, Vol. II. Comprehensive Psychiatry, 1976, 17:135-152.

Grand, S., Freedman, N., & Steingart, I. A study of the representation of objects in schizophrenia. Journal of the American Psychoanalytic Association, 1973, 21:399-434.

Ivey, M. & Bardwick, J. M. Patterns of affective fluctuation in the menstrual cycle. Psychosomatic Medicine, 1968, 30:336-348.

Money, J., Hampson, J. G., & Hampson, J. L. Hermaphroditism: Recommendations concerning assignment of sex, change of sex, and psychologic management. Bulletin Johns Hopkins Hospital, 1955, 97: 284-300.

Silbergeld, S., Brast, N., & Noble, E. P. The menstrual cycle: A double-blind study of mood, behavior, and biochemical variables with Enovid and a placebo. Psychosomatic Medicine, 1971, 33:411-428.

Stoller, R. J. Sex and gender: The development of masculinity and femininity. New York: Science House, 1968.

Schedule 1

Questionnaire Regarding Oral History

NAME_____   DATE_____

1. Do you know whether you were bottle or breast fed as an infant?
   A. _____Breast
   B. _____Bottle
   C. _____Both breast and bottle
   D. _____Don't know

2. How long were you on the breast and/or bottle?
   _____ 0- 3 months
   _____ 4- 8 months
   _____ 9-12 months
   _____13-18 months
   _____19-23 months
   _____24 or more

3. Have you had any dental or gum problems?
   _____When? _____What kind? (Please mention specifically)

4. Have you had any oral injuries, blemishes, diseases, or oral
   surgery?
   _____Yes _____No _____When? _____What kind?

5. When you're nervous do you tend to eat?
   _____More? _____Less? _____Eating habits do not change

6. Did you ever chew your finger nails? _____Yes _____No
   _____Often _____Little _____Not at all

7. Do you still bite your nails? _____Yes _____No
   _____Often _____Little _____Not at all

8. Do you chew pencils or toothpicks?
   _____Often _____Little _____Not at all

9. Do you have difficulty talking freely with (Please circle)
   Friends, Parents, Students, Teachers, Employers, Intimates?

10. Did you ever stutter or stammer? _____Yes _____No
    If so, was it _____Mild _____Moderate _____Severe

11. Do you like tart foods as much as sweet flavored ones?
    _____Yes _____No

12. Do you get a lot of cold sores or canker sores in or around the mouth?

_____Rarely _____Once in a while _____Often

13. Do you smoke cigarettes, cigars, or a pipe? (Circle which one)

_____Yes _____No

14. If you do smoke, how often?

_____Daily _____Weekly _____Monthly _____Not at all

15. Do you chew tobacco? _____Yes _____No

_____Often _____Little _____Not at all

16. Do you smoke marijuana? _____Yes _____No

17. How often have you used marijuana in the past 12 months?

_____Not at all
_____Daily
_____Several times a week
_____Several times a month
_____About once a month
_____Less than once a month

18. How often have you used alcohol in the past 12 months?

_____Not at all
_____Daily
_____Several times a week
_____Several times a month
_____Once a month
_____Less than once a month

19. Do you usually drink?

_____Wine _____Beer _____Whiskey _____Gin _____Other

20. On the average, how many drinks do you have when you drink?

_____One _____Two _____Three _____Four _____More than four

21. When you're nervous do you tend to smoke?

_____More _____Less _____Not at all

22. Do you have any other oral habits, problems, difficulties, or taboos that have not been mentioned so far? ___Yes ___No

Please specify_____

Schedule 2

Classification of Oronasal Functions and Activities

NAME_____   DATE_____

A. Oral functions and activities

B. Oral anatomical references

C. Nonfood objects or substances placed on lips or in mouth

D. Food references and references to other substances ingested

E. Speech references

F. Oral diseases

G. Words referring to taste, appetite, smells, hunger, thirst

H. Nasal functions and activities

I. Nasal anatomical references

ACTION, FANTASY AND LANGUAGE: DEVELOPMENTAL LEVELS OF EGO

ORGANIZATION IN COMMUNICATING DRIVES AND AFFECTS

Sebastiano Santostefano

Harvard University Medical School

Cambridge, Massachusetts

Laboratory studies were conducted in an attempt to operational-
ize and explore the developmental interrelations among action, fantasy, and language behaviors conceptualized as ego modes which regulate and communicate drives and affects. These studies, and the developmental model they suggest, were used as a lens through which the
analysis of a latency boy was examined, in order to gather longitudinal data that explore the model further. The laboratory data and
the analytic case are related to theoretical questions concerning
personality development and to analytic technique with children.

INTRODUCTION

     In addition to the stress psychoanalytic theory has placed upon
the instinctual life of an individual, emphasis since the 1940's has
been given to ego apparatuses by which instinctual tensions are mastered. In these writings, the construct ego is viewed as a set of
behavioral-cognitive structures which channel, selectively regulate,
control, and render socially adaptive and appropriate expressions of
drives and affects. Moreover, in this view, organizational modes of
ego behaviors such as activity, fantasy, and language are distinguished
and seen as following a developmental course (Hartmann, 1958; Ekstein &
Friedman, 1957; Freud, 1965; Schafer, 1973, 1976). Stated broadly, the
psychoanalytic view of ego modes proposes that, early in development,
the individual is fused to objects in his environment, responds immediately in action, and in socially inappropriate ways (little reality
testing). With differentiation of self from world, and with the growing capacity to delay, the individual gradually articulates himself
from the environment, postpones action, and develops the capacity to
employ fantasy and language as substitutive modes to achieve the same
end.

While this hypothesis has received support from clinical observations made in the treatment situation, it has not been subjected to systematic study in the laboratory. Accordingly, I became interested in devising experiments that would test the proposed developmental progression of action, fantasy, and spoken language as ego modes expressing drives. To accomplish this, it was necessary first to construct operational definitions of each mode, of maturation within a mode, and of developmental shifts from one mode to the next, so that appropriate laboratory methods could be constructed.

This task, I felt, would be facilitated if experimentally based advances in cognitive development were integrated with clinically based concepts of psychoanalytic ego psychology. Werner, Piaget, and their students propose that, with development, the individual gradually articulates himself from the environment and develops the capacity to employ substitutive means to achieve the same end, and to accept alternative goals as satisfying the same mean. Because of this availability of multiple means and alternative goals, the individual is free from the demands of the immediate situation, having now the capacity to express cognitive behavior in more delayed, planned, indirect, and organized terms. Applied to cognitive development, cognitive activity is dominated first by sensorimotor behaviors; with further development, perceptual-ideational activity emerges from this action base and dominates; then, conceptual-representational cognitive activity emerges from this action base and dominates and finally, conceptual-representational cognitive activity emerges and dominates the functioning of the developmentally mature individua

The cognitive-operational concepts of alternative means and ends of self-object distance, and of delay, if applied to the issue of communicating drives, enables us to define further, in more operational terms, developmental change within ego modes of action, fantasy, and language. For example, consider a five-year old boy who punches his infant sib, and later covers him with bath powder from head to foot. Both behaviors would be viewed as alternative means for expressing aggression towards the same goal. Punching is more direct (there is person-person contact with the goal) and shows little delay. Sprinkling powder is less direct (there is some physical distance between the boy and his sib), and more delayed (it takes some time to shake the powder from the can). The concept of directness and delay, then, can be operationalized to distinguish systematically and developmentally between _forms_ or _means_ by which ego modes express drives.

Similarly, consider a five-year-old boy who punches his infant sib and punches a toy belonging to his infant sib. The child is now using alternative ends or goals (sib and toy) to satisfy the same mean. As a goal, the sib represents directness and little delay, and the toy more indirectness and delay. The same operational concepts of directness and delay, then, can also be used to distinguish among goals used to satisfy the same drive. Lastly, a five-year old

boy could punch the toy belonging to his infant sib, fantasy punching his sib, or shout, "I'll smash you," a series of modes (action,
fantasy, and language) that could be distinguished in terms of revealing different degrees of directness and delay.

By integrating, in this fashion, the organismic view of cognitive development with psychoanalytic hypotheses of ego modes of action, fantasy, and language, a developmental scheme could be formulated and used to guide the construction of test methods and questions for experimental study. At this point, we turn first to a
brief review of a developmental model of ego expressions of drives
and affects. Following this, test methods devised based on this
model, and some findings obtained with them, are discussed.

DEVELOPMENTAL MODEL OF EGO MODES FOR EXPRESSING DRIVES AND AFFECTS

(1) Action, fantasy, and language systems of responding (i.e.,
modalities) represent alternative means for expressing the same drive
or affect.

(2) The transition from action, to fantasy, to language responses, as alternative means for drive expression, is determined by
two simultaneously occuring, and complementary, regulating processes:
(a) differentiation and subsequent distancing of the individual from
the drive-satisfying goal-object; and (b) differentiation and subsequent distancing of the motoric-action modality from the goal object. The young child should be characterized more by motoric expressions of drives, and less by fantasy and language. Gradually,
the action system becomes integrated within and subordinated by the
fantasy system which emerges. With further development, fantasy and
action expressions become subordinated by, and integrated within, the
language system which dominates. Thus, early modalities are not replaced by later developing systems, but remain potentially active so
that, at each point in development, they codetermine subsequent structures which develop to express drives.

(3) Development within each modality also follows a transition
from lack of differentiation to articulation and integration. At an
early stage of development, the individual shows direct, immediate,
and less socialized drive expressions within a modality, while the
more developed individual shows detoured, delayed, controlled and
socially approved forms.

(4) In the developmentally mature individual, all three modalities are potentially available. Changes in environmental conditions
and expectations, and/or shifts in the emotional-psychological state
of the individual, could cause him to revert, temporarily, to a developmentally more primitive modality for expressing motives, or to a
more primitive level within a modality (regression), or to higher levels (progression).

(5) These propositions are qualified by the following assumptions: (a) The behavioral modalities specified by the proposed
model (i.e., acting upon objects; constructing mental images or
fantasies of action, and speaking language) appear in development
long before each is used as an effective instrument for expressing
drives; (b) Developing increased capacity for delay, constructing
multiple means for expressing a motive, and using multiple goal objects towards which expressions are directed, enables the individuals
to meet environmental expectations economically, while satisfying
unique motivational needs, sparing him the frustration of having his
discharge blocked, and the task of constructing anew each opportunity
for discharge; (c) Motoric, fantasy, and language structures used to
express drives are acquired through learning from, identifying with,
and internalizing the standards of parents and other ego ideals (Schafer, 1967); (d) Poor coordination between the environment's restrictions and opportunities and the child's capacity for delay and for
constructing means-ends alternatives results in the formation of deviant (pathological) structures of motive expression (e.g., fixation
in the action mode; premature dominance of fantasy); (e) Lastly,
several formal characteristics distinguishing the three modalities
should be noted. Action expressions of a drive involve physically
manipulating a drive-satisfying object. Fantasy expressions are less
direct, since the individual now "manipulates" an image or symbol of
the goal rather than the goal itself. Fantasy is also more delayed,
since contact with the actual goal is postponed at least for the duration of the fantasy. The language modality is distinguished by its
use of socially shared words and symbols that are directed to reality
(unlike the private symbols of fantasies). Moreover, a spoken word
does not physically resemble its referent, whereas an image in fantasy
does, literally or symbolically (e.g., the spoken or written word,
"stab," bears no resemblance to the act of stabbing).[1]

LABORATORY STUDIES OF THE DEVELOPMENTAL RELATIONS AMONG ACTION, FAN-
TASY, AND LANGUAGE BEHAVIORS

Methods of assessment

When this conceptual model is used as a guide to construct laboratory methods, it becomes clear that test procedures should be devised which assess levels of behavioral expressions within each of
the three modalities, and which also assess the relative dominance
of one over the other. Moreover, the model emphasizes that the tests
constructed capture three particular characteristics of behavior:
degree of directness, degree of delay; and degree of social appropriateness. We will consider here as illustrations only methods develope

---

[1]These distinctions among modalities by psychoanalytic ego psychology
have some relation to those proposed by Piaget between signs and symbols, and by Bruner between enactive, ikonic, and symbolic stages of
representation. (See Rapaport, 1967.)

to assess expressions of the aggressive drive.[2]

Three tests were devised to assess aggression in each modality:
the Miniature Situations Test to assess the action mode; the Structured Fantasy Test to assess the fantasy mode; and the Continuous
Word Association Test to assess the language mode. In addition,
two tests were devised to assess the relations among the three ego
modalities. The Action Versus Fantasy Test was constructed to assess whether action behaviors or fantasy behaviors dominate in the
expression of drives. The Action Versus Fantasy Versus Language Test
was constructed to assess whether action, fantasy, or language behaviors dominate in the expression of drives. The methods were constructed and scaled with a common rationale. Within each behavioral modality, immature genetic levels were defined by direct and immediate action, fantasy, or language behaviors. More mature genetic levels were
defined by indirect and delayed action, fantasy, or language behaviors.
With procedures assessing multiple modalities simultaneously, action
behaviors were viewed as most direct and immediate, fantasy behaviors
as less direct and more delayed, and language behaviors as most indirect and delayed. To permit statistical analysis of the test responses observed, numbers were assigned to each behavioral expression,
a low number to behaviors that are the most direct and the least delay, and high numbers to behaviors that are the most indirect and delayed.

The Miniature Situations Test. With this procedure, the child
is told that he will be given three games to play, that he will play
all three, and that he should perform first the game he wants to play
most, and then perform the others accordingly. He is urged to make
his choices as quickly as possible, and encouraged to make use of
the feelings he experiences when confronted with each set of materials. He is told that there are no right or wrong answers, that
children play all the games, and that the examiner is interested in
the games the child feels like playing. Each of the five structured
play situations that make up the test are viewed as containing three
levels of aggressive actions, from direct and impulsive to indirect
and delayed. For example, with one, the child is presented with
three sheets of paper and a pair of scissors. One of the sheets has
a line drawn across the center. The child is asked to tear the first
sheet of paper, to crumple the second, and to cut the third in half
carefully along the line. The examiner records the sequence in which
the child performs each action, the affects the child reveals, and
the spontaneous comments the child makes. Following each item, the
examiner conducts an inquiry in an attempt to gather the child's associations.

---

[2]The author has reported elsewhere methods developed along the same
conceptual lines to assess expressions of oral drives. These same
reports describe the several procedures in detail and validating data
(Santostefano, 1965a and b, 1968, 1970, 1971).

The Structured Fantasy Test. With this procedure, four pictures are placed before the child. One of the pictures constitutes the beginning of a story or fantasy which the examiner provides. The child is told that the other pictures show three possible events that could follow. It is further explained that all three are possible, that the child should select, first, the picture that shows what he imagines most likely happens, and then to select the other pictures accordingly. For example, with one item, the child is told, "This boy found a dog with a hurt paw. What do you imagine happened to the dog? Did another dog bite his paw; did a porcupine stick the dog's paw with needles, or did the dog step on a stone?" After the child makes his selections, the examiner conducts an inquiry in an attempt to gather the child's associations to the fantasy.

Continuous Word Association Test. With this procedure, the examiner asks the child to say aloud every word that comes to mind, after hearing the stimulus word, and until the examiner says, "Stop" (after 60 seconds). To assess expressions of the aggressive drive in the language mode, the stimulus word "knife" is used. It is assumed that this word arouses the aggressive drive, and that the words associated and spoken by the child represent language expressions of aggression. The words that the child speaks are rated as aggressive or nonaggressive in their content. To evaluate the aggressive words associated in terms of genetic levels, a low numerical score is assigned to words that convey direct, forceful acts of aggression, the consequences of such acts, and intense emotional states (e.g., kill, blood, scream), and higher numerical scores are assigned to words which describe attenuated, delayed, indirect aggressive acts (e.g., chip, peel).

Action Versus Fantasy Test. With this procedure, test materials are arrayed behind two screens. With one item, the examiner locates a toy bulldozer and a tower of blocks behind one screen, and behind the other, a picture of a worker operating a bulldozer and toppling a building. The child is told, "You can knock down a building of blocks with a toy bulldozer, or you can look at a picture of someone knocking down a building with a bulldozer and imagine what's going on." When the child completes his response, the examiner conducts an inquiry to gather associations stimulated by the game.

The Action Versus Fantasy Versus Language Test. This procedure parallels the preceeding test, and includes the language mode as an alternative means of expressing aggression, in addition to action and fantasy. Three screens are set before the child. Behind one are play materials the child can use to perform an aggressive act; behind the other is a picture of someone performing that aggressive act, and behind the third is a microphone into which the child speaks a word expressing that aggressive act.

Study I: Age Differences in Action, Fantasy, and Language Expressions of Aggression (Eichler, 1971)[3]

One study was designed to test the hypothesis concerning developmental differences in expressing aggression within each mode and between modes.   The five procedures were administered to 72 boys, 24 at each of three age levels: six, eight, and 10 years.   All of the children were Caucasian and had no known physical or psychological difficulties.   They were of average or better intelligence as assessed by formal testing (Mean I.Q. for each group approximately 109), and they represented both high and low socioeconomic families.   The children were administered the tests individually in a clinic office, and the sequence of items within each test and the sequence of tests were counter-balanced for each age group.

Let us first consider the age trends observed within each of the three modalities assessed.   With the Miniature Situations Test, six-year-olds more often performed the direct, immediate aggressive actions first; for example, they tore paper first, then crumpled paper, and later cut paper with a pair of scissors.   The 10-year olds more often performed the more indirect, delayed actions first (e.g., they cut the paper first, then crumpled, and later tore the paper), and the eight-year-olds fell between.   The age trend was statistically significant.

With the Structured Fantasy Test, the six-year olds and the eight-year-olds completed the fantasy stories by selecting first pictures that conveyed direct, impulsive aggression.   The 10-year olds tended to select first pictures that conveyed more indirect, delayed expression of fantasied aggression.   The age trend was also statistically significant.

With the Continuous Word Association Test each age group associated the same number of words to both the stimulus word "knife" (used as the aggressive stimulus) and to the word "tree" (used as the control stimulus).   At each age level, then, both stimulus words stimulated the same number of associated words.   Moreover, an age trend was observed with the older child showing a greater capacity to verbalize associated words.

We can now ask the question, does the stimulus word "knife" arouse more associated words which convey aggression than the control word, "tree?"   We found that each group associated significantly more aggressive words to the stimulus word, "knife," than to "tree," supporting the stimulus word knife as effective in arousing language expressions of aggression.   (Each age group associated only about 15%

---

[3]This study was conducted by Eichler (1971) under the writer's supervision as a doctoral thesis.   The reader is referred to Eichler's report for a more complete discussion of the findings.

aggressive words to the stimulus "tree.") Moreover, the older the
child, the greater the number of aggressive words associated to
knife. The age differences were statistically significant.

The aggressive words associated to "knife" by each child were
assigned a developmental ranking, as discussed above, to distinguish
words that convey direct, immediate aggression from words that convey indirect, delayed aggression. The rankings assigned were averaged according to the total number of words the child associated.
We found that although six-year olds associated fewer aggressive
words, the words they verbalized conveyed more direct and impulsive
aggression (e.g., "kill," "smash"). The 10-year-olds, who associated
the greatest number of aggressive words, associated words that conveyed more indirect, delayed expressions of aggression (e.g., "chip,"
"peel"). The eight-year-olds fell between these two groups. The
age differences were statistically significant.

The results with the word association test indicate that the
language mode as an instrument of drive expression is less differentiated in the younger child (fewer aggressive words associated and
verbalized), and is developmentally primitive in organization (the
few words spoken express aggressive tensions in more direct and less
delayed terms). In contrast, the older child showed a more differentiated language mode (many aggressive words associated and verbalized) which, however, is organized in terms of expressing words
that convey delayed, indirect aggressive expressions.

Taken together, the findings with the three procedures support
the psychoanalytic proposition that each ego modality, action, fantasy
and language, follows a developmental progression from more direct,
less delayed behavioral expressions of drives characterizing the
younger child, with more indirect, delayed behavioral expressions
characterizing the older child.

Let us now turn to the question of the relative dominance of
modes at each age level. When given the option of expressing aggression in the action mode or in the fantasy mode (Action versus
Fantasy test), both six-year-olds and eight-year-olds tended to behave through the action mode rather than the fantasy mode. The 10-
year olds showed a tendency for expressing aggression relatively
more often through the fantasy mode rather than the action mode.
When all three behavioral modes are made available, action again dominated as the mode by which six-year-olds expressed aggressive tensions, language dominated more in the expressions of 10-year olds, and
eight-year olds fell between. The trends were statistically significant.[4]

---

[4]These age trends concerning the relations among modalities reached
statistical significance if the order in which the tests were administered is taken into account.

In summary, the findings obtained with procedures assessing multiple modalities support the psychoanalytic hypothesis that early in development the more direct, immediate modality, action dominates in the expression of drives. With development, the more delayed, indirect fantasy mode emerges as dominant, and with further development, language emerges as dominant.[5]

Taken together, this first study provided support for the proposition that aggressive behaviors communicated by means of one modality, or communicated by means of one rather than another modality, define levels ordered in terms of developmental principles of delay and directness.

Study II: The Influence of Action and Fantasy Experiences (Treatments) on Action and Fantasy Ego Modes (Blaisdell, 1972)[6]

From these findings, we turned to study whether progressive and regressive changes might occur, following an aggressive experience, in the ego mode an individual typically uses to express aggression. Specifically, we wondered, if a child showed a tendency to communicate drives through the action mode, what is the influence on the developmental organization of both his action mode and his fantasy mode, if he engages in aggressive actions as a treatment experience? And, what is the influence if he engages in aggressive fantasies as a treatment experience? Similarly, if a child showed the tendency to express drives through the fantasy mode, what is the effect on the developmental organization of both his action mode and fantasy modes if he experiences treatment methods that primarily activate either fantasies or actions?

To select children who tended to express aggression in action or in fantasy, the Action Versus Fantasy Test was administered first to a large number of first and fifth graders. Boys who performed five actions, of the five presented by the test (and no fantasy choices), were accepted as representing an "Action-Oriented" group. Boys who performed four or five of the fantasy choices (and none or only one action) were accepted as representing a "Fantasy-Oriented" group. Ten first graders and 10 fifth graders were located to meet these criteria for each of the groups, resulting in a total sample of 40 children.

---

[5]This report concerns only the sequence of test behaviors observed at each age level. I am reserving for future reports a discussion of the associations children produce at each age level following their engaging the test materials. In general, younger children associated more to harsh superego-related experiences, while older children to experiences that reflect an ego-investment in outer reality and industry.

[6]This study was conducted by Blaisdell (1972) under the writer's supervision as a doctoral thesis. The reader is referred to Blaisdell's report for a more complete discussion of the findings.

About a week following the selection, the child was administered
the Miniature Situations Test to assess the developmental level at
which aggression was expressed in the action mode, and the Structured
Fantasy Test to assess the level at which aggression was expressed
in the fantasy mode. Then each child participated individually in
one of two experimental "treatment" conditions. Half of the Action-
Oriented subjects and half of the Fantasy-Oriented subjects were
randomly assigned to an "action treatment" condition, and half of
both groups to a "fantasy treatment" condition.

In the action treatment condition, the child was invited to perform various aggressive acts on materials (e.g., punching a Bobo clown
for one minute, breaking sticks, striking a sheet of unbreakable glass
with a hammer). With the fantasy treatment condition, the child was
seated in a chair and asked to view a film of the Lewis-Schmelling
1930 boxing match and magazine pictures portraying violence. The
children were asked to watch the film and pictures, and to imagine
what was going on. The duration of each treatment condition was
about 20 minutes. Immediately following the experimental treatment,
each child was readministered the Miniature Situations Test and the
Structured Fantasy Test.

By comparing the child's test performance before and after the
treatment condition, one could explore whether or not a child shifted
in the action and fantasy modes towards expressing more direct and
impulsive aggression or toward more indirect and delayed aggression.
We observed the following. Action-oriented boys, after experiencing
the action treatment condition, shifted in the action mode towards
more indirect and delayed action behaviors. At the same time they
showed a regressive shift in the fantasy mode, expressing more direct and impulsive aggressive fantasies. Fantasy-oriented boys,
after experiencing the fantasy treatment condition, regressed in the
action mode, expressing more direct and impulsive aggressive behavior.
At the same time, they shifted progressively in the fantasy mode, expressing more indirect, delayed aggressive fantasies. In other words,
when the treatment experience was concordant with the child's ego
tendency, the action-oriented boy showed a progressive shift in the
action mode and a regressive shift in the fantasy mode, while the
fantasy-oriented boy showed a regressive shift in the action mode and
progressive shift in the fantasy mode. With both action-oriented
and fantasy-oriented children who experienced a treatment condition
discordant with their ego tendencies, a progressive shift was observed in both the action and fantasy modes.

Although the experimental treatment experience occurred over a
brief period of time, and although the assessments were cross-sectional, the findings nonetheless bring attention to several questions. What mode should the content of treatment emphasize for a
child given his ego orientation? Our preliminary observations suggested that a treatment process that is initially concordant with

the child's dominant mode may be more effective. For example, one could speculate that if an action-oriented child engages in treatment initially permitting action behaviors, ego development in the action mode would be promoted. At the same time, the fantasy mode would regress providing the child with opportunities to master drive tensions in fantasy and to differentiate the fantasy mode.

Further, if a child expresses drives over a long period of time primarily in the action mode, does this mode gradually acquire new, more differentiated structures of delay, indirectness and alternative means and ends? Do these new structures of the action mode then give rise to fantasy dominant, and eventually to language as dominant? Are the same drives and issues expressed in each mode, and are these drives and issues progressively mastered as they are expressed and worked through first in action, then fantasy, and then in language behaviors?

THE ANALYSIS OF A LATENCY BOY: A CASE ILLUSTRATION OF ACTION, FANTASY, AND LANGUAGE AS DEVELOPMENTAL LEVELS FOR EXPRESSING AND WORKING-THROUGH DRIVES AND CONFLICTS

To explore these questions and to extend the observations made in the laboratory, I turned to the psychoanalytic treatment of children as a way of gathering longitudinal in-depth data. Psychoanalytic observation would also permit an exploration of one key aspect of the proposed model; namely that identification with ego ideals is the source for acquiring new structures of delay and indirectness within modalities.

Accordingly, in reviewing observations recorded immediately after each analytic session, I focused my attention with the case reported here on three interrelated questions which derive from the foregoing discussing: (1) If the action, fantasy, language behaviors the patient showed are plotted, do these behaviors reveal a sequence which supports the laboratory findings of a developmental line from action, to fantasy, to language expressions? (2) Given the proposition that ego structures of delay and alternative means and ends are acquired from identification with ego ideals, can we observe behavioral evidence that the patient developed new ego ideals which relate to the acquisition of new action, fantasy, and language structures that organize and express drives more adaptively? (3) Are the child's neurotic conflicts and fixations restructured and resolved as they are expressed progressively in action, in fantasy, and in language modes? These questions, then, served as the lens through which the analysis of a seven-year old boy was examined. Given this focus, I am omitting the child's history and other details of the analysis, including my interventions, save for those that are characterized.

Albert was presented for analysis at the age of seven years. During the previous three years he had shown increasingly hyperactive, impulsive, stubborn, destructive behaviors, and marginal school performance in spite of his high intellectual and verbal skills. From the view of the second study discussed above, he represented an action orientation.

I saw him twice a week for seven months in psychotherapy to prepare him for analysis. During this time, his play was frantic, aggressive, and sometimes destructive (e.g., he played war games, drew pictures of planes with huge guns, and threw play material around the treatment room, sometimes at the office window and lamp shades). He was preoccupied with particular classmates who broke rules, damaged property, and the like, reflecting his tendency to project his impulses. My responses included: physically restraining him when needed, redirecting him to act aggressively in more indirect ways (e.g., punching a bag), teaching him competitive games, and joining him in industrious play (building model battleships). We also worked on his main anxiety about treatment--that his "secrets" would be discovered.

Following this period of psychotherapy, the frequency was increased to four sessions per week. An examination of the first four years of analysis suggested six distinct phases, defined by the ego mode that dominated the child's behavior, the ego ideals that developed, and the repetition of his neurosis and fixations (see Table 1). As we trace the analysis in terms of our preselected questions, we will observe that Albert first organized and expressed superego and ego ideal issues in the action mode before giving expression, also in the action mode, to the severe anal neurosis and fixation which were crippling his emotional development and blocking his wish for phallic adjustment. As ego ideals developed and became influential, this whole pattern repeated itself in the fantasy mode, and again in the language mode.

To facilitate reporting these phases, several terms are employed: Macroactivity is used to indicate that the action mode dominates, and the child moves his body in elaborate and differentiated ways through the total space provided by the playroom. The action may be accompanied by fantasy and language but these modes are subordinate to the activity. Microactivity is used to indicate that the child's body is more or less stationary, and he is engaged in miniature activity that is confined to a few square feet of space. Microactivity is usually dominated by some elaborate fantasy that accompanies the miniature actions. Macrofantasy is used to designate an elaborate fantasy that is accompanied by little or no activity. Although the fantasy is communicated with words, the language mode is subordinate to, and operates in the service of the fantasy. Macrolanguage is used to indicate that the dominant ego mode involves spoken words about objects and events in reality, past or present. The conversation may be

Table 1

Phases of Mode Dominance (Action, Fantasy, Language)
In The Analysis of A 7-year-Old Boy

PHASE	1. Macroactivity: 6 months	2. Macroactivity: 7 months	3. Macroactivity and Microactivity:4 months
ISSUES	Ego and Id differentiated Ego and Superego differentiated Ego and Superego gain strength	Ego ideal introduced Superego less archaic Anal neurosis expressed in action	Ego ideal and superego vs. Id continued Phallic wish expressed in action
ACTIVITY	Ratman (bad forces) battles Batman (good forces) Ratman, King of Ratland, joins Batman in pursuit of bad rats	King's Highest Servant takes captured bad rats to King for punishment Punishments differentiated to fit crimes General Bolthead gathers tail glands in his anus Highland Rat Police capture rats stealing tail glands	Spear carved for King's Protector Guard Paper airplanes constructed for contest
CHARACTERS	Rats	Rats	Rats and Humans

PHASE	4. Macrofantasy with Microactivity: 7 months	5. Macrofantasy with Microactivity and Language: 7 months	6. Language with Fantasy and Action: 12 months
ISSUES	Anal neurosis and phallic wish expressed in fantasy Ego ideal and identity elaborated	Anal neurosis and phallic wish expressed in stories. Superego and punishment	Castration anxiety Discussion of anal behaviors and fantasies Superego and the law
ACTIVITY	Savage rats battle Highland Police for Wamba Club "Ass Monsters" live in wild house (sheet of paper); scientist and Dracula, a "human monster," control them Dracula stopped from becoming member of Silver Stallion Squadron David Barcelona (a new religion) pursues monsters for scientist	Telling stories of "Teddy's" "ass club" (AC) and its activities Telling stories of fathers who discover ass club and punish children Teddy struggles to go from "ass phase" to the "dink phase"	Writing essay about sharks Shooting galley with air rifle Rating sexy pictures Discussion of past anal activities and fantasies Listening to Point of Law radio program
CHARACTERS	Rats; Monsters; Human Monsters	Humans	Patient and analyst

accompanied by some fantasy and activity but these are subordinate
to, and in the service of communicating reality-related drives, issues, and conflicts through spoken words.

First phase of macroactivity: 6 months. With the start of
analysis, I focused on Albert's anxiety about revealing his secrets
to me and on strengthening the alliance. Soon he introduced a game.
He lay on the floor pretending he was a "captured person with secrets," and that his hands and feet were tied. He asked me to pretend I was a giant rat attacking him from "the hole in the wall"
which he designated was the large diamond-shaped design on a blanket
hanging from the playroom wall. I played the part, lunging forward,
snarling and growling. Albert rolled and twisted on the floor, sometimes screaming.

In the weeks which followed, Albert prescribed one attack after
the other, sometimes 20 or 30 in one session without interruption.
The attacks were elaborated into various forms of torture (e.g.,
whipping, chopping off fingers, stretching on the rack; boiling in
oil). Occasionally he paused between attacks to ask questions about
the different methods of torture used at different times in history,
and in different countries. In terms of the conceptual scheme being
studied, we should note that Albert gradually prescribed that the
analyst hold a puppet which would do the attacking, a development
that would be seen as a shift towards indirectness--that is, from
the analyst's body to a puppet. In the course of these hundreds of
attacks, during which Albert squirmed his total body, I introduced
the notion that these various characters are "evil forces" that attack and harass the victim who is a "good force."

Albert responded in subsequent sessions by playing that the analyst was the evil force battling Albert, the good force. He articulated my role further and labeled it "Ratman." Ratman is the "King
of Ratland" in charge of "infinity rats," and of all of the "evil
forces in Ratland." Albert labeled the role of the good force, "Batman." If Batman gained control over King Rat, and all the rats he
ruled, he could make them do good, instead of bad.

Interventions at this time included: it must be difficult for
Batman to fight off all these enemy forces alone; having to fight
against these forces must exhaust Batman and leave him with little
energy to do anything else; the analyst could help Batman find out
who these enemies are and find allies who could aid Batman in his
battle against them. As was the case during preanalytic psychotherapy, Albert would respond by shouting, "Shut up! Let's just
play the game and not talk like that!"

The influence of these interventions, however, appeared over
several sessions. Albert introduced play activity which suggested
the beginning differentiation of ego and id, and the introduction of

superego issues, as well as suggesting a deepening of the therapeutic alliance. Albert, as Batman, joined the analyst who was Ratman, in pursuit of "bad rats" throughout Rat Land. Batman and Ratman crawled about the playroom in a partnership, and eventually captured the "bad rats."

Second phase of macroactivity: 7 months. The next phase of macroactivity is marked by three significant developments. The superego became more differentiated and less severe, and an explicit ego ideal figure is introduced for the first time. Following this growth in superego and ego ideal, Albert appeared to have the ego strength to regress libidinally and express his severe anal neurosis. In doing so, Albert still made predominant use of the action mode.

As the play activity unfolded, Albert assigned himself a new role, the "King's Highest Servant" who assisted the king in punishing "rat executioners" for crimes they committed, and because they were trying to capture the king. As the Highest Servant, Albert captured rat executioners, presented them to the king for punishment, and detailed the crimes they committed. Albert was very uncompromising in what he called a crime. "A crime is a crime, even stealing a stone off the streets of Ratland is a crime." Albert insisted the king behead any bad rat who dared to steal a stone, and many rats were beheaded (played by Albert).

At this point, the analytic work attempted to develop the superego, from primitive to more advanced forms, by looking for opportunities to play out the notion that punishment should fit the crime. As each bad rat was brought in by the Highest Servant for punishment, the King (analyst) with the Highest Servant (Albert) gradually wrote up a long list of various crimes, each requiring different punishments. Over many weeks a code of laws was written for Ratland.

With gains in ego, superego, and ego ideal functions, achieved in expressions through the action mode and in macrospace, Albert, at this point in the analysis, gave organized expression, still within the action mode, to anal conflicts and fixations that were formidable barriers to his development.

He introduced a new character "General Bolthead," who is armed with "a big gun" (a car vacuum cleaner Albert had brought to the office). With the analyst at his side, Bolthead crawled around the floor through a labyrinth of underground corridors. General Bolthead fought one bad rat after the other who attacked him. After defeating each rat, Bolthead cut out the "tail glands" from the anus of each defeated rat and placed them in his own anus. Bolthead also sat on volcanoes (Albert squated over a pillow), and with his anus, sucked up millions of tail glands that were located in the volcano. All the other rats were envious of Bolthead's many tails and tail glands.

This activity suggested the psychological independence Albert's
anus had achieved, and revealed the fusion of oral, anal, and phallic
stages. The activity also suggested that, in addition to apparent
anal fixations, Albert's libidinal organization also showed regression from phallic anxieties.

Following the anal activity of Bolthead, the material shifted to
superego and ego ideal taming these impulses. However, arachaic
qualities, observed earlier in the superego play, were absent now.
Moreover, new ego ideals appeared and were integrated and coordinated
with superego. Albert introduced an elite, revered corps of "Highland Rat Police" who pursued rats that stalked the streets of Ratland
to suck blood and glands of other rats. It is against Ratland law to
steal glands. Here, as a Highland Policeman, Albert would march about
the playroom with a military posture, and firmly and efficiently capture bad rats and take them to headquarters.

Phase of macroactivity with episodes of microactivity: 4 months.
For the next four months, the material continued to include ego ideal
and superego issues versus id forces. In addition the material
shifted, for the most part, to phallic issues concerning power, competence, and castration fears, with anal issues subordinated. While
this shift could be seen as a defense against the anxiety associated
with the intense, anal activities and fantasies in which Bolthead
had been engaged for many weeks, it could also be viewed as revealing Albert's phallic ambitions which were kept beyond his reach by
his neurosis. From the viewpoint of the conceptual model proposed
in this report, the modalities employed by Albert now included both
macroactions with fantasies relatively subordinated and microactions
(actions subordinated) with fantasies more dominant.

Albert interrupted the Highland Police activity when he asked
for a jacknife and a piece of wood. For several sessions, he sat
relatively still and carved a four foot spear. With it, he played
being the "King's Protector Guard" and a "Roman Soldier." Each of
these involved macroactivity and the total playroom.

In this phase, Albert also asked me to show him how to make
paper airplanes, and he constructed many. He introduced a "contest."
We glided airplanes in the treatment room, timing which one remained
"up" the longest. Here Albert also wondered, "at what age can you
have a gun?"

Phase of macrofantasy with microactivity: 7 months. The next
phase is characterized by a sustained period in which fantasy dominates served by microactivity. Albert remained still, lying on the
floor, manipulating play materials relatively little. Simultaneously,
fantasies become increasingly elaborated and differentiated. Critical
for the focus of this report, we should note that during this phase

id, superego, and ego ideal issues, as well as anal conflicts which
were expressed to this point primarily in macroaction, are expressed
again in this phase primarily in the higher fantasy mode assisted by
microactions. Moreover, the fantasy mode gradually undergoes change
bringing the issues closer to reality. The content of the fantasies
progressed from rats, to monsters, to human monsters.

Albert took a set of plastic "monster" figures out of his cup-
board. Over the next months, he sat on the floor with the monster
figures before him, and moved them about very little, and only within
the space of about two square feet. Gradually he evolved the following themes: the plastic monsters are "dirty, wild savages;" they
spit, urinate, defecate, and wallow in filth; they are stupid, and
have no language. I placed a sheet of construction paper on the
floor and suggested that the monsters live "in here." Albert placed
the monsters on the paper calling it "the wild house," where they "do
dirty things." Albert then selected one of the more human-looking
figures and called it "a scientist who owns the monsters." I placed
the plastic container in which the figures are kept next to the wild
house and suggested that the scientist lived in there. I also suggested that since the scientist owns the monsters, he determines
what the monsters do. Albert elaborated the fantasy further.

He selected another toy monster, "Dracula," who was a "human
monster," and who helped the scientist control the monsters. Dracula's house was represented by another sheet of construction paper
placed next to the scientist's house, and alongside of the wild
house. Albert also introduced a "punishment chamber," a fourth sheet
of construction paper, where monsters were punished when they went
against the scientist's wishes, and especially when they attempted
to break into Dracula's house to make it "dirty." Punishment usually
included intense heat which burned the filth off the monsters. Gradually, Albert identified each monster, giving special attention to
"Ass Monster" and "Finger Monster." When in the wild house, the
Finger Monster loved to stick his finger in the anus of another monster and in his own. The analyst, as the Scientist, asked the Finger
Monster if he ever wanted to be free from the wild house.

Following this, Albert introduced new ego ideal elements. He
invented an elite "Silver Stallion Squadron."[7] This squadron consisted of strong, intelligent soldiers (played by the analyst) who

---

[7]The writer is grateful to Dr. Bernard Rosenblatt for suggesting the
possible ego-ideal determinants of Albert's choice of these labels.
There are as many letters (22) in "Silver Stallion Squadron" as in
the analyst's first and last names. Moreover, the letter "S" begins
each word (Silver Stallion Squadron) and also the three names that
make up the analyst's first and last names.

lived in and guarded "the treasury" filled with silver rods and bul-
lets. Dracula, played by Albert, disguised himself to become a member of the squadron because he and the scientist wanted silver rods.
(Here Albert expressed his hope of leaving the wild house of the
anal stage and achieving the phallic stage.) Dracula was given tasks
to master in order to qualify for membership in the squadron. Although Dracula accomplished the tasks, he was discovered by members
of the Squadron. Dracula (now played by the analyst) is taken to the
judge (played by Albert) who denies Dracula membership because, "although you are clean you are not honest, but a monster in disguise.
A member of the Silver Stallion Squadron must be honest."[8]

In interpreting this play activity, we could speculate that although Albert is under the pressure of the wish to get into the treasury (and have the phallus), he himself renounces dishonesty suggesting
that his superego (the focus of the first two years of the analysis)
was now sufficiently organized to provide prohibition from within
against obtaining the phallus surreptitiously. The material also
suggested that Albert unconsciously accepted the goal that the re-
formation of Dracula was necessary before he could be admitted into
the treasury and obtain the phallus.

Albert next introduced a new ego ideal he called David Barcelona.[9] David is strong, honest, intelligent, and a leader of the
Silver Stallion Squadron. He is not a Christian and not a Jew, but
he is a "new religion." He is also from both the "old and new," because he was born from 11:45 p.m. to 12:15 a.m. on the last day of
the old year and first day of the new year. David Barcelona, and
his friend, hunt savages and monsters made by the scientist.

Phase of macrofantasy with microactivity and language: 7 months.
Following this, Albert made continued use of fantasy but assisted increasingly by the language mode. That is, from the view of the model
guiding this report, superego and id issues, his anal neurosis and
phallic ambitions are expressed again in fantasies, but now the fantasies are related even closer to objects and events in reality.
Bringing a jacknife he borrowed from his father, and borrowing another

---

[8] Note, that in this theme, Albert changes roles and designates himself
as the person who denies membership to the dishonest Dracula.

[9] The name David Barcelona, and the two religions assigned to him, appear to relate to the patient's Jewish background and the writer's
Italian background. Given this assumption, the ego ideal being
formed now integrates aspects of Albert's family heritage and the
standards represented by the analysis.

from the analyst, Albert asked the analyst for help, and carved a
series of swords, each one more large, and more decorative, than the
last. As we carved, Albert asked the analyst to tell him about Teddy
(a fictitious character) and "the worst thing he ever did?" I encouraged Albert to author "stories" about Teddy's experiences. Over
the months, Albert's stories included:

Teddy would stand nude before a mirror, holding another mirror
behind him so he could look at his buttocks. In that way he would
get "all kinds of ideas and feelings."

Teddy made huge, decorative cakes from his feces, and forced
his sibs to eat them. He counted the number and length of each piece
of feces, and assigned "stars" to the best ones. He and his sibs
would take turns watching each other having bowel movements.

Teddy wrote a newspaper called the "Ass Times" which contained
descriptions of "different asses," descriptions of bowel movements,
and pictures of "the perfect ass." Albert drew a number of pictures
and constructed a newspaper.

Teddy organized an "Ass Club." The fathers discover their
children during club meetings, punished them severely (e.g., whipping,
dipping the children in hot oil, chopping off their fingers). Note
the similarity with the torturing done by rat executioners at the
start of the analysis.

The focus of my remarks, during this story telling, was that
for Teddy, what he did, wanted to do, and imagined doing were all
tangled together, that Teddy felt this tangle was so bad he deserved
the most severe punishment.

The analyst also introduced the concept that Teddy was in the
"ass phase." Albert developed some understanding of this discussion,
commenting, for example, that for Teddy, "his ass was the most important part of his life." I also pointed out that all boys go through
an ass phase, that this is followed by a "dink" phase (a label most
often used by Albert). Albert noted that Ted is "stuck in the ass
phase, but wants to climb up." To illustrate, he used the diamond-
shaped design on the blanket which, in the first phase of the analysis, he had designated as the hole from which rats attacked. The
outline of the diamond is formed by steps. Albert pointed out that
Teddy must climb one step at a time to get to "Penis Peak," the top
of the diamond. "There are no short cuts." Teddy is stuck or slips
back to a previous step because he "sometimes still does his ass
things."

Phase of macrolanguage alternating with and assisted by fantasy
and activity: 12 months. In the last phase covered by this report,
the ego mode of language dominated. Instead of acting out rats,
and fantasizing monsters, and Teddy, Albert now began to talk about,

for the most part, real persons and events, past and present. Moreover, while he continued to work through the struggle between superego, ego ideal, and id impulses, Albert showed a major libidinal
shift from the anal conflicts and impulses which pervaded the previous years to phallic-oedipal strivings and the accompanying castration anxiety.

   Following the stories of Teddy's struggle to reach Penis Peak,
Albert ushered in this phase by becoming very involved in preparing
an essay about sharks, a topic he had selected to satisfy a school
assignment in science. Over many weeks, he used the analytic sessions
to draw pictures of sharks, and to write chapters on the habits and
physical anatomy of sharks, giving particular focus in our discussions
to reports of sharks attacking humans.

   Following this project, he became involved in several lines of
activity, shifting from one to another, but sticking with each for a
number of sessions. He constructed a shooting gallery using a large
cardboard box and paper cutouts of animals. He asked the analyst to
provide a bee-bee gun, and the two of us took turns shooting in competition. He brought "playboy" pictures to the office, and joined
the analyst in playing "judge," rating each picture in terms of several issues; for example, "how vulgar are they," "which one is the
most artistic," "which one is the most animalistic." He also introduced discussions about his own anal activity and fantasies of the
past. At first he made only fleeting references to them, and then
gradually returned to them adding more details and raising questions.
He could talk about these behaviors and fantasies for brief periods
without anxiety and guilt escalating and crippling him, and we made
several connections between his behavior, fantasies and concerns,
and our past work with General Bolthead and Teddy who was stuck in
the ass phase. He noted his growing interest in girls. He discussed
"girlfriends" he liked in his class, brought pictures of girlfriends
to the sessions, and asked many questions such as the age at which
a boy could kiss a girl, touch a girl, have intercourse with her,
and so on. Another activity involved listening to a radio program
called "Point of Law" during sessions, and discussing whether the
ruling issued by the judge in the legal case described was appropriate

CONCLUDING REMARKS

   This report addressed the psychoanalytic hypothesis that in organizing and communicating drives and conflicts, the action mode
dominates first in development, that with ego growth the fantasy
mode emerges, integrating actions, and that with further development
both of these modes are subordinated and integrated into the language
mode which emerges and dominates. This report also addressed the
related hypothesis that the process of internalizing ego ideals plays
a critical role in this progression. The demands of ego ideals to
delay and detour impulses, and to find opportunities for expression

permitted by reality, were proposed as the stimulus for ego reorganization from the direct, impulsive action mode, to the more delayed
and indirect fantasy mode, to the language mode which accommodates
most to the requirements of reality.

I presented experimental cross-sectional data that supported the
basic developmental principle of ego changes within and between modes.
I also presented experimental data that relates to regressive or progressive restructuring of action, fantasy, and language behaviors as
a function of laboratory experiences.

To explore the hypothesis longitudinally, to study directly the
proposed role of ego ideals, and to determine whether psychic conflicts are repeated and worked-through in one mode and then another,
I examined the analytic process observed with a latency boy. Over
the course of four years, the patient organized and expressed id,
ego, superego, and ego ideal issues first primarily in macroactions.
That is, he moved his body through the total space of the playroom to
express impulses, issues, and conflicts. The same impulses and conflicts were then organized and expressed in macrofantasy. In this
phase, fantasies dominated, assisted by miniature actions, performed
within microspace. The important distinction here, is that the expression and working through of impulses and conflicts took place
within fantasies, the details of which extended far beyond the refined, miniature actions that were, for the most part, incidental
to the activity depicted by the fantasies. This was followed by a
phase of macrolanguage, when the patient repeated expressions of the
same impulses and conflicts, but now primarily by talking about objects and events in reality, past or present.

In terms of the hypothesized role ego ideals play in this progression, we observed the interplay, in point-counterpoint fashion,
between the formation and elaboration of ego ideals and a shift in
ego modes. The construction, elaboration, and assimilation of new
ego ideals usually was associated with a progressive shift in ego
mode from action, to fantasy, to language.

Lastly, two additional broad conclusions could be drawn from a
review of the six phases described. We observed that in this interplay between ego ideals and ego modes, severe anal neurotic conflicts and fixations were beginning to be surrendered by the patient
with libidinal development proceeding to the phallic stage. Furthermore, issues and conflicts that were unconscious, and expressed primarily in actions, gradually became more conscious as they marched
through fantasy expressions, ultimately gaining expression in the
language mode.

The expression of unconscious conflicts in action is a familiar
issue in psychoanalysis. Freud first gave direct attention to the
unconscious communication of "chance actions" in his studies of

psychopathology of every day life (Freud 1901). Later he pointed
out that chance actions which the patient performs while on the
couch seemed to suggest some unconscious conflict which only later
became conscious as a result of analytic work. These actions were
considered in terms of the concepts of acting-out and repetition
instead of recollection (Freud 1914), and in terms of the concept
of action, ideation and affect as alternative pathways for discharge
(Freud 1915).

Of the attention given this issue since Freud's writings, the
recent investigations and creative formulations by Mahl of what he
has termed the "A-B Phenomenon" are especially relevant to the focus
of this report (Mahl, 1967, 1968, 1976). Mahl has observed and described how miniature actions which an adult patient shows throughout therapy, occur first as expressions of some issue. These microactions are later followed by verbalizations of that same issue.
Mahl proposes that microactions may be the first stage of some issue
or impulse becoming conscious, and that this sequenced progression
is critical to the therapeutic process.

The work by Mahl and earlier psychoanalytic workers have tended
to articulate two modes, action and thought. In this report I have
brought particular attention to the possible theoretical and clinical
value of distinguishing between three ego modes (action, fantasy, and
language) as alternate pathways for discharge, to the developmental
progression of these modes, and to the role this progression plays
in ego restructuring. I have also brought attention to the possible
value of not viewing all actions simply as actions and thought as an
alternative expression, but of distinguishing among actions, and
fantasies, and spoken thoughts in terms of the degree of delay and
directness they reveal. Distinguishing among forms of actions,
fantasies, and spoken thought should be of considerable assistance
in charting ego development within a mode and the mastery of conflict.

These hypotheses, and the child analytic data presented, also
suggest a thesis concerning technique in child psychoanalytic therapy.
If language and thought are embedded in and emerge from actions, then
cognitive constructs and statements by the therapist about impulses,
wishes, and conflicts have a greater potential for restructuring the
patient's behavior if the analyst's constructs are embedded in, and
related to, an experiential progression from action, to fantasy, to
language shared by both the child and the analyst.

From this thesis it would follow that the _form_ and _content_ of
an intervention by the analyst (that is activity, versus fantasy,
versus cognitive concepts and constructs), and the timing of such
interventions are important. When should the analyst respond with
some action, and when with a fantasy, and when with a spoken concept
about a reality event or object? In phasing-in interventions, the
goal would be to facilitate therapeutic progression from action

without thought to thought without action, so that all modes (action, fantasy, and language) are available to the child in integrated, flexible, mobile, adaptive, and growth-fostering ways.[10]

Lastly, when applied to child treatment, the model proposed suggests that the steps along this pathway should not be hurried or partially bypassed by the analyst insofar as the psychological make-up of the child and analyst permit. The model also suggests that ideally cognitive constructs and schema (insights, awareness, understanding) which emerge as a result of analytic work, should have deep and wide-spread roots at the developmentally lower level of a well elaborated fantasy-representational mode, and at the still lower, developmental level, of action. Without these roots, which tie together and integrate the three modalities, insights (words and concepts) would float detached, as intellectualizations and psychologizing, fantasies would be deprived of their fulfillment in reality-related experiences, and actions would be robot-like without the breadth, psychological economy, and meaning provided by thought and fantasy.

REFERENCES

Blaisdell, O. Developmental changes in action aggression and in fantasy aggression. Unpublished doctoral dissertation. Boston University, 1972.

Eichler, J. A developmental study of action, fantasy, and language aggression in latency boys. Unpublished doctoral dissertation. Boston University, 1971.

Ekstein, R. & Friedman, S. The function of acting out, play action, and play acting in the psychotherapeutic process. Journal of the American Psychoanalytic Association, 1957, 5, 581-629.

Freud, A. Normality and pathology in childhood: Assessments of development. New York: International Universities Press, 1965.

Freud, S. (1901). The psychopathology of everyday life. In J. Strachey (Ed.), The Complete Works of Sigmund Freud. Standard Edition, Vol. 6. London: Hogarth Press.

Freud, S. (1914). Remembering, repeating and working through. Further recommendations on the technique of psychoanalysis, II. Standard Edition, Vol. 12. London: Hogarth Press, 1958.

---

[10]In terms of psychoanalytic treatment with adults, this proposal urges us to study systematically, for example, whether and when the "acting out" of adolescent or adult patients (that is, repeating in action rather than remembering) might be a necessary action phase in the service of ego restructuring which leads to fantasy and language phases and brings conflicts to consciousness.

Freud, S. (1915). The unconscious. Standard Edition, Vol. 14. London: Hogarth Press, 1957.

Hartmann, H. Ego psychology and the problem of adaptation. New York: International Universities Press, 1958.

Mahl, G. Some clinical observations in nonverbal behavior in interviews. Journal of Nervous and Mental Disease, 1967, 144, 492-505.

Mahl, G. Gestures and body movements. Research in Psychotherapy, 1968, 3, 295-346.

Mahl, G. Body movement, ideation and verbalization during psychoanalysis. Paper presented at the Downstate Series Symposium in Research in Psychiatry: Communicative Structures and Psychic Structures, January, 1976.

Rapaport, D. The collected papers of David Rapaport. M. Gill (Ed.), New York: Basic Books, 1967.

Santostefano, S. Construct validity of the miniature situations test: I. The performance of public school, orphaned, and brain damaged children. Journal of Clinical Psychology, 1965, 21, 418-421. (a)

Santostefano, S. Relating self-report and overt behavior: The concepts of levels of modes for expressing motives. Perceptual and Motor Skills, 1965, 21, 940. (b)

Santostefano, S. & Wilson, S. Construct validity of the miniature situations test: II. The performance of institutionalized delinquents and public school adolescents. Journal of Clinical Psychology, 1968, 24, 355-358.

Santostefano, S. Assessment of motives in children. Psychological Reports, 1970, 26, 639-649.

Santostefano, S. Beyond nosology: Diagnosis from the viewpoint of development. In Herbert E. Rie (Ed.), Perspectives in child psychopathology. New York: Aldine-Atherton, 1971.

Schafer, R. Ideals, the ego ideal, and the ideal self. Psychological Issues, 1967, 5, 129-176.

Schafer, R. Action: Its place in psychoanalytic interpretations and theory. The Annual of Psychoanalysis, 1973, 1, 159-196.

Schafer, R. Emotion in the language of action. Psychological Issues, 1976, 9, 106-133.

ISSUES POSED BY SECTION 5

Benjamin B. Rubinstein

New York Psychoanalytic Institute

New York, New York

Although the papers we have heard this morning are only indirectly concerned with the problem of communication, I take the lib-
erty, before discussing the papers themselves, to say a few words
about this concept. It seems that it is not always understood the
same way. While some people apparently have no difficulty saying
things like "Unconsciously the patient communicated to the analyst
his wish to be loved," to others this statement is confusing. These
others--and I happen to be among them--believe that the essential
meaning of the statement can be expressed by saying that the patient
behaved in a way that led the analyst to infer an unconscious wish
on his part to be loved. This is not just quibbling about words.
If we want to form an idea about the processes involved, we will arrive at entirely different hypotheses depending on whether we, as
our starting point, take the first or the second of the two expressions mentioned.

Man emits a great many signals, some of which are picked up by
his fellow men. A number of these are meant to be picked up, while
others are not. Only the former qualify as communications. The
well-known communication theorist MacKay (1972) and the linguist
Lyons (1972) agree that an item of information emitted by a person
is a communication only if the person in question has intended to
emit it. Information that is emitted unintentionally, MacKay refers
to as a symptom. Thus, if a person, to affirm something, nods his
head, his head nodding is a communication. But if he smiles, and
if his smile is what we call genuine, he obviously does not smile in
order to communicate to people around him, say, that he feels friendly.
His smiling is an expression of this feeling, a symptom of his enter-
taining it.

355

To take another example. While the contents of speech normally are communicative, the so-called paralinguistic features of speaking, its tempo, rhythm, pitch, etc., and some types of bodily movement associated with it, although either manifestly or potentially informative, do not qualify as communications. Ordinarily a person does not intentionally speak in a low, slow monotone to communicate to others that he feels sad. Among the movements I have in mind are the hand-arm movements--partly paralleling the paralinguistic features of speaking--Freedman (1972) has labeled speech-primacy movements and the fidgety movements associated with hesitation pauses in speech described by Dittmann (1972).

This should be fairly clear. However, as I will indicate at the end of the discussion, on closer scrutiny, the distinction--following MacKay and Lyons--I have tried to make, is less clear than it seems.

Let me turn now to the papers we have just heard. I will begin with the paper by Dr. Santostefano. This author has derived much of his inspiration from traditional psychoanalytic theory. That being so, he is not intent on testing the theory but, for the most part, merely on using it. It is thus legitimate to ask how well it has served him.

The paper is in two parts, a report on a series of experiments and a report on the psychoanalysis of a seven-year old boy. Because it is tied in with what to me is a rather ambiguous aspect of the experimental study, I will not consider the analysis. In the experimental part, Dr. Santostefano set himself the task to determine the kinds of aggressive behavior that characteristically occur at different developmental stages. He used, as his subjects, a number of boys at each of three age levels, 6, 8, and 10 years, respectively. Two sets of tests were administered, and a third set was given to a different group of subjects.

I will consider only what seemed to be the most basic and least equivocal of the tests. They were the ones first presented, and were designed to determine the preference of the subjects for particular types of aggressive behavior in each of two modalities: action and fantasy, and, in addition, their aggressive proclivity in the language modality.

Closely following psychoanalytic theory, Dr. Santostefano based the action and fantasy tests on two principal assumptions: namely, that an aggressive drive pressing for discharge is present, and that factors are also present that cause the discharge to be delayed and indirect. I will refer to these factors as discharge constraining factors. A further assumption is that their emergence is partly a function of maturation and partly of learning. Among them, Dr. Santostefano mentions, specifically, concern for social acceptability.

The assumption that the aggressive drive is continually present in an active state is implicit in Dr. Santostefano's statement to the effect that the tests provide <u>opportunities</u> for the discharge of "aggressive tensions." This, it seems to me, is a gratuitous assumption. It fits the facts as well, if not better, to describe the tests as <u>inviting</u> the subjects, if they should feel like it, to behave aggressively. If we accept this formulation, our concept of the test situation changes radically. It is now not just a question of providing outlets for aggressive discharge and of determining whether the discharge constraining factors, as the theory requires, make for greater delay and indirectness with increasing age. The question is, rather, whether the tests do or do not stimulate aggressive behavior and, if they do, what kind of aggressive behavior they stimulate.

In both the action and fantasy modality, the subject is presented with a number of tests, each comprising three items supposedly stimulating aggression as modified by different degrees of delay, indirectness, and concern for social acceptability. The subjects are required to indicate in a special way the item they prefer in each of the tests. To make my point, I must briefly describe a few of them.

In one of the action modality tests, the subject has to indicate his preference by doing one of the following: stab a toy soldier with a knife, hit it with a stick, or tie its legs with a rope. In another action test, he has to smash a lamp bulb with a hammer, or hammer a nail into a board, or turn a screw into the board with a screw driver. In one of the fantasy tests, the picture of a boy whose baseball team has just lost a game is shown. The subject is then asked, with the aid of additional pictures, to imagine whether the boy, in his frustration and anger, is most likely to take his baseball bat and smash the windshield of a car, or dent its fender, or perhaps just let the air out of the tires.

While, roughly speaking, most of the 6-year olds chose to stab the toy soldier, to smash the light bulb, and to imagine that the boy would be most likely to smash the windshield of the car, most 10-year olds chose to tie the legs of the toy soldier, to turn the screw into the board, and to imagine that the boy would be most likely to let the air out of the tires. It thus does seem plausible that in the 6-year olds, at least some of the tests, in one way or another, had in fact aroused their aggression. We must, however, not overlook the fact that the aggressive items were also the simplest which, at least in some of the tests, may have influenced the choice. To decide this question, Dr. Santostefano's free association session after each test may be of help. The results of this part of the study, however, he has not yet published, so we cannot tell.

In the case of the 10-year olds, the situation is more complicated. It is important to remember that in each test, the subjects

had to make a choice between the three items offered to them.   There
are at least three possible reasons for why they may have made the
choices they did in fact make: (1) their aggression was aroused,
but the discharge constraining factors made the subjects in the tests
choose the most delayed, indirect, and socially acceptable of the alternatives offered; (2) the aggression of the subjects was not
aroused but, since they <u>had</u> to make a choice, they chose the most
innocuous of the available alternatives; and (3) without their aggression having been aroused, the subjects chose the alternative
that, to them, seemed the comparatively most interesting and/or challenging in the sense of requiring greater skill and coordination than
the other items. This last possibility, of course, seems most plausible in tests like the <u>smash-the-bulb or hammer-the-nail or turn-the-
screw</u> test. It is important to note that if it should turn out that,
at least in certain cases, aggression has not been aroused, at least
in these cases the categories of delay and indirectness have no meaning. We have reason to believe that there indeed may be such cases.
How adequate is it, for example, without the imposition of Dr. Santostefano's theoretical presuppositions invariably to classify turning
a screw into a board with a screw driver as an act of delayed and indirect aggression? The free association sessions might be of help
here. But as long as we do not know, we are justified, I think, in
being skeptical.

It seems that primary unquestioning acceptance of psychoanalytic theory and casting the results of the tests exclusively in its
terms, has blinded Dr. Santostefano to other possible interpretations
of these results. Accordingly, he has not been able to appreciate
that, since there are a number of possible interpretations, the interpretation that is consistent with the theory cannot be assigned
more than a certain, perhaps fairly low, degree of probability. I
may mention that examination of the reported results with a continuous word association test, which is meant to tap the language modality, leads to the same conclusion. It follows that the theory has
not served Dr. Santostefano at all well. In fact, it has served him
rather poorly in that, as just indicated, it has led him to overlook
possible interpretations of his data that to a theoretically unbiased
observer seem at least as plausible as the one he has chosen.

Dr. Mahl's paper raises problems of a different sort. The paper
focuses on what Dr. Mahl calls the A -->B phenomenon that he has
studied for some time now. Briefly, this label applies to a particular behavioral sequence occurring during psychoanalysis, the most
commonly observed sequence being that the patient performs an action
or movement of some kind or assumes a special posture that, in retro-
spect, is seen to express, often symbolically, an idea he later expresses verbally. The idea may be a memory, a wish, or a more or
less specific attitude, as in some of the cases of Freud's and Dr.
Mahl's own which he cites.

This is the basic A -->B phenomenon. Dr. Mahl also recognizes
a number of variants. Thus, instead of observing an overt motor activity, the analyst may, in one way or another, become aware of muscular tensions in some part of the patient's body that seem either
preparatory to action, or in some other way related to the idea that
later is expressed verbally. It also happens that dreams and waking
imagery, apparently reflecting a feature of the A-event, are inter-
posed between A and B; or an A-event and an image may each, in its
way, be seen as representing the partial fulfillment of a wish that
is expressed verbally at a later date. Dr. Mahl points out further
that short-term A -->B sequences at times appear to be links in what
he refers to as a long-term A -->B process.

As Dr. Mahl describes them, the A -->B sequences, at least in
some cases, appear to become integral parts of the analytic process.
In his report of the early phase of his analysis with the patient he
calls Edward, the role played by A -->B sequences seems comparable
for the analyst's understanding of what is going on to the role played
in classical analysis by the analysis of dreams and parapraxes. Dr.
Mahl does not, however, use the phenomenon as a technical tool in
conducting his analyses. To avoid influencing its occurrence, he does
not even call it to the attention of the analysand.

Let me return to the basic A -->B phenomenon. The underlying
hypothesis is, of course, that there is an actual, not merely an apparent, connection between the motor activity and the subsequent verbalization. Assuming the reality of the connection, Dr. Mahl speaks
about the nonverbal event as literally anticipating the verbal one.
In certain cases, particularly when the interval between the two events
is short, the claim that there is in fact a connection between them,
seems quite persuasive. But when the interval grows longer--and Dr.
Mahl has registered intervals of several weeks--the persuasiveness
may wear thin. An important factor, obviously, is the nature of the
formal relationship between the events, on the basis of which the connection is inferred. If a movement observed at time A, by virtue of
some quite peripheral attribute they have in common, is seen as symbolizing an idea expressed verbally at time B, and if A and B are
weeks apart, then we may wonder whether there really is an intrinsic
connection between the movement and the idea. Theoretically there
may well be. The question is how to demonstrate that there probably
is. The difficulty seems even greater with some of the variants I
have just referred to.

Apparently Dr. Mahl relies heavily on interlocking chains of
inferences from a number of observations. This is the usual way of
clinically confirming clinical hypotheses, often thought of as confirmation by what is called the consistency criterion. The difficulty with this method is that the observations that are used are
selected, and the individual inferences are drawn and related to each

other according to mostly tacit rules--the validity of which, precisely because they mostly are tacit, is not questioned. But, even
if we assume their validity, can we also assume that they are always
used the same way?

The fact that we operate with vaguely defined or completely
undefined rules makes it incumbent on us to determine to which extent we, as analysts, agree with one another. In reading the report
on Edward's analysis, I found some of the claims reasonable enough,
while others seemed unconvincing. There is, however, still another
point to be made. It is not sufficient merely to agree or disagree.
That is done in most clinical case seminars. There are degrees of
acceptance between yes and no and, furthermore, with more than two
judges, there are different extents or degrees of agreement. Both
can be measured. One way is to use a group of analysts as our instrument. We can thus instruct each member of the group, on the basis of
the available material, to assess the probability (according to an
agreed upon scale) of a set of interpretations; for example, some
of the long-term A -->B interpretations Dr. Mahl has referred to today, and then determine the degree of agreement on the assessed probability of each interpretation. We will thus get both the assessed
probabilities of the interpretations and a measure of the agreement
on these assessed probabilities. This way may be one of deciding
scientific questions by majority vote. But at least for now, we have
no better instrument.

I have elaborated this point partly because the phenomenon Dr.
Mahl calls attention to, if not new, has not before been emphasized
to the degree he has done, and partly because--infusing new life into
a half-forgotten theory of Freud's--he has constructed on this basis
a quite original theory on the nature of unconscious mental processes
as well as on the transitional stages on their way to becoming conscious. The theory is interesting and deserves to be taken seriously.
But this involves a strict critical evaluation of its clinical, i.e.,
its empirical, base, perhaps along the lines I have tried to indicate.
Already at this point, however, I feel inclined on essentially impressionistic grounds to acknowledge that it is an important theory, although a partial one. I can appreciate Dr. Mahl's view--his evidence
for which I have not presented--that processes directed toward primitive sensory goals and their associated motor processes form part of
unconscious mental events. I cannot, however, see how waking imagery
and dreams, and finally verbal expression, arise from processes of
this kind. Dr. Mahl's solution is to posit what seems like an active
spatially laid out full A -->B sequence that eventually unfolds in
the temporal dimension. He is careful to point out that this is
merely a tentative solution. There are many details to be worked
out here. Until that is done it is best to withhold judgment.

I will only say a few words about the paper by Drs. Gottschalk
and Uliana. Having observed, in an analytic patient a correlation

between lip fingering and speech characterized by "memories and associations of a supportive type," and between hand position at the
sides and more negative speech content (1974, p. 288f), Dr. Gottschalk asked himself whether the expressed feelings induced the hand
positions and movements, or whether, the other way around, the feelings were induced by the movements and positions. In a previous,
carefully planned and executed experimental study focusing on the
relationship between expressed hope and lip fingering, Drs. Gottschalk and Uliana, under strictly structured laboratory conditions,
found evidence in favor of the second of these alternatives. Their
method was essentially to ask the subject, in the presence of one of
the authors, to speak for five minutes about any interesting or dramatic life experience under two conditions, (1) while fingering his
lips, and (2) with hands at his sides.

   The authors have now extended their study and found marked individual differences in the effect of lip fingering on speech content. I will take two examples. While lip fingering in some subjects induced generally hopeful and pleasurable feelings, in others
it had the opposite effect. Subjects who had been breast fed and
who had not chewed their finger nails were mostly in the first group.
But so were the subjects who had scored low on Luborsky's social assets scale and who thus had experienced some kind of "psychosocial
deprivation" in childhood. If, as the authors suggest, the effect
of lip fingering may be related to early experience, the relationship
cannot be a simple one.

   The second example is the finding that subjects with the highest shame anxiety score, when fingering their lips, on the average
showed an increase in certain negative feelings, while the opposite
effect was noted in subjects with low shame anxiety scores. The
authors point out that children who finger their lips and nose are
often ridiculed by their parents, and that the subjects of the first
of these groups may well, as children, have been through some such
experience. Intuitively this makes sense--and the authors claim no
more than that.

   One thing, it seems to me, we can learn from studies of this
kind is that psychoanalytic problems can be approached with rigorous experimental techniques. The results so far may be merely suggestive. But they are suggestive in a different way than simple
clinical observations. They lead not only to further questions, but
also to new experimental methods by which answers to these questions
may eventually be found. As Drs. Gottschalk and Uliana emphasize,
these studies may also alert the clinician to look for lip fingering
and other body-focused movements, and thus put him on a trail that
may lead to the uncovering of significant past experience. Dr. Mahl's
paper clearly underscores this point.

I have a question about the method. Both lip fingering and hand position at the sides, each for five minutes at a time, are enforced by the experimental conditions. The enforced position and movements obviously prevent the free flow of speech-primacy and other hand-arm movements that otherwise might occur, and in any event may act as constraining factors. It would be odd if the constraint had no effect, but maybe it does not. In any case, the question seems worth pursuing. Another question, arising from the one just posed, is whether in regard to their effects, the enforced position and movements are comparable to similar movements and positions that occur spontaneously in the treatment situation.

The basic point Drs. Gottschalk and Uliana make in their paper carries an implication that is at odds with the particular concept of communication I tried to outline in the beginning of this discussion. The paper calls our attention to the unintended, clearly unconscious effect of certain movements on the contents of speech, i.e., on what we take to be intentionally emitted information. Suddenly the boundary between what is and what is not intended becomes blurred. One way out is to regard intention as a particular kind of experience on the part of an agent that, on the basis of certain signs, an observer may also attribute to him. According to this view, it is not contradictory to claim that an intended verbal expression, because of partly unconscious determiners, may carry at the same time some unintended information; in other words, that the verbal expression may be simultaneously both a communication and a symptom.

Without expressing it in these words, we as psychoanalysts are of course conversant with this way of thinking. But generally we are not able to demonstrate the phenomenon in the rigorous manner Drs. Gottschalk and Uliana have done. We should note, on the other hand, that the indicated view does not permit us to speak about unconscious communication. Being a particular kind of experience, intention, as I indicated earlier in a general way, obviously cannot be unconscious.

It is the conceptual point that creates the difficulty. To regard a verbal expression as at times being both a communication and a symptom is a drastic solution. It treats the problem of intention in much the way the problem of freedom of will is usually treated by determinists. Its main advantage is that it allows us to use our terms in a consistent manner. But there may be other ways of achieving this end. One is not to take MacKay's definition of communication too seriously. That is what Tavolga (1974, p. 68), writing primarily about animal communication, suggests.

REFERENCES

Dittmann, A. T. The body movement–speech rhythm relationship as
a cue to speech encoding. In A. W. Siegman & B. Pope (Eds.),
Studies in dyadic communication. New York: Pergamon Press, 1972.

Freedman, N. The analysis of movement behavior during the clinical
interview. In A. W. Siegman & B. Pope (Eds.), Studies in dyadic
communication. New York: Pergamon Press, 1972.

Gottschalk, L. A. The psychoanalytic study of hand–mouth approximations. In Psychoanalysis & Contemporary Science, Vol. 3.
New York: International Universities Press, 1974.

Lyons, J. Human language. In R. A. Hinde (Ed.), Non-verbal communication. Cambridge: Cambridge University Press, 1972.

MacKay, D. M. Formal analysis of communicative processes. In R. A.
Hinde (Ed.), Non-verbal communication. Cambridge: Cambridge University Press, 1972.

Tavolga, W. N. Application of the concept of levels of organization
to the study of animal communication. In L. Krames, T. Alloway,
& P. Pliner (Eds.), Nonverbal communication. New York: Plenum
Press, 1974.

SECTION 6
COMMUNICATIVE STRUCTURE IN THE PSYCHOANALYTIC SITUATION

INTRODUCTION

In this concluding section, we shall be dealing with the "stuff" of psychoanalysis as this is manifest in the verbal dialogue between patient and therapist. In this setting, we can see played out in the "intimate separation" between the patient and analyst, the communicative derivatives of the basic dialogue between parent and child: the cyclical and repetitive variations in wish and defense balance, self- and object-representation, and distance and intimacy, which are the end products in the ontogeny of psychological structuralization.

The three papers in this section are similar in that they all focus upon verbal communication, each attempting to specify, in methodologically rigorous fashion, the process of distilling latent meaning from manifest verbal communication. The contributions differ from one another in the methodology employed and the units chosen for study. In terms of methodology, the papers present three novel approaches to the psychoanalytic process: measurement of process via the computerized assessment of word frequencies; measurement of process via the patient's representation of relationship themes; and, finally, measurement of process via the interaction between distancing and intimacy themes. Thus, these papers reflect the current "state of the art" in the area of content analytic research into the psychoanalytic process.

While Spence does not deal with verbal communication in the psychoanalytic situation per se, he does focus on the way words can reflect an unverbalized biological substrate in the doctor-patient interaction. His data are the verbal utterances of patients undergoing cone biopsy for suspected cervical cancer. From computer content analysis, Spence was able to isolate discrete marker words which predicted positive or negative biopsies. Moreover, those patients who were highly defensive about the possibility of having cancer, produced many more of these predictor words than did those patients who were overtly fearful about this possibility. The fact that selected words appear in the language of patients who are subsequently diagnosed as having cancer raises a host of theoretical issues concerning the function of psychic defense and the process by which ideas are transformed into communicative utterances. In this regard, Spence's paper constitutes a link to the work described by Shevrin and Silverman in Section 4 of this book.

Luborsky's work gets at the central idea that, in the analytic
situation, there occurs a re-evocation of the internalized object
relationships of the earliest period in childhood. He does so via
his method of analyzing relationship themes occurring in the content
of patients' communications. He then attempts to distill from these
themes, what he terms the "core conflictual relationship," that is,
the repetitive basic wish vis-a-vis the object, together with the
patients' anticipated consequence of the enactment of this wish. The
implication to be drawn from such "core conflictual relationships" is
that they represent highly organized and internally structured relations to significant objects which, in their repetitive manifestations, recapitulate the basic self-object interactive schemata of
early childhood development. As such, Luborsky's approach highlights,
once again, the line of interactive regulatory processes detailed in
the work of Sander, Kaplan, and Dittmann.

Horowitz' work also deals with relationship themes. Yet, his
tenet is that psychoanalytic communication, seen as a recapitulation
of a phase of development, reflects a continuing process of engagement and disengagement. The themes that Horowitz examines in the
patient's communication--closeness (C type themes) and distancing
(D type themes)--reflects this internalized interaction process. By
focusing upon the concomitant changes in the evocation of these two
classes of themes over the course of treatment, he could note an
orderly sequence: D type behavior precedes C type behavior. The
sequence of intimacy and distancing, and the necessity for distancing
to precede intimacy, is reminiscent of the chase and dodge situation
described by Beebe and Stern. Likewise, it is also reminiscent of
the phenomena depicted by N. Freedman in his examination of bodily
activity in communication, involving the alternating of body-focused
movements (used for distancing) and object-focused movements (used
for sharing).

Each of the contributions to this section demonstrates how words
may be used to illustrate the vicissitudes of psychic structure:
whether in the interplay of wish and defense, object relatedness, or
the forging of self and object schemata in the process of working
through the transference. The ability to objectively and reliably
identify communicative structures offers a powerful tool for the
study of meaning in the analytic situation. Those presented here
are but a few of the structures necessary for analytic communication. Indeed, Arlow adds others, e.g., metaphor and illiteration, in
his discussion of these papers. But, the work presented in this section underscores the rich potential of utilizing communicative structures to objectively identify those psychic structures at work in
one of the subtlest of human interchanges--the psychoanalytic situation.

MEASURING A PERVASIVE PSYCHIC STRUCTURE IN PSYCHOTHERAPY: THE CORE

CONFLICTUAL RELATIONSHIP THEME [1]

Lester Luborsky

University of Pennsylvania

Philadelphia, Pennsylvania 19104

I'll first tell the story of the preparation for tracking a whale-sized theme, "the core conflictual relationship theme," and then tell its method. The idea surfaced recently after a long search for the curative factors in psychotherapy (Luborsky, in press). It took shape as part of the perspective gained after seeing the consistent results of the three largest multivariate predictive psychotherapy studies: the Chicago Counseling Center Project (Fiske, Cartwright & Kirtner, 1964), the Mitchell et al. Arkansas Project (1973), and the Penn Psychotherapy Project (Luborsky et al., in progress).

The first of these, the Fiske et al. (1964) study, like most predictive studies of this kind, mainly examined patient factors as measured before treatment. They found, in agreement with the Penn Psychotherapy Project, that patient factors before treatment only occasionally reached significant levels of prediction, and the variance accounted for by these variables was very limited (about 9% or 10%). The Mitchell et al. (1973) study, in agreement with the Penn Psychotherapy Project, revealed that 5-minute segments of sessions early in treatment are generally unable to provide significant levels of prediction of the outcomes of psychotherapy (contrary to the early significant results of the Rogerian studies[1954, 1957]based on client-centered psychotherapy). In the Penn Psychotherapy Project, the patient-therapist match, as estimated from before-treatment measurements

[1]This study was supported in part by USPHS Research Grant MH 15442 and Research Scientist Award MH 40710 to Dr. Luborsky, and by the Eastern Pennsylvania Psychiatric Institute, Philadelphia.

The author wishes to thank Marjorie Cohen for her assistance in the preparation of this paper.

on both participants, likewise provided at best a few variables predicting with correlations of .3 to .4 (at <.05 level of significance). Evidently pretreatment information on the patient and therapist, or even 5-minute segments of initial sessions, are not the place to look for factors which would predict a large share of the outcome variance.

About five years ago, I began to examine curative factors that might be found in larger facets of the treatment itself such as the designated form of the treatment. A large-scale review of comparative treatment studies (Luborsky, Singer & Luborsky, 1975) revealed that the form of the treatment, whether group, individual, short-term, long-term, client-centered, or behavioral, usually did not make much difference in the percentage of patients benefiting: the differences in percentages of patients benefiting between the compared treatments were usually insigificant statistically. At this point, I reasoned, similarly to Rosenzweig (1936), that since a variety of different treatments showed benefits, there must be some potent common elements in the differently designated treatments that are responsible for their benefits. One of the most promising was the prominence in all of them of the patient's experiencing a helping relationship.

It was this re-realization of the centrality of the helping relationships that gave me the impetus to take the plunge into the sea of tape recordings of the complete treatments of 73 patients collected as part of the Penn Psychotherapy Project. A first paper (Luborsky, in press a) gave a partial report on interrelations of types of helping relationships and the outcomes of psychotherapy.

It seemed good research strategy to cast a net, wide enough to catch a reasonable sample of relationship patterns, both helping relationships and other typical relationships. One could then describe the patient's typical relationships and examine how the helping relationships fit into these. It was these experiences, in attempting to describe each person's patterns of relationships, that led me to what I came to recognize as a deep psychic structure: the core conflictual relationship theme.

The aims of the present report are: (1) To develop the core conflictual relationship theme method for objectively identifying each person's relationship themes in psychotherapy, and (2) To further examine interconnections among types of core conflictual relationship themes, helping relationships and outcomes of psythotherapy.

PROCEDURES

Several procedures needed to be devised for selecting more versus less improved patients, for sampling the psychotherapy sessions,

for developing methods of evaluating the relationship patterns, especially types of helping relationships and types of conflictual relationship themes. I was guided by a trio of principles: clinical
meaningfulness, parsimony, and reliability.

Selecting extreme groups of more versus less improved patients.
The tape recordings of the psychoanalytically oriented psychotherapies
of the 73 patients in the Penn Psychotherapy Research Project were the
data base (almost entirely patients in the nonpsychotic range). Rather
than transcribing tapes for all patients, focusing on small extreme
groups was much more feasible. The 10 most improved and the 10 least
improved of the 73 patients were selected on the two most reasonable
outcome measures: Residual Gain and Rated Change. It is the first
of these which will be used in the present report.

Residual Gain is a composite of measures provided by the patient
(Lorr Status Questionnaire, Symptom Checklist, MMPI-Es, Hs, Hy), and
by the clinical observer (Prognostic Index Adjustment Items, Health-
Sickness Rating Scale), both initially, and at termination (with the
patient measures and the clinical observer measures weighted equally).
Residual Gain is a component of the difference between initial and
termination composite measures; it is the gain scales relative to
other patients starting at the same initial level. It correlated
.76 with Rated Change.[2]

The patients in each extreme group were markedly different not
only in outcome according to our main criterion, Residual Gain, but
also for the other measures--the therapists' ratings, the patients'
ratings, and the clinical observers' ratings, as well as on the reasons for termination as stated by the therapist (Luborsky, in press
a). The mean number of sessions was only slightly greater for the
high improvers. For the present report we further restricted the
extreme groups of 10 each to those patients who had at least 25 sessions, since our main interest was in intensive treatment. For the
Residual Gain criterion there were, then, seven high gain patients
and eight low gain patients.

---

[2]Rated Change is a combination of ratings of change made by patient
and therapist independently, weighting each equally. Since substantial agreement was obtained between patients' and therapists' ratings--
something that has not been typical in other studies--a combined measure could be obtained. This outcome measure, Rated Change, actually
correlated highly (.68) with the Raw Gain; that is, the difference
between pre- and post-treatment adjustment scores. For the Rated
Change extreme groups, there were eight improvers and seven nonimprovers who had 25 or more sessions; six highs and seven lows
were extremes by both criteria.

Selecting a sample of sessions. Next, a sample of the sessions
was reviewed for each of these subgroups--for each patient it was
two early sessions and two late sessions. The two early sessions
were Sessions 3 and 5 usually, and for the late sessions, it was
the session at the point at which 90% of the sessions had been completed, and the session before that one. For each session, it seemed
sufficient to use only the first 20 minutes as a way to reduce the
work. The first 20 minutes seemed preferable to a random segment in
the middle, since by taking a sample from the beginning, the judge
would know everything that had happened in the session up to that
point.

Scoring the types of helping alliances. A list of signs of
various types of helping alliances was compiled into a scoring manual (Luborsky, in press a). The signs were selected largely on the
basis of clinical judgment. Type 1 includes evidence of the patient's
feeling that he is being helped; Type 2 includes evidence of the patient's feeling that he and the therapist are doing the job of the
treatment as a joint endeavor, and that he is acquiring the skills
himself. Two judges independently read the four 20-minute segments
for each of the patients, noting every time these signs appeared.
One of the two judges was kept blind as to whether the patient was
an improver or nonimprover, and whether the session was early or
late. Only those signs were used, which were caught by both judges.

Determining the core conflictual relationship theme.[3] My interest initially had been in understanding the conditions leading
to the development of helping relationships. As part of this, I
wanted to identify more general relationship patterns to see how the
two concepts might fit with each other. Possibly, for example, certain types of core relationship patterns would be more conducive to
the development of helping alliance relationships.

(1) The first step in estimating the core relationship theme is
to locate "relationship episodes" in the 20-minute segments. These
are the present and past specifically described interactions with
people, both outside of the treatment or with the therapist. Every
one of such relationship episodes is marked off in the transcript.
(The focus is on interactions with specific people, since ratings
based upon transference as expressed to specific "objects" in a segment of the transcript were found to be rateable with higher interjudge agreement than transference ratings based upon the entire segment [Luborsky et al., 1973].)

These episodes were usually easily identifiable and separable.
Occasionally, the limits were unclear when an episode could be seen

---

[3]The procedure and results of this new method have been briefly described earlier (Luborsky, in press a).

as a subepisode of a larger sequence. The agreement in selecting
episodes was very high for the larger, well described interactions
with objects; it was not as good for the brief, vaguely described
interactions. Focusing on these episodes, reduced the data to be
inspected and, even more importantly, highlighted relationship behaviors that were of most interest.

(2) All relationship episodes, regardless of object, were inspected in sequence in order to find the consistencies in their theme.
This was done first for all the relationship episodes in the two early
sessions (the first 20 minutes of each). Then it was done again, in
identical fashion, for all the relationship episodes in the later two
sessions (first 20 minutes of each).

This inspection job is a high level clinical exercise. The main
key to finding the consistencies is reading and rereading the episodes.
The first ones in each 20 minutes are easier to understand after having
read the later ones; the episodes in the early sessions became easier
to understand after having read the episodes in the later sessions.
The redundant themes within the across episodes will then gradually
appear in a saltatorily accreting sequence of eurekas. It does not
matter that a few episodes are opaque or do not seem to fit--these
drop out, since our focus is only on those whose themes repeat themselves. The redundancy of the theme is a mark of where the main conflict lies.

Methods for estimating interjudge agreement on core conflictual
relationship formulations. Without guidelines for formulating theme
statements, they might differ considerately for each clinical judge.
A method for improving agreement was therefore tried. Each judge
made an independent theme formulation according to a standard structure which seemed appropriate for such clinical analyses.

The structure might be described as a single tree with branching
subthemes. The main trunk of the tree is composed of the wish, need,
or intention, and the branches are the consequences as in Figure 1.
The judge can write in the object of the wish, need or intention.
The consequences can be divided into two main types, external and
internal, and for each of these the main ones are listed in the order
of the judge's expectation of their frequency.

After each judge makes his formulation of the core conflictual
relationship theme, the components of the theme are scored for each
of the relationship episodes. Scoring of the theme can be done independently by other judges who are asked to rate the degree to which
each component of the theme applies to each relationship episode.
Each judge's theme formulation can be applied separately to the episodes, or--more economically--a single "tree" can be made by grafting
on any unrepresented subthemes of the several judges. Then, this combined tree can be scored for the relationship episodes. Each limb of

Wish, need, intention   Consequence

A. I want (general theme)*   1. Negative external response
   from (object) but
                                          a._____*
         a._____
                                          b._____
         b._____
                                          c._____
         c._____
                             2. Negative internal response

                                          a._____

                                          b._____

                                          c._____

                             3. Positive external response

                                          a._____

                                          b._____

                                          c._____

                             4. Positive internal response

                                          a._____

                                          b._____

                                          c._____

*List in order with the most frequent at the top

Figure 1: The suggested format for the core conflictual
          Relationship Theme formulation

the tree receives a frequency in terms of the mean number of relationship episodes in which it is found (for each session, and for the
whole treatment). In summary, this method has three main steps:
marking off the relationship episodes, reviewing these and creating
a theme formulation, and then scoring the theme components for each
of the relationship episodes.

     The first description of the core conflictual relationship theme
method (Luborsky, in press a) was based on my own theme formulations.

The present, more sophisticated version of the method adds independent judgments on the degree to which each limb of the theme structure applies to the episodes. The results include both the overall frequencies of the theme in the episodes throughout the treatment, and the separate frequencies for the early sessions versus the late sessions. This quantification reflects the degree of pervasiveness of each patient's theme; that is, the proportion of the relationship episodes in which the theme's components are evident.

An alternative method was not used, although it had the appeal of seeming to be more natural; having theme formulations done independently but unguided by the structure in Figure 1 for the theme formulations. Such a method provides valuable clinical data, but is hardly susceptible to reliability analyses. Even this more sophisticated addition would have some of the same limitation; embedding the formulations in a larger list of formulations from other patients, and having them judged by means of paired comparisons in terms of the degree of similarity of each pair. By this method one could then establish the degree to which themes derived from the same patient are considered to be similar.

RESULTS

Finding #1: A core recurrent relationship theme was detected when the relationship episodes were abstracted according to the suggested procedure.

The reader should examine the brief samples of data and scores provided (in Figure 2 and 3, and Tables 1 and 2) for two sample patients: Ms. DR, an improver, and Ms. BJ, a nonimprover. These two patients were in the extreme groups according to both of the outcome measures described, that is, Residual Gain and Rated Change. Only samples of two patients will be chosen since, although the conclusions can be best understood by starting with the basic data--that is, the four 20-minute segments--these are inevitably too lengthy to be included in entirety--they range from a minimum of 10 to 13 or 14 typewritten pages for each segment.

As noted in the procedure, the judge reads and rereads the transcripts, but is instructed to focus on the relationship episodes which have been marked off in pencil on the transcript. The judge is instructed to search for the theme formulation which fits the most relationship episodes. The structure of the theme is presented to him as drawn in Figure 1. That structure requires that the judge try to find a wish, need, or intention in relation to an object and the expected consequences of trying to get these satisfied. After the core theme is discerned then, typically, a branching of subthemes becomes apparent. Even though I occasionally refer to one core theme, when it is both pruned and grafted to fit the largest number of relationship episodes, it flourishes into a tree of meaningfully related themes. It is my assumption that the most frequent

components found in the relationship theme--usually there are only
one or two substantial limbs on the wish side, and one or two on the
consequence side--deserve the designation of a core conflictual relationship theme.

Patient #6, Ms. BJ, aged 21, came to the University Student
Health Service for what she called a "nervous breakdown." It started
after speaking to her boyfriend to try to find out why he had given
her up. Relationships with people had been difficult for her to maintain, and it was hard for her to know what goes on in her relationships. Her thinking appeared loose, and she was extremely distract-
ible. She showed some suspiciousness and suicidal tendency. One of
her symptoms was what she referred to as an indiscriminate openness,
an inability to say "no," which resulted in promiscuity.

The initial relationship formulation for Ms. BJ was, "I want to
show that I 'open up' to (object) but I usually get negative reactions
"Negative" is being used in the sense of responses which mean, to the
patient, an interference is to be expected with satisfaction of her
wishes. Actually, inspection of Figure 2 shows several subthemes on
each side of the "but." Of the subthemes on the "wish" side, "1 A"
seems to be the most frequent. "1 A" refers to the wish to show that
she gives openness, friendliness, or affection (or tries to withhold
this wish). Two less frequent subthemes are, "I want to get friendliness or affection," and, "I want to get from others money or other
help." (These may well be synonyms to the patient for her expression
"open up.") The "I want" is probably alternatively expressed in, "I
have to or must...," "I should...," or "I do...." On the consequences
side, the patient experiences most frequently the negative external
response or negative internal response, or both of these. The negative internal response, which seems most frequent, is a feeling of
being passive and helpless (designated in Table 1 as "2 b").

Another subtheme sometimes occurs on the wish side: The patient
may speak about someone else's wanting to open up; most often it is
her mother. When her mother tries to show affection, for example, she
suffers the same consequence as the patient. This subtheme can be
scored as "B," referring to someone else instead of "A," referring to
the self.

In one relationship episode, there is an unusual twist (Table 1,
Session 5, Episode #4). The patient manages to avoid the usual "but"
by altering the expression of the need. She describes one relationship in which she was able to have her wish without any immediate bad
consequences. The instance is the one in which she arranged it so
that both she and the "guy" kept cool and unemotional about the relationship; i.e., she did not show that she "opened up." However,
she did not succeed ultimately because she said he then tried to
dominate her. (Such instances may have special value to the patient

Table 1: MS. BJ #6

Relationship Episodes and Scores for Each Episode

Relationship Episode (abbreviated)	Object Judges	Wish Need Intent	External Response	Internal Response
Session #3				
1. "I have to talk about everything" (1A) (in treatment to the therapist) and get it all out. But when it comes out "I can't put anything together"(2b) and "I get worse instead of getting better." (2b)	Treat- ment (and thera- pist) LL FL TW RK	1 A 4* 1 A 5 1 A 3 1 A 4		2 b 4 2 b 5 2 b 4 2 b 4
2. "Everytime that I show that I like somebody, (1A) they've never liked me." (1a)	Boys	1 A 4 1 A 5 1 A 3 1 A 3	1 a 4 1 a 5 1 a 3 1 a 4	-- -- 2 N 4 2 a 4
3. "We (family) are isolated"--we ask and we give and we do not show our posi- tive feelings. ("You don't even let on your feelings.")	Family	1 A 4 1 A 4 1 A 3 1 A 2	1 a 3	2N4, 2d3 (2b5)2d5 2b2,2a1 2b3
Session #5				
1. "I want to get the relationship back on a friendly basis" (1A) (with AJ) but "he completely clammed" (1a) and he is "really scared to have people close to him" and "(his lying) really got me upset." (2b)	Guy(AJ)	1 A 5 1 A 5 1 A 2 1 A 5	1a4,3N2 1a5 1a3,1b2,3N2 1N3,3N4	2 b 4 2b4,2a3 2b2,2N3 2b4,2N4

Table 1 Continued

Relationship Episode (abbreviated)	Object Judges	Wish Need Intent	External Response	Internal Response
2. "I didn't want (2N) to be nice" (to the guy with the busted leg yet I let him stay overnight in the apartment) but "he wouldn't let me out of bed," "then he dragged me (1b) out of bed" and "I got really mad," but there was nothing really that I could do except sort of put up with him." (2b)	Guy	1 A 2 1 A 2 1 A 1 1 A 5	1 b 4 1 b 5 1 b 3 1 a 5 ?b	2 b 5 2 b 3 2b2, 2b3 ---
3. (I wanted not to be with this guy) but "he wouldn't let me out of his apartment."	Guy (not let her out)		1 b 5 1 b 5 1 b 4 1 a 5	2 b 3
4. "Although I slept with him" I did not show my warm feelings (for Sweet Fred). "I didn't want him to think I was his true love," and "he was cool about it" and "I was very happy (but later the same Sweet Fred "started dragging me up the street to his apartment.")	Sweet Fred	? 1 A 5 1 A 5 1 A 2 1 A 4	1b5, 3N2 1 b 3 1b4, 3N2 1 b 4	2 b 2 ? 2b2, 2a3 2 N 4
Session #42 1. "I really can like people but they do not reciprocate," "but when they don't reciprocate I get upset."	People	1 A 4 1 A 4 1 A 4 1 A 5	1 a 4 1 a 4 1a3, 1b3 1a5, 1b4	2 b 4 2 b 3 2 b 2 2 b 4

#	Statement	Object			
2.	I give (advice) to Helene and she accepts it, "but I can never get close enough to people ... so they respect my opinion."	Helene	1 A 4	3N3,1a5?	2 b 3
			1 A 4	3 N 2	2 b 2
			1 A 3	3 N 2	2 b 2
			1 A 5	3 N 5	2 b 3
3.	(Crying) "I don't want to be just an isolated person." "I care about people" but "then I always get the feeling that nobody cares about me."	People	2,1A4	1 a 4	(2a5)2b3
			2 A 5	1 a 5	2 a 3
			2 A 4	1a4,1b3	2 N 5
			2 A 5	1a4,1b4	
4.	"They (guys in the movie) think I'm stupid" and "I really felt dumb." "I don't want to "write them all off."	Guys in Movie	2 A 2	1 a 5	2a5,2d3
			2 A 2	1 a 5	(2a4)2a2,2b3
			2 A 2	1 a 4	2 a 4
			2 A 5	1 a 5	2 a 3
5.	"I don't seem to be getting any better and you (therapist) seem to be getting worse" that is, I'm not getting what I need from the therapist. "I just want to give up. I want everyone to keep away from me."	Therapist	3 A 5	1 a 4	2d4,2N5
					(2d5)2b5
			A 3		2a3,2b3
			3 A 5	1 N 4	2d5,2a5

*Table 1 is a sample of the core conflictual relationship theme components as scored by four independent judges. Each judge reads the entire episode (not the abbreviated one above) and scores the components in the theme formulation created by the independent team (Figure 2). In Table 1, for example, the first judge (LL) coded the wish component in Session #3, Episode 1, as "1a4"—he judges the patient to have expressed "1a," a wish to show that she opens up and shares (by "talking about everything"). The "4" refers to a rating of "4" on a 1 to 5 scale of intensity. The other three judges identify the wish component similarly. All four judges agree that there was no evident external response but that the internal response was to be judged "2b," that is, a negative internal response having to do with inability to cope. The next episode whose object was "boy" was similarly rated by the four judges as containing the wish component "1A," having to do with opening up in the form of showing liking. All four judges agreed that the external response was most prominent here. In general, this sample indicates that the judges were able to identify a highly frequent wish component and a highly frequent consequence component.

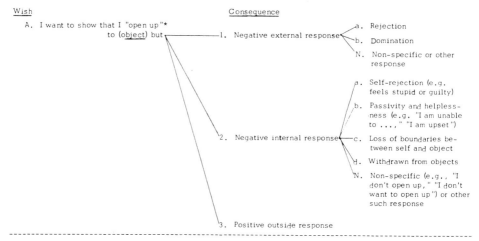

Wish   Consequence

A. I want to show that I "open up"*
   to (object) but ─────────────── 1. Negative external response ── a. Rejection
                                                                      b. Domination
                                                                      N. Non-specific or other
                                                                         response

                                                                      a. Self-rejection (e.g.
                                                                         feels stupid or guilty)
                                                                      b. Passivity and helpless-
                                                                         ness (e.g. "I am unable
                                                                         to ...," "I am upset")
                          2. Negative internal response ──────────── c. Loss of boundaries be-
                                                                         tween self and object
                                                                      d. Withdrawn from objects
                                                                      N. Non-specific (e.g., "I
                                                                         don't open up," "I don't
                                                                         want to open up") or other
                                                                         such response

                          3. Positive outside response

*Includes:

   1. I want to show that I give (openness, friendliness or affection) ("I have to ..." or "I do ...")

   2. I want to get closeness or liking (or I do get ...)

   3. I want to get from others money or other help

Figure 2:   The Core Conflictual Relationship Tree of Subthemes of Ms B.

and therapist since they suggest one possible solution on which to
build more satisfactory types of relationships.)

The second patient, #49, Ms. DR, aged 47, was a successful
fashion designer who sought treatment because of depression and
suicidal tendencies, and a wish to be able to break off an unsatisfactory relationship with a married man. She had two adopted children from an earlier marriage. She was very competent in her job, and
had many old and deep friendships. At least by the time of the later
sessions she seemed able to get some satisfaction of her wish expressed in her main theme, that is, to show that she was okay in all
the senses listed below.

The theme for Ms. DR (Figure 3) is quite different in its components from the one described for the first patient. It is, "I
need to be given reassurance that (or I want to demonstrate that) I
am okay (or better than others, or special). Three main branches
are evident on the consequence side:

1.   A negative external response, "I can't get it from (object),"
or "I don't get it from (object)."

2. A positive external response, "I do get it from (object),"
"I am appreciated by people."

3. A positive internal response, "I am okay," "I am more than
okay," "I am number one," "I give a positive response to myself by
proving my capabilities."

Again, for the general statement of the wish, need, or intention
there are several related subthemes. These are: "I am mentally okay,"
"I am sexually okay, that is, I am not a lesbian," "I am professionally
okay."

Finding #2: Independent scoring of the theme components in each
of the relationship episodes were found to agree moderately well.

The initial theme formulations had been done by one judge for
all 15 patients. Beginning with the two patients who are used here
as examples, independent theme formulations were attempted. The
theme formulation, which was actually used thereafter for scoring
the episodes, was a slightly modified one, based upon variations or
additions by other judges.[4] For example, although the initial theme
formulation for Ms. BJ was by Judge LL, it was modified by one addition from the formulation by Judge FL (that is, "1 b," Domination).
The combined theme formulation[5] was then used to score the relationship episodes by the four judges independently. A sample of scores
for the subthemes for the two patients are presented in Table 1 and
Table 2.[6]

---

[4]The four judges were Dr. Lester Luborsky, Dr. Frederic J. Levine,
Dr. Thomas Wolman, and Dr. Richard D. Kluft. When this group completes its work on 15 patients, a report with more quantitative results will be prepared.

[5]In future uses, the method of obtaining the theme formulation was to
have each of the four judges make an initial theme formulation, and
then to compare these and add any subthemes into a combined theme
formulation. It is this combined theme formulation which was to be
applied back to the relationship episodes. We had considered using
each of the separate theme formulations to apply back to the episodes,
but the additional time involved made it seem impractical.

[6]The precis of the "relationship episodes" listed in the first column
of Figures 2 and 3 are the work of Judge LL and were not made available to other judges. They are provided in Figures 2 and 3 as illustrations of the relationship episodes. They are paraphrases made up
as much as possible from direct quotes.

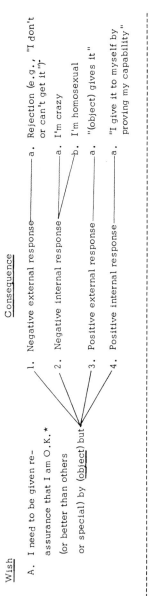

Wish

A. I need to be given re-
assurance that I am O.K.*
(or better than others
or special) by (object) but

Consequence

1. Negative external response ——— a. Rejection (e.g., "I don't
                                        or can't get it")·

2. Negative internal response ——— a. I'm crazy
                                    b. I'm homosexual

3. Positive external response ——— a. "(object) gives it"

4. Positive internal response ——— a. "I give it to myself by
                                      proving my capability"

* 1. I am mentally O.K.

2. I am sexually O.K., i.e., not homosexual

3. I am professionally O.K., i.e., customers appreciate me or I am "number one" with them

4. I am appreciated by people, i.e., they think I am "number one" compared to other
   women (especially Jackie, and "I am as good as you (T) or better")

N (a non-specific example of the general category)

Figure 3:   The Core Conflictual Relationship Tree of Subthemes of Ms DR

Table 2: MS. DR. #49

Relationship Episodes and Scores for Each Episode

Relationship Episode (abbreviated)	Object	Judges	Wish Need Intent	External Response	Internal Response
Session #3					
1. I want to be told I'm okay (1A) (by the test report) but I'm scared that I'm not. (2N)	Thera-pist	LL	1 A 4	1 a 4	?? a 4
		FL	1 A 4		2N3,4N2
		TW	1 A 4	1 a 4	
		RK	1 A 5	1 a 5	2 N 4
2. I want to get a mark of special favor (4A) or recognition ("the center cut of cake") from Jackie but she won't give it.	Jackie		4 A 4	1 a 4	
			4 A 4	1 a 5	2 N 4
			4 A 3 (3)	1 a 4	
			4 A 3	1 a 3	2 N 3
3. I have to win Morris in the competition with Jackie but ...	Jackie		4 A 3	1 a 3	2 b 3
			4 A 4		2 N 3
			4 A 4		
			4 A 4	1 a 4	
Session #5					
1. I think I am a good decorator (3A) (I want you to know that) and that people appreciate me. (3a)	People (and Self and T)		3 A 3	3 a 3	
			3 A 4	3a5,4a3	
			3 A 4	3 a 4	4 a 2
			3 A 5	3a5,1a4	2 N 4
2. I am afraid that I am very sick psychologically (and that my test report will show that).	Therapist (and Self)		1 A 3	1 a 3	4 N 4
			1 A 3		
			1 A 4	3 a 2	2 a 2
			1 A 5	1 a 3	2 N 3
3. I wanted to be invited for Passover by my relatives (brother and sister and friends) but no one did.	Relatives (bro. & sis.., esp. sis.).		4 A 3	1 a 3	
			4 A 4	1 a 4	4 a 2
			4 A 4	1 a 4	
			4 A 4	1 a 5	

Table 2 Continued

Relationship Episode (abbreviated)	Object Judges	Wish Need Intent	External Response	Internal Response
4. I sold a lot today. (3A) I'm very successful in my work (and I want the therapist to know it).	Her client and T.	3 A 3 3A4,1A2 3, 4 A 4 3 A 4	3 a 4 3 a 5 3 a 4 1 a 4	4 a 3 4 a 4 4 a 3 4 a 3
Session #88 P: "You know you can't leave the city and let me run around loose--it's dangerous." T: "Why?" (Paraphrased: It's your fault I quit my job, not mine.)	Therapist	4 A 4 A 4	1 a 4 1 a 4 1 a 4	
I work hard and more reasonably than anybody at work. They don't appreciate it and they mess things up.	People at store and T.	3 A 4 3 A 5 3 A 4 3 A 5	1 a 3 1a5,3a2 1 a 4 1 a 4	4 A 5
I try to do a good job and she (Blanche, the switchboard operator) stops me and doesn't appreciate me, and the assistant manager sides with her.	Girl at switchboard (Blanche?)	3 A 4 3A5,4A5 3 A 3 3 A 4	1 a 3 1 a 5 1 a 4 1 a 4	?4 a 4 4 a 5
Session #89 1. When Dr. F. asks her whether she "had quit her job and set up independently" she says, "I want to tell you something, Dr. Freud," meaning (paraphrased): I did right and am successful going on my own.	Therapist	1 A 3 1,4 A 4 4 A 3 1 A 4	1 a 4	4 a 3 4 a 2 4 a 2

Table 2 Continued

Relationship Episode (abbreviated)	Object Judges	Wish Need Intent	External Response	Internal Response
2. You think I left my job because of problems with women but you are wrong and I'm right. (Later in this episode she gets him to agree.) P: "It's people. It's not just women." (That she must have respect from.) T: "All right."	Therapist	1 A 3 1A4,4A5 1 A 3 1 A 3	1 a 3 1a3,3a4 1 N 4 1a3,3a2 1 a 3	4 a 4 ? 4 a 5 4 a 4
3. I was able to maintain my opinion and to say "no" and then they came around to my view.	A divorced woman (a friend)	4 B 3 A 3	3 a 3 3 a 5 1 a 5 1 a 3	4 a 3

An examination of the two tables, despite the brevity of the samples, illustrates the moderately good agreement by the four independent judges.

Finding #3: The core conflictual relationship themes appear to be similar across virtually all types of objects.

The fact that the core conflictual relationship theme applies to all kinds of objects suggests that a pervasive psychic structure is being tapped by the method. However, the sample of objects is relatively small because of the small sample of relationship episodes from each patient. If a larger number of episodes from each patient were surveyed, themes which are more distinctive for subclasses of objects might appear. (Future work using an enlarged sample is planned.)

Finding #4: The same core conflictual relationship theme was identifiable in both the early and later sessions.

The scoring of the relationship episodes in both the early and the later sessions is listed in Tables 1 and 2. For each of the two patients, a high-frequency core theme was located in the early sessions, and the same theme was again located in the later sessions. The same perseveration of type of theme in early and late sessions was found for all 15 patients (from the theme formulations of one judge). For Ms. BJ, the theme components seem to be very similar in the early sessions and in the later sessions; for Ms. DR the theme components are also similar early and later, but there is a greater emphasis on a positive internal response in the later sessions.

Finding #5: An obvious difference between the early and late sessions appeared for all patients, both high and low improvers: Although the content of the core relationship theme was similar early and late, in the later sessions it became more deeply experienced in the relationship with the therapist.

Ms. BJ (whose theme was her wish to "open up" despite internal and external penalties) had no instances in the early sessions in which she experienced that theme in relationship to the therapist, although she had been afraid that treatment would make her worse. In the later sessions, she did experience that theme strongly in relation to the therapist. For example, the therapist asked her, "What are you crying about?" Patient answered angrily, "I don't know because I don't seem to be getting any better and you seem to be getting worse."

Ms. DR, in the early sessions, was already demanding reassurance that she was okay. But then in the later sessions she escalated her experiencing of the theme by acting out a similar demand in her job. Then she presented the therapist with her behavior in quitting her job when the demand was rejected, and insisted on and appeared to receive his okay and acceptance.

Finding #6: Although the core conflictual relationship theme in the early sessions is similar to that in the later sessions, the high improvement patients showed a major difference from the low improvement patients in terms of a greater sense of mastery of the theme.

Ms. BJ, the low improvement patient, was experiencing the theme not only outside the treatment but also in the relationship with the therapist but with absolutely no sense of mastery of it.

Ms. DR showed the same type of theme in the later sessions, but became relatively more secure that she was okay. This does not mean that the conflictual relationship theme was worked out[7] in the sense that she understood it and resolved it, but later in treatment, she felt that it was not in her way, possibly because of the help she experienced from the therapist and her consequently raised morale. (It should be emphasized that if it were not for the focus provided by the core relationship theme, it might have been difficult to locate her improvement, since at the time of the two later sessions she was involved in an acting out of what seemed to be oedipal transference material.)

Finding #7: The core conflictual relationship themes for these 15 patients showed considerable diversity.

At first, the high level of abstraction of the theme, which is required by its having to fit across so many relationship episodes, led to concern that the theme formulations would not differ much from one patient to another. But, in fact, all of them are distinctive even though some are of similar types. The core themes for the two patients who have been described, for example, are quite different. (The degree of distinctiveness of the core themes can be shown by applying the core theme of each patient to relationship episodes of other patients. This step should show that each core theme makes a comfortable fit with only one patient--the one for whom it had been tailored.)

LOOKING BACK AT THE LINEAGE OF THE CONCEPT AND OF THE METHOD

The Lineage of the Concept of the Core Conflictual Relationship Theme

What is the phenomenon which underlies the core conflictual

---

[7]Does this imply that if the therapists had been more attentive to the core conflictual relationship theme and helped the patient work it through, then mastery would be greater? Probably "yes" for these two cases, although mastery does not mean awareness--note that Ms. DR had little.

relationship theme concept? Such a massive structure could hardly
have gone unnoticed; related concepts deriving from the phenomenon
must exist. The fact that the same theme is discovered both in the
early sessions and in the later sessions for improvers and for nonimprovers, strongly suggests that what has been uncovered is worthy
of being considered a pervasive psychic structure with a slow rate
of change. By far, the best candidate as a cognate is the main transference theme. I have not spoken much so far about transference
since, in the early history of this study, I was not trying to make a
measure of transference, but rather was trying to classify types of
relationship patterns. I am tempted now to consider these two concepts two sides of the same spade; but I must resist it, for it is an
empirical matter to determine how these two concepts relate to each
other. I have described an empirical method for deriving the core
conflictual relationship theme. No such method exists for deriving
the transference pattern and showing consensus on its content. (Although there are several studies showing a moderate agreement on the
amount of transference expressed [Luborsky et al., 1973; Luborsky et
al., 1975; Graff & Luborsky, 1976]), psychoanalysts have been the
only ones who have concerned themselves with the importance of the
transference. Their clinical approach typically yields one main
transference pattern with one or two variants. In almost every psychoanalytic article in which a patient's treatment is described, a
formulation is given of the transference pattern, yet none offers
independent formulations. Even in the Menninger Foundation Psychotherapy Research Project (Kernberg et al., 1972) where both the
initial and termination evaluations required a formulation about the
transference patterns, it was done unsystematically by consensus of
the research team.

Psychoanalysts' formulations are guided by a variety of definitions, most of them containing the same components as this sample one
by Curtis (1973): "Transference is the revival in a current object
relationship, especially to the analyst of thought, feeling, and behavior derived from repressed fantasies originating in significant
conflictual childhood relationships." This definition suggests that
the comparison of transference patterns with core conflictual relationship themes might be best done for those themes which are simultaneously present: (1) in relation to the therapist, (2) in relation to important archaic objects, and possibly also (3) in relation
to current important objects. It seems likely that if the theme is
present for all three of these, it is likely to be generally present
in all relationships and, therefore, appear as similar to the main
core conflictual relationship theme. In any case, I expect the comparison will show considerable overlap in transference pattern statements and core conflictual relationship theme statements.

Analysts, beginning with Freud, have been impressed with recurrent
conflictual patterns, which is another similar concept to the core conflictual relationship theme. Freud (1914) described the compulsion to

repeat or "repetition compulsion" which is evident in the transference
and resistance. The mechanisms of defense were considered by Freud
(1937) to be modes of reaction which are repeated throughout the person's life. French and Wheeler (1963) put forward the idea of a single
"nuclear conflict" in each patient. Similar also is the concept of
"residual trauma" (Blos,1941), a recurrent conflictual pattern which
is evident from time to time throughout a person's life and even after
psychoanalysis is completed.

The recurrence of a single main overwhelming theme was elaborated
by Arlow (1961, 1969a, 1969b). In his 1961 paper, for example, page
377, "Fantasies are grouped around certain basic instinctual wishes
and such a group is composed of different versions or different edi-
tions of attempts to resolve the intrapsychic conflict over these
wishes." In the 1969b paper, page 47, "The organization of these
fantasies takes shape early in life and persists in this form with
only minor variations throughout life. To borrow an analogy from
literature, one could say the plot line of the fantasy remains the
same although the characters and the situations may vary." The last
sentence states vividly what is measured by the core conflictual
relationship theme method. Dr. Arlow (in his discussion of my paper)
views the core conflictual relationship theme as one offshoot of a
more basic substrate composed of unconscious fantasies. Actually
both may be a product of highly overlearned patterns of relationships
to internal and external objects. From that point of view, both the
unconscious fantasies and the core conflictual relationship theme are
expressions of these overlearned relationship patterns which get expressed when wishes are activated toward objects.

Recurrent patterns persisting even after the analysis have been
noted; for example, Pfeffer (1963), "In analysis repetition is not
eliminated but the content and substance of what is repeatable is
changed." Similarly Schlessinger and Robbins (1975) described the
follow-up of a patient which illustrates the perseveration of conflictual themes with the addition "of a self-analytic function as the
significant outcome of the analysis." Finally, Graff and Luborsky
(1976) compared two relatively more successful analyses with two
relatively less successful analyses by means of the trend of daily
post-session therapists' ratings of amount of transference and resistance. Transference was even more evident in the later stages
of the more successful analyses, suggesting that the concept of a
reduction in the amount of the transference in a successful analysis
(Ekstein, 1956) has to be reformulated.

After coming to the idea of a core conflictual relationship
theme, I realized that I had been there once before in my research
on the symptom-onset theme. The symptom-context research showed
that there is a particular theme for each patient which appears before recurrent symptoms in psychotherapy and psychoanalysis. This
theme is recurrent within each patient, but different from patient

to patient (Luborsky, 1967; Luborsky and Auerbach, 1969). In the
1967 paper, I noted the similarity of this symptom-onset theme to
the themes evident in the patient's dreams and other material in
the same session. It would be no great surprise, though it has not
yet been shown, if the symptom-onset theme for each patient were
found to be the same as the core conflictual relationship theme.

The Lineage of the Core Conflictual Relationship Theme Method

In essence, it is the only clinical-quantitative method--based
on the clinical procedure of listening for redundancy and based on
scoring of transcripts of psychotherapy--which is aimed at finding
the unique core conflictual relationship theme for each patient.
The analysis is guided by the principle of finding the relationship
theme which fits the most relationship episodes. After the core
theme is formulated by independent judges, the components of the
theme are then scored for every relationship episode. In that way,
it is possible to specify the extent to which the theme formulations
apply, and what components of the theme formulation might change or
remain the same over time.

One method, which has some general currency in academic psycholog
which may tap a similar phenomenon, is the Kelly Role Construct Repertory Test (1955). Kelly believes that the construct discerned for
each person is highly stable and likely to remain the same during
treatment. Someone should try both methods, and see the extent to
which they do capture the same theme. In general, though, it is fair
to conclude that with the possible exception of the Role Repertory
Construct Method, academic psychology has neglected the phenomenon
which is caught by the core conflictual relationship theme method.
Clinicians readily see such a phenomenon they designate as transference because they are willing to rely upon the results of their
clinical method of observation. The academic psychologists miss
seeing it for lack of a method.

From the Mount Zion San Francisco Psychotherapy Research Group
has come an approach which bears one important resemblance to our
method: After thoroughly examining some of the early sessions, some
important themes are selected. These are then scored independently
through large segments of the treatment (Sampson et al., 1972; Horowitz et al., 1975). Mayman & Faris (1960), and Mayman (1968) have
devised a clinical system for finding relationship paradigms in
early memories and dreams.

Much less similar to the core conflictual relationship theme
method are the scores of content analysis schemes which are available for application to psychotherapy (Marsden, 1971). Some begin
with word counts and build these up into meaningful constellations
(e.g., Dahl, 1972); some begin with thematic analyses of phrases and
build up from there (e.g., Gottschalk & Gleser, 1969, and TAT based

systems, e.g., Aron, 1949). All of them are based upon looking for
evidences of preset categories which apply across all patients, rather than catching the supraordinate theme for each patient. (Murray et al., 1938 came close, but never developed one of his original
ideas--the "unity theme"--for scoring unique supraordinate themes.)
None of these approaches relies upon the degree of clinical inference about relationship themes which is part of a psychotherapist's
usual task. The present system starts with the kind of high level
clinical inference which the psychotherapist takes as his basic data,
and works back down to the patient-therapist exchange to examine its
degree of fit.

LOOKING TO THE FUTURE OF CORE CONFLICTUAL RELATIONSHIP THEME RESEARCH

How Recurrent and Pervasive is the Core Conflictual Relationship Theme?

During the treatment: The data reveal a pervasive theme within
the treatment--it appears both in the early and later sessions. All
of the results in the present paper came from small samples of the
sessions--only two 20-minute segments early in the treatment, and two
20-minute segments later in treatment. At first, working with such
a reduced sample of the psychotherapy seemed like spearing fish in
murky waters. After more experience, it seemed that the outlines
of the phenomenon being stalked were so broad that the danger of
coming home empty-creeled seemed minimal.

Nevertheless, in later reports, consistency of the patient's
theme in other sessions will be explored. The same analysis could
be made for four different 20-minute segments from the same patients;
for example, for Sessions 2 and 4, and two other later sessions. Not
only would this provide information on the degree to which the same
theme formulation emerges from other sessions--a kind of crossvalida-
tion within each patient--but also it would provide a larger sample
of relationship episodes so that differences in relationships to
different objects can be examined.

Before the treatment: Since it is such a durable theme, it is
likely to have been present in similar form before the treatment. A
bit of data based upon a tape-recorded hour-long prognostic index
interview just before the treatment, as well as a five-minute speech
sample just before the treatment, gave some indication that the same
conflictual relationship theme was present earlier. These data imply
further that the core conflictual relationship theme established
during treatment is not just a function of the particular match of
patient and therapist, although it must be colored by it. (In one
therapy there were two therapists, and it would be of interest to
do the theme analysis for both.) For the patient's distant past, we
have only some early memories reported by the patient in the sessions.
It would be of tremendous value to learn whether the core conflictual

relationship theme was present in the archaic family relationships.
(The best that could be done by direct observation would be to take
a group of young children and establish theme statements, possibly
on the CAT, and redo the test much later in life. A more feasible
alternative might be to find some data in the longitudinal studies
of several decades ago, and follow up a sample of these people. However, these data were not collected as part of psychotherapy sessions.[8])

After the treatment: It would be desirable to have follow-up
data on these subjects--further sessions several years later (as
was done by Pfeffer, 1963, and Schlessinger & Robbins, 1975). Consistency would probably remain.

How are the Core Conflictual Relationship Themes Related to Helping
Alliances and to the Outcome of the Psychotherapy?

I had originally gotten into the exploration of relationship
themes in order to learn the place of the helping alliance relationship within the larger pattern of the person's typical relationship
themes. I will present here the available results of the interrela-
tionship of these two concepts, and in turn with the outcome of psychotherapy.

1. The type of core conflictual relationship theme does not
appear to be related to either the presence of a helping alliance
type of relationship or to the outcome of psychotherapy.

2. The positivity of the expectations from objects, as reflected
in the relationship episodes, does appear to be somewhat related to
the development of helping alliances and to the outcome of psychotherapy. (I should examine separately the patient's expectations
from the therapist and expectations from other objects. I expect
these two will be positively correlated, implying that the relationship with the therapist is part of a set of expectations from objects
which is characteristic of the person. I should also consider Orne's
concept of "anticipatory socialization" for psychotherapy (Orne &
Wender, 1968), since it is clear that in at least one study (Hoehn-
Saric, et al.,1964) anticipatory socialization increases general

---

[8]Nevertheless, it is of interest to note the considerable temporal
consistency of some trait items. Block (1975) for example, reported
on rated CQ items (California Q -sort items) which show consistency:
"is a genuinely dependable and responsible person" correlates .58
in the male sample from junior high school to senior high school, and
.53 from senior high school until adulthood: or for females the CQ
item "basically submissive" correlates .50 from JHS to SHS, and .46
from SHS to adulthood. Possibly, if the most highly intercorrelated
cluster for each person was given a score at each time point, it woul

positivity of expectation from the treatment and has a positive effect upon the outcomes of psychotherapy.)

3. The most striking association is that between helping alliances and the outcome of psychotherapy. In our sample, there is a
major difference between improvers and nonimprovers in the development of helping alliances--improvers show very early development of
helping alliances, that is, already in Sessions 3 and 5 (Luborsky,
1976a). Several factors probably contribute to this finding:

(a) The improvers show slightly greater initial positivity
of expectations from objects, including the therapist. The patient
may size up the therapist as a person who can be helpful or even a
loved object; for example, Ms. DR, who had tried two previous therapists and not responded well to either one, decided in the first interview that the present therapist was someone she liked. She expressed this evaluation, and related positive expectations in a variety of ways, one of them being that the therapist had narrow feet
and her lover had narrow feet. Within Sessions 3 and 5, she indicated
that she already was feeling helped (helping alliance, Type 1). She
had reduced taking the tranquilizers, and had been able to begin to
give up her lover, which had been one of the initial aims of her
treatment. By contrast, Ms. BJ, in the early sessions, made no comments indicating positive benefits of the treatment and, in fact, indicated that the requirements of the treatment which involved talking
and expressing one's feelings would have a bad effect upon her.

(b) The therapists of the improvers may show more behaviors
related to the encouragement of the development of the helping alliance. (A manual has been constructed for scoring therapists' behaviors which facilitate or inhibit the development of helping relationships, Luborsky, 1976a.)

Now that the theme-tracking equipment has been constructed, further uses for it may be considered: (1) It may have some utility for
guiding therapists in identifying the main theme in the initial sessions. In some forms of short-term treatment (Sifneos, 1972; Malin,
1963), such rapid formulation is of value as the consistent focus of
the therapeutic effort; (2) It may help in evaluating the outcome
of treatment. The main theme can be compared initially and near
termination, especially in terms of the degree of mastery of the
main theme at the two points. We saw that this helped in identifying the area of improvement for Ms. DR who otherwise might be considered by some clinicians to be only in a state of resistive acting
out.

---

be somewhat more like the core conflictual relationship theme. It
would be of interest to see whether such a cluster for each person
would have a recognizable kinship with the core conflictual relationship theme.

In sum, the proposed content analysis methods should serve as helpful "sonar" equipment for tracking the core conflictual relationship theme of each patient. With this equipment, there is little reason to fear that clinicians will miss the massive structure, which is its intended target, or even disagree much about its shape, as I hope I have demonstrated with the two patients presented here. Among its most distinctive characteristics are: Its generality across relationship episodes and across different types of objects, its presence early and later in treatment, its tendency to be more deeply experienced within the patient-therapist relationship later in the treatment, and its shift toward being mastered for those patients who improve.

REFERENCES

Arlow, J. Ego psychology in the study of mythology. Journal of the American Psychoanalytic Association, 1961, 9:371-393.

Arlow, J. Unconscious fantasy and disturbances of conscious experience. Psychoanalytic Quarterly, 1969, 38:1-27. (a)

Arlow, J. Fantasy, memory, and reality testing. Psychoanalytic Quarterly, 1969, 38:28-51. (b)

Aron, Betty. A manual for analyses of the thematic apperception test. Berkeley, Calif.: Willis E. Berg, 1949.

Block, J. Recognizing the coherence of personality. Unpublished manuscript, July, 1975.

Blos, P. The adolescent personality. A study of individual behavior for the commission on secondary school curriculum. New York-London Appleton-Century-Crofts, 1941.

Curtis, H. Toward a metapsychology of transference. Paper read to American Psychoanalytic Association, New York, 1973.

Dahl, H. A quantitative study of a psychoanalysis. In R. R. Holt & E. Peterfreund (Eds.), Psychoanalysis & Contemporary Science, Vol. 1. New York: Macmillan Company, 1972.

Ekstein, R. Psychoanalytic techniques. In D. Brower & L. E. Abt (Eds.), Progress in clinical psychology, Vol. 2. New York: Grune & Stratton, 1956.

Fiske, D. W., Cartwright, D. S., & Kirtner, W. L. Are psychotherapeutic changes predictable? Journal of Abnormal & Social Psychology 1964, 69:418-426.

Freud, S. (1914). Remembering, repeating and working through. In
J. Strachey (Ed.), Standard Edition, Vol. 2. London: Hogarth
Press, 1955.

Freud, S. (1937). Analyses terminable and interminable. In J.
Strachey (Ed.), Standard Edition, Vol. 23. London: Hogarth Press,
1964.

French, T. & Wheeler, D. R. Hope and repudiation of hope in psychoanalytic therapy. International Journal of Psychoanalysis, 1963,
44:304-316.

Gottschalk, L. & Gleser, G. The measurement of psychological states
through the content analysis of verbal behavior. Berkeley: University of California Press, 1969.

Graff, H. & Luborsky, L. Long-term trends in transference and resistance: A quantitative analytic method applied to four psycho-
analyses. Journal of the Psychoanalytic Association, in press.

Hoehn-Saric, R., Frank, J., Imber, S., Nash, E., Stone, A., & Battle,
C. Systematic preparation of patients for psychotherapy. 1. Ef-
fects on therapy behavior and outcome. Journal of Psychiatric
Research, 1964, 2:267-281.

Horowitz, L. M., Sampson, H., Siegelman, E., Wolfson, A., & Weiss, J.
On the identification of warded-off mental contents. Journal of
Abnormal Psychology, 1975, 84:545-558.

Kelly, G. A. The psychology of personal construct, Vol. 1. New York:
Norton, 1955.

Kernberg, O., Burstein, E., Coyne, L., Appelbaum, A., Horowitz, L., &
Voth, H. Psychotherapy and psychoanalysis: Final report of the
Menninger Foundation's Psychotherapy Research Project. Bulletin of
the Menninger Clinic, 1972, 36:1-275.

Luborsky, L. Momentary forgetting during psychotherapy and psycho-
analysis: A theory and research method. In R. R. Holt (Ed.),
Motives and thought: Psychoanalytic essays in honor of David
Rapaport. New York: International Universities Press, 1967.

Luborsky, L. Helping alliances in psychotherapy: The groundwork for
a study of their relationship to its outcome. In J. L. Claghorn
(Ed.), Successful psychotherapy. New York: Brunner/Mazel, in press.
(a)

Luborsky, L. Curative factors in psychoanalytic and psychodynamic
psychotherapies. In J. P. Brady, J. Mendels, M. Orne, & W. Rieger
(Eds.), Psychiatry: Areas of promise and advancement. New York:
Spectrum, in press. (b)

Luborsky, L. & Auerbach, A. H.   The symptom-context method: Quantitative studies of symptom formation in psychotherapy.   Journal of the American Psychoanalytic Association, 1969, 17:68-99.

Luborsky, L., Graff, H., Pulver, S., & Curtis, H.   A clinical-quantitative examination of consensus on the concept of transference.   Archives of General Psychiatry, 1973, 29:69-75.

Luborsky, L., Crabtree, L., Curtis, H., Ruff, G., & Mintz, J.   The concept "space" of transference for eight psychoanalysts.   British Journal of Medical Psychology, 1975, 48:1-6.

Luborsky, L., Singer, B., & Luborsky, Lise.   Comparative studies of psychotherapies: Is it true that "Everybody has won and all must have prizes?"   Archives of General Psychiatry, 1975, 32:995-1008.

Luborsky, L. & Mintz, J.   Psychotherapy: Who benefits and how. (Book in progress.)

Malan, D. H.   A study of brief psychotherapy.   London: Tavistock Publishing, 1963.

Marsden, G.   Content analysis studies of psychotherapy: 1954 through 1968.   In A. Bergin & S. Garfield (Eds.), Handbook of psychotherapy and behavior change.   New York: Wiley, 1971.

Mayman, M.   Early memories and character structure.   Journal of Projective Techniques, 1968, 32:303-316.

Mayman, M. & Faris, M.   Early memories as expressions of relationship paradigms.   American Journal of Orthopsychiatry, 1960, 30:507-520.

Mitchell, K., Bozarth, J., Truax, C., & Krauft, C.   Antecedents to psychotherapeutic change.   An NIMH Final Report, MH 12306, March, 1973.

Murray, H. A.   Explorations in personality.   New York: Oxford University Press, 1938.

Orne, M. & Wender, P.   Anticipatory socialization for psychotherapy: Method and rationale.   American Journal of Psychiatry, 1968, 124: 88-98.

Pfeffer, A.   The meaning of the analyst after analyses: A contribution to the theory of therapeutic results.   Journal of the American Psychoanalytic Association, 1963, 11:229-244.

Rogers, C. R.   The necessary and sufficient conditions of therapeutic personality change.   Journal of Consulting Psychology, 1957, 21: 95-103.

Rogers, C. R. & Dymond, R. F. Psychotherapy and personality change. Chicago: University of Chicago Press, 1954.

Rosenzweig, S. Some implicit common factors in diverse methods of psychotherapy. American Journal of Orthopsychiatry, 1936, 6:412–415.

Sampson, H., Weiss, J., Mlodnovsky, L., & House, E. Defense analyses and the emergence of warded-off mental contents: An empirical study. Archives of General Psychiatry, 1972, 26:524–532.

Schlessinger, N. & Robbins, F. The psychoanalytic process: Recurrent patterns of conflict and changes in ego. Journal of the American Psychoanalytic Association, 1975, 23:761–782.

Sifneos, P. E. Short-term psychotherapy and emotional crisis. Cambridge, Mass.: Harvard University Press, 1972.

Requests for reprints should be sent to Dr. Luborsky, 207 Piersol Bldg., Hospital of the University of Pennsylvania, Philadelphia, Pa. 19004.

LEXICAL DERIVATIVES IN PATIENTS' SPEECH:

SOME NEW DATA ON DISPLACEMENT AND DEFENSE

Donald P. Spence

Rutgers Medical School

Piscataway, New Jersey 08854

During an hour toward the end of the first six months of her analysis, a patient of Paul Gray's "began to speak of her success at overcoming shyness at work. She said this was allowing her, during the past several days, to persuade her boss that the company could, in fact, pay her way to a neighboring state for a week during the coming month for research purposes which would be valuable for the company" (Gray, 1973, p. 479).

Gray goes on to compare three possible responses to this announcement: (1) Point out how the trip would interrupt the analysis; (2) Suggest that such an impulse should be analyzed before it is carried out; (3) Show its relation to surrounding material. In this instance, it followed a statement of disappointment over the difficult location of the analyst's office. The sequence of thoughts, difficult location and the impulse to take a trip, suggest that the problem of location could be solved by simply not coming, and solved in a way that would spare the patient the discomfort of expressing her feelings to the analyst.

More abstractly, we can conceptualize the comment about the trip as a displacement of her negative feelings about coming to the office. Rather than expand on these feelings, the patient alludes to them by talking about the trip. The analyst is sensitive to the displacement by virtue of its contiguity in time and, by analyzing the displacement, can bring to the surface her negative feelings about the office, and perhaps similar feelings about the analysis as well. Notice how the displacement occurs on the heels of a conflict; we would expect this from our theory of defense, and our concept of the primary process. When expression along one path is blocked, we would expect to find a substitute expression; and, we would also expect some kind of transformation or disguise.

I have given you one example, and we might feel somewhat tentative about exploring this sequence any further at this point. But suppose we had noted, over the course of many sessions, how a mild negative statement (or an implied negative comment) was immediately followed by thoughts of moving away. We would feel fairly sure that the connection was more than accidental; we have moved from one contiguous pairing to many. If we were to keep systematic track of every negative transference comment and every reference to moving away, we would be able to determine the proportion of times they were paired as a function of their combined occurrences. If each session were scored for each category, negative feeling and moving away, a positive correlation over sessions would indicate the co-occurrence of these two classes of events, and the larger the correlation, the stronger the relationship. Thus, the size of the correlation can be used to indicate the amount of displacement.

You notice that I said every occurrence--an important qualification. To keep complete track of both events over a large number of hours would be an impossible task for a clinician, but a very reasonable one for a machine. If you allow that a computer is a kind of machine, and allow that a computer can be programmed to recognize words, you see how it might be possible to use the computer to actually uncover displacements, to discover more than the clinician heard in the first place.

There is a second reason why computers are the tool of choice, and it has to do with the linguistic distinction between surface structure and deep structure. As you know, the surface structure refers to the specific words which are used to make up a sentence, their order (syntax), and their content (semantics). Deep structure refers to the meaning conveyed by these words. We almost always attend to the deep structure and ignore the surface structure, as I can show by the following examples:

1. If I make a statement like "Do you have your watch on?," you will, almost without thinking, respond by telling me the time. I could have made that request in any number of ways; the actual words I use (surface structure) are largely immaterial to the conveyance of the meaning.

2. Verbal learning experiments, such as the recent study by Bransford and Franks (1971) and others, recently summarized by Jenkins (1974), show that if Ss are given a list of sentences to learn, and then later are asked to go over a second list to determine whether each sentence did or did not appear on the first list, they are equally likely to label a sentence with equivalent meaning as one of the target sentences as they are one of the target sentences. In other words, differences in surface structure are almost impossible to detect. Suppose the target sentence was, "The car pulling the trailer climbed the hill." Subjects tend to be almost certain that

they have also heard the sentences, "The car was old," and, "The old car climbed the steep hill." In fact, neither sentence had appeared. They have attended to deep structure, as we all do, and ignored the particular words of the surface structure.

3. Quite interesting things happen when we reverse the usual procedure. If I make the statement "Do you have your watch on?," and you answer "Yes" (attending to surface structure), I would feel frustrated and misunderstood, even though you have made an accurate response. Examples like this show how overtrained we are to attend to deep structure and ignore surface structure.

4. There is one class of events, however, in which we quite intentionally turn things around, and I am referring to clinical listening. We frequently pay just as much attention to the specific words used by our patient, the surface structure, as we do to his meaning, or intended meaning. Slips of the tongue provide an obvious example; when they occur, our attention is suddenly shifted from the deep structure (what he was trying to say) to the surface structure (what he accidentally said). But the same shift may take place in more subtle contexts. Suppose a patient makes the statement: "I can't stomach another fight with my boss." We would begin to suspect that these fights have made his stomach hurt. We draw that conclusion by listening carefully to the surface structure, and experience has taught us that language use is not random but, on the contrary, what we like to call over-determined. Given a certain intended meaning (deep structure), we have many ways in which to map this meaning on to the actual form of the utterance, and the choice of ways is determined by such nonrandom forces as wishes and feelings.

Here is where the computer comes into its own. For the very reason that it is grossly insensitive to deep structure (why, for example, it proved such a failure in language translation), it is highly sensitive to surface structure. If we feel that important information is contained in the specific words people use, and if we feel that this information can even be recognized out of context (as in the preceding example with stomach), then the computer is our tool of choice. It keeps perfect track of word occurrence and co-occurrence, and allows us to investigate contingencies in very thorough fashion. From the data on contingencies, we can make some statements about displacements.

Let me turn to some actual examples. We have samples of natural language from women who, at the time of the interview, were at risk for cervical carcinoma. They had come to the hospital for diagnostic cone biopsies because of local irregularities detected by their regular doctor. The interview took place before the results of the biopsy

were known. Thus, both patient and doctor were blind to the actual
outcome.[1]

     First, we asked two judges to rate each interview for the degree
of concern shown by the patient about her current condition on a 7-
point scale. The scale ranged from complete denial, as gathered
from statements like "There's nothing wrong with me," to open worry
and concern; statements like "I'm sure I have cancer." The interviews were unlabeled as to age (a good predictor of cervical carcinoma), or later diagnosis. Reliability between judges on 62 cases
was very high (r = .94); disagreements appeared on only 8 cases,
and these did not exceed two points on a 7-point scale. These disagreements were resolved by discussion.

     I should point out here that the rating of concern was unrelated
to the biopsy findings (r = -.02); in other words, we are measuring
something about the patient's cognitive style, her way of handling
the fact that she is at risk for cervical carcinoma. As you well
know, patients have different mechanisms for handling that kind of
stress, and the most frightened patients are not always the sickest
(hypochondriacs, in fact, often live quite long and unhappy lives).
I want to come back to the cognitive style somewhat later, because
it has a bearing on the form and manifestation of displacements.

     The lack of correlation between concern and diagnosis also
tells us something else; namely, that these patients were not consciously aware of the presence of a malignancy. They knew that they
were at risk, but did not know that they were actually ill. Yet our
theory, and in particular the literature on prodromal markers,
would suggest that at some other level, these patients actually did
"know" and the word is in quotes that they were carrying the disease.

     To find evidence for such knowledge, we looked for displacements
of the underlying symptom. To use the contingency rule I discussed
before, a viable displacement would have to be highly correlated
with the diagnosis; that is, it should appear in the patients found,
by cone biopsy, to actually have cancer, and it should not appear
in the controls. And to qualify as a displacement, it should also
show some relation to cancer. But since we expect transformations
to appear, almost by definition, the relation might be quite distant. Therefore, the semantic link between a possible lexical
marker and cancer should not be a primary consideration because we
want to be willing to accept a wide range of transformations. For
the purposes of this discussion, I will define as a displacement
any word that significantly discriminates between cancer patients
and controls at better than the .05 level.

-----

[1]I want to express my appreciation to Dr. Arthur Schmale of the
Rochester University School of Medicine for giving me access to
this material.

Now a few words about the relationship between displacement and defense. In the General Introduction to Psychoanalysis, Freud made very clear the relation between defenses (which he called censorship) and displacement. "The second achievement of the dream work is displacement... we know that it is entirely the work of the dream censorship" (quoted in Gill, 1963, p. 99). He reasoned that displacement was needed to allow unconscious derivatives to bypass the censorship and appear in the dream; displacement also allowed the dream to be remembered. It follows that the extent of displacement is, in part, a function of what Holt would call the defense-demand of the unconscious idea. Derivatives which do not arouse anxiety, for example, would not invoke the censorship and the need for displacement; derivatives with a high loading of defense-demand would produce a wide range of displacements. We can also assume that the degree of disguise can be used, very roughly, as an index of defense-demand. Highly transformed derivatives are, we assume, transformed for a purpose, to evade the censorship or, to use more modern language, to make them more ego-syntonic.

Applied to our sample of patients at risk for cervical cancer, this formulation would suggest the following. The patients who deny any concern over the outcome of the biopsy are, we would think, denying the danger and indicating that the threat of cancer is ego-dystonic and potentially quite disruptive. If derivatives of the cancer theme did appear, we would expect a fair amount of transformation would be necessary before they would appear in consciousness. This very disguise would make them difficult to detect, but our machine approach, which takes advantage of contingencies, might come up with some interesting specimens.

What about the patients who are overtly afraid? We might expect one of two possibilities to occur. On the one hand, their lack of defense would suggest that no transformation was necessary; that references to the cancer theme (and perhaps even the word "cancer") would appear early and often. On the other hand, the easy discharge of their anxiety might rob the cancer derivatives of much of their force. If the patients are freely abreacting, it seems possible that no derivatives would appear. Careful study of the interviews made it seem as if the first possibility was more likely; all patients, even those rated overtly concerned, were quite clearly under control with their feelings held in check. In either case, our method for looking for contingencies should give us some useful specimens which we can apply to the two possibilities.

Our method takes the following form. First, we selected, from each interview, only the patient's statements. (Changes in language of the interviewer raise interesting questions in their own right, and will become the subject of another study.) Patient speech, for each interview, was then broken up into separate words, sorted alphabetically, and stored on computer tape. Then a special program

was designed which allowed us to compare cancer cases with controls
and determine, for any word of interest, the extent to which it could
discriminate between the two groups; in short, the correlation between marker variable and diagnosis. Because of our assumptions
about the interaction between defense and displacement, we made separate analyses of the two groups of patients, dividing them according
to their score on the 7-point defense scale.

Our search for displacements was guided by Schmale's theory of
hopelessness/helplessness and its relation to serious illness. In
a number of papers, Schmale and others have pointed out the relation
between this cluster of feelings and the onset of serious and/or
terminal illness. Recent widows, for example, are more likely to
fall ill in the six-month period following their husband's death
than are a sample of matched controls; old people are more likely
to die after their birthday than before. There are many other
statistics of a similar kind. In general, the patient's feelings
that no alternatives are open seems often to precipitate either a
worsening of the medical picture, or the onset of disease. Schmale
and his colleagues tend to conceptualize the problem in terms of a
set of correlated systems. A breakdown on the level of subjective
feelings, as manifested by an increase of hopelessness and helplessness, seems to be a fairly good predictor of a breakdown in the body's
immune system. As a result, the host becomes more vulnerable to whatever infectious agents may be present in the local environment.

To examine their theory more intensively, Schmale and Iker (1966)
collected a series of women who were being referred to the Rochester
Hospital for a cone biopsy for suspicion of cervical carcinoma. Women were selected by their own physician because of repeated Class
III Pap smears revealing cells which were suspicious, but not diagnostic of, cancer. Sixty-two women were studied (40 came from the
first series reported in Schmale & Iker, 1966; 22 were subsequently
added) ranging in age from 21 to 52. Each woman was interviewed at
length with an attempt to cover both current feelings and background
development. The following criteria were used by Schmale for judging
hopelessness: devotion to causes with little or no feeling of success
or pleasure; feelings of "doom," feelings of frustration and loss,
etc. All interviews were recorded before the results of the biopsy
were known to either patient or interviewer. Interviews tended to
last about one hour. The interviewer (Schmale, in all but one case)
attempted to predict, from the assessment of hopelessness which he
made on the basis of the interview, the outcome of the biopsy.

The correlation for 62 cases was .44, significant but not overwhelming. Nevertheless, it seemed promising, and strong enough to
support another, more intensive examination of the data--which brings
me to the present study. And I think it should be clear that our
model, although similar, differs in several important respects. First,

we did not restrict ourselves to looking only at hopelessness. Second, we assumed that the defensive style of the patient would, as I indicated above, have an important effect on the form and distribution of the lexical markers. Third, we were assuming less in the way of conscious awareness. We felt that some markers might be present which, although present in the patient's speech, were actually uttered out of her awareness; subtle changes in the surface structure for example, of the kind I described earlier. And fourth, because of their fringe position, these markers might not be detected by the interviewer; therefore, we might actually do a better job with a computer analysis than did the original clinical judge.

We began our search by looking at words from the following six categories: Distress (from the Harvard dictionary, developed by Stone and collaborators, 1966, and chosen because it contained synonyms of helplessness); Attempt, also from Harvard, and seen as the opposite of helplessness; Follow, from Harvard and closely related to helplessness; Death, from Harvard, and related to a significant aspect of any cancer and, in particular, to the popular stereotype of cancer; and Illness, from Psychodict and also related to cancer. You will notice that our choice of categories covers a range from highly cancer-specific (Illness), through close connotations of cancer (Death), to more distant connotations (the remaining categories which touch on significant aspects of helplessness and hopelessness).

The critical details of our search are presented in Table 1. After we picked a given category, we first checked each word in the category against all words in our sample of patient speech. Only if a given word appeared two or more times in the total corpus was it retained for further search. Over all, 39% of the dictionary words appeared in our corpus, reducing the pool of possible markers from 468 to 181. This reduction stems, in large part, from the fact that we are dealing with spoken language which, quite characteristically, uses many fewer different words than written language.

One word is far and away the best predictor from our original pool of 181 candidates, and it is the word "death." It appears significantly more often in patients with a positive biopsy than in controls (t = 3.2, p <.001). No other single word does nearly as well in discriminating cancer patients. Cancer patients use the word "death" with an average rate of 2.42 times per 10,000 words, compared to the average rate for control patients of .45 times per 10,000 words, more than five times as often. The norm for spoken English, taken from a smaller sample of 200,000 words (Howes, 1966), is .45 per 10,000 words, almost exactly the rate shown by our control patients.

How is it used? In one of three ways--as a concrete reference to the patient herself ("I have a fear of death"); as a concrete

Table 1

Source of Words which Discriminate between Cancer and Control Patients

Category	Source	No. Words	No. Words in Corpus (2 or More Occurrences)	%	No. Significant/ Afraid t > 1.5	No. Significant/ Defended t > 1.5	Total
Death	Harvard-83	108	36	33	5	7	12
Distress	Harvard-31	124	70	56	4	9	13
Illness	Psychodict-23	113	29	26	3	2	5
Attempt	Harvard-50	38	9	24	0	0	0
Follow	Harvard-47	44	22	50	0	2	2
Passive	Psychodict-50	41	15	37	0	0	0
		468	181	39	12	20	32

reference to some other person, living or dead ("He died a natural
death"); or as a metaphor ("I almost froze to death"). Concrete
self references account for 10% of the total of 50 instances; concrete other references account for 30%, and metaphor accounts for
60%. Concrete self references are clearly in the minority which
suggests that the concept of her own death is incidental rather than
focal in the patient's speech; we might guess that the patients are
not aware of its significance as a marker word (whether the interviewer was aware is another question, to be taken up in a later
study).

Only 10 words beside "death" discriminate between cancer patients and controls with a t better than 2.0. (The words are "black,"
"complains," "depend," "difficulty," "disgusted," "fall," "fractured,"
"infections," "screaming," "worried.")

To enlarge our sample of markers, and to investigate in more detail the question of how the type of marker depends on the defensive
style of the patient, we divided our sample according to defensive
style, and searched separately for defended and afraid patients. We
rejected any word whose discrimination level ("Student's" t) fell
below 1.5, significant for 30 cases at slightly better than the .20
level. (We set our cutoff purposely low to allow us to look at a
wide range of markers.) And, to simplify the analysis, we used only
positive markers, that is, words which appeared more often among the
cancer patients. Twelve markers met this double criterion for the
afraid patients, and 20 for the defended patients. It should also
be explained that in all comparisons, we are talking about rate of
occurrence for a given marker per 1000 words, enabling us to compare subjects with different amounts of verbal output.

The two sets of words are presented in Tables 2 and 3, along
with the discriminant level ("Student's" t) for each word, and a
rating of Relatedness which I will explain later. The two lists
are arranged in decreasing order of significance, and the line shows
where the level changes from significant (t > 2.0, p < .05) to nonsignificant (t < 2.0, .20 < p < .10). There are significantly more
words above the line in the defended group of patients (p < .02,
Fisher exact test). This difference does not reflect a difference
in the number of words spoken by the two groups of patients (Defended, mean = 5827; Afraid, mean = 6076), nor the differences in
number of different words (Defended, mean = 868; Afraid, mean = 869).

Look more closely at the markers for the afraid or undefended
patients. The only two significant markers are the words "cancer"
and "death"--clearly denotative, clearly related to the illness,
and showing a minimum amount of transformation or displacement.

Now look at the markers for the defended patients, and, again,
study only those above the line. Only the word "death" is clearly

Table 2

Significant Marker Words for Defended Group

Word	Discriminant Level (t)	Relatedness (1=none; 7=most)
Dark	3.35	4.0
Disgusted	2.85	5.2
Screaming	2.84	5.2
Difficulty	2.68	5.7
Conflict	2.36	5.3
Depend	2.35	4.6
Drop	2.35	3.2
Tense	2.35	5.7
Accept	2.15	5.0
Strain	2.10	5.4
Black	2.04	---
Death	2.01	6.9

(All words above this line are each significant,
 p <.05, two-tailed t test)

Fractured	1.83	3.0
Complains	1.83	5.4
Confused	1.80	5.0
Infections	1.76	4.8
Crying	1.71	5.8
Winter	1.70	2.5
Finish	1.55	5.1
Unhappy	1.53	6.3

Correlation between Discriminant Level and
Relatedness: r = -.06, N.S.

denotative. Some, like "screaming" and "tense," are partially related to the theme of cancer, but are not likely to appear as responses to cancer in a word association test; and others, like
"black" and "dark," are primarily connotative. Both of the significant markers for the afraid patients (100%) are denotative; only one
out of 12, or 8% of the significant markers for the defended patients
are denotative. In other words, not only did we turn up more significant markers from our original pool of 181 words in the defended

Table 3

Significant Marker Words for Afraid Group

Word	Discriminant Level (t)	Relatedness (1=none; 7=most)
Cancer	2.74	6.8
Death	2.40	6.9

(All words above this line are each significant,
p < .05, two-tailed t test)

Word	Discriminant Level (t)	Relatedness
Painful	1.98	6.3
Worried	1.89	6.2
Fall	1.82	3.5
Black	1.74	---
Bitter	1.57	5.8
Ached	1.57	6.0
Bled	1.55	5.3
Complains	1.54	5.4
Infections	1.54	4.8
Alcoholic	1.51	4.0

Correlation between Discriminant Level and
Relatedness: $r = .61$, $p < .05$.

patients, but those which did appear tend to primarily connotative rather than denotative.

Despite their weak link to cervical cancer, we are tempted to conclude that the markers in the defended group are transformations of the original cancer theme. Notice first that the word "cancer" does not appear as a marker in this group; its t value is not only nonsignificant (-.18), but in the wrong direction as well, showing that it is used more often by control patients. Notice, second, that the word "death" is much less significant ($t = 2.0$) than some of the more connotative words such as "dark" ($t = 3.3$) and "disgusted" ($t = 2.8$). Third, 12 words discriminate significantly between cancers and controls.

One way to account for these data is to assume the need for disguise or displacement is much greater in the defended patients.

As a result, the derivatives which we can identify by machine, are less obviously related to cancer. We know from their interviews that the defended patients are at great pains to show that although they may be at risk in the eyes of their referring doctor, they do not feel at risk in any subjective sense. It stands to reason that these patients, with their heavy use of denial would screen out any obvious reference to the likelihood of cancer or the fear of death. Despite these, and other defenses, the patients in this group who are diagnosed as having cancer still show significant differences in their language, as compared to the controls. The answer, in part, lies in the use of displacement. These markers are so well disguised that they are, with very few exceptions, almost completely ego-syntonic

At this point, you might ask whether we can really justify the assumption that the significant marker words are, in fact, derivatives of cancer. First, are they meaningfully related to cancer? We asked a sample of 102 judges to give us associations to the word "cancer," and the response "death," our single best marker, is clearly the most popular associate. It appears in 70% of our total sample of 102 judges, followed by the second choice, "lung" at a fair distance (45%). Only one of the other marker words appeared as an associate ("black"). To get around this problem, we asked a subset of the same sample of judges to scale each of our marker words on a 7-point scale, ranging from highly related to terminal illness (7), to unrelated (1). (See Tables 2 and 3.) All of our significant markers score 3 or better, with an average score of 5.4 out of a possible 7. Even more striking evidence appears when we look separately at the two types of patients. In our afraid patients, the extent to which a marker discriminates between cancer patients and controls is highly correlated with the extent to which it is related to terminal cancer. Thus the markers "death" and "cancer" are the two best markers for this group of patients, and they are scaled 6.8 and 6.9 by our sample of judges. Less significant markers are judged less related to terminal illness; overall, the correlation between level of discrimination (t) and judges' estimate of relatedness is .61, p <.05. In other words, the judges' estimate is a fairly good predictor of the likelihood that the word will be a successful marker.

When we go to the defended patients, the relationship disappears; the correlation between marker discrimination and judges' rating falls to near zero. Again, we begin to suspect that additional transformations are set in motion, and that the highly defended patients censor the appearance of clearly related markers because they are too directly threatening, using more ambiguous indicators instead. This fact, if true, raises the question of what principle can be found which will characterize the marker words in the defended patients? They do not seem to be categorized along a dimension of relation to terminal illness. Do they belong to a particular part of speech, to a particular part of speech, to a particular part of the sentence, in other words, to a particualr syntactic category? Can we find a rule which we can apply to future samples to isolate their marker words? This is a problem for future research.

. . .

What are the implications of these findings for the Schmale theory of hopelessness/helplessness? Our single best predictor of cancer, the word "death," is perhaps the ultimate in hopelessness/ helplessness. But once we move to other markers, we find a sharp difference among our two sets of patients, with the difference apparently mediated by defense. In our less defended patients, we can scale words for their relation to terminal illness and find reasonably good predictors of cancer. Many of these words also fall along a hopeless/helpless dimension (e.g., "painful," "worried," "bitter," etc.). But among our more defended patients, the picture changes. They use more disguised derivatives, and some of their markers seem to violate Schmale's law (e.g., the word "accept"). Thus we would conclude that the Schmale formulation works reasonably well with patients who are overtly fearful and subjectively feel at risk, but it does not account for the markers in the more defended patients.

We would expect that the interviewer, in the original analysis of these interviews, would have more difficulty with the defended patients because their defense screens out the emergence of hopeless/helpless markers. We correlated the interviewer's prediction of the diagnosis with the actual diagnosis, separately for the two groups of patients, and found that he was slightly more successful with the afraid patients than with the defended patients (correlations = .44 and .37, respectively). Thus, the interviewer seemed somewhat less sensitive to manifestations of hopelessness among the defended patients, but in both cases, he was able to discriminate significantly between cancers and controls.

How does our hit rate compare with the original interviewer? Using our best set of marker words for the defended patients, we find we can successfully predict 90% of the cases (compared to a 70% hit rate for the original interviewer). Our overall correlation with diagnosis is .80 (p < .001); we miss only three patients out of 30.

Turning to the afraid patients, and using their best marker words, we find hit rate is 81% (compared to an original hit rate of 72%) and our overall correlation = .70, p < .001. Worth noting is the fact that whereas the original interviewer did somewhat better with the afraid patients, our procedure, using marker words, does somewhat better with defended patients.

What happens when we combine the two approaches? In the defended group of patients, the correlation between the combined predictors of interviewer and computer, and the criterion, is .80; the computer accounts for 64% of the variance and the judge adds almost nothing. In the afraid patients, the multiple R is .75, with the computer accounting for 49% of the variance and the judge adding 7%. It is interesting that the judge contributes significantly to the assessment of the undefended patients, perhaps because their lack of defense gives him additional clues he can put to use. Defended patients, on the other hand, are more screened over and offer fewer clues.

                                        . . .

The emergence of the word "death" as a significant marker in the speech of our diagnosed cancer patients has some interesting linguistic implications. In the first place, it does not emerge (with one or two exceptions) as an aspect of the patient's intended meaning; very few of our patients are talking about their own death. Instead, it appears in the surface structure, adrift, so to speak, in a sea of words, and probably goes unnoticed by both speaker and listener. It is safe to say that if we had each of these interviews translated into another language, few, if any, of the translations would contain references to death. It is merely a word, not a central idea, and therefore would become a victim of the transparency of language.

Nevertheless, it is not a random event. Just as Mosteller and Wallace (1964) were able to show that the use of function words like "although" was significantly greater in a sample of writings by Madison than in a sample by Hamilton, so it seems as if word usage in our cancer patients is significantly different than among our controls. How can these differences be explained? By what process do these markers emerge in the word stream? To say that they are overdetermined would simply beg the question. We need to be more precise. At what level of awareness do they present themselves to the speaker for acceptance or rejection?

To begin with, we know that spoken English uses substantially fewer different words than does written English, and this difference probably reflects the greater pressure for response--silence in spoken language is a very public sin (the radio and TV people even call it "dead air"). So the speaker is under greater pressure to find words to fill an intended frame, to convey an intended concept. Second, as Becker (1975) and others have shown, people speak much of the time in clichés, and a good part of their discourse is padded out with stock phrases. In choosing one of these phrases, the speaker usually doesn't have the time to inspect it word for word. Rather, he inserts it in the thought stream as it occurs to him, and takes the chance that the pieces will mesh with what has gone before (note the frequency of mixed metaphor in casual conversation).

Put these facts together, and you will realize that the speaker is probably very little aware of the precise words he is using, and certainly less aware than a writer. So we have a situation in which key markers could emerge in the word stream without the speaker being aware of them at all. But we still have to explain where they come from in the first place. And despite their status on the fringe of awareness, we have to explain why the highly defended patients are still able to screen out the more telling markers. Are they monitoring their word stream that carefully?

Consider the two markers "death" and "cancer." The first is a significant discriminator in both samples; the second discriminates only in afraid patients. The first shows eight different usages in Webster's Unabridged and over 100 separate quotations in Bartlett's; the second shows five different usages in Webster's and only two quotations in Bartlett's. There are, it would seem, many fewer ways to use (and therefore disguise) the word "cancer" in spoken English than the word "death," and perhaps for this reason, it is more subject to conscious control and more likely to be screened out by our more defensive patients. I am assuming that the word "cancer" is less likely to be in the fringes of awareness, unlike the word "death" which lends itself to many expressions and can therefore appear as an incidental member of the surface structure. The word "cancer," if used at all, tends to be used with a purpose to express some central idea. Therefore, it stands to reason that we see censorship at work with "cancer" where we didn't see it operate with "death."

Which brings us to the question of the disguised derivatives. If our hypothesis is correct, the marker words used by our defended patients will have more multiple meanings than those used by our afraid patients, enabling them to be used in incidental contexts and expressing incidental meanings. In addition, we would suspect to find a relationship between the disguised derivatives and the more direct, supporting the fact that one was used in place of the other.

Let's take the second question first. Going back to the words scaled for relevance to terminal illness, we made up two sets of predictors--those which fall between 6.2 and 5.2, highly relevant to illness, which we will call Level I predictors; and those which fall below 4.8, which we call Level II. We then computed category scores for each patient for each category, and computed correlations between each category, the word "cancer" and the two words "death" and "cancer." Correlations were computed separately for cancer patients and controls and are presented in Table 4.

First, we see that within the control patients, there is no relationship between the direct markers ("death" and "cancer") and the disguised markers, either Level I or Level II. And this is what you might expect. Where there is no disease process to supply the

Table 4

Correlations between Different Types of Marker Words

Cancer Patients

	"Cancer"	Level I	Level II
"Death" and "Cancer"	.91	.13	-.27
"Cancer"		.08	-.34
Level I			.17

Control Patients

	"Cancer"	Level I	Level II
"Death" and "Cancer"	.97	.00	-.06
"Cancer"		.07	-.02
Level I			-.12

link between direct and indirect derivatives, there is no reason to
think they would be related. Now look at the cancer patients. The
most interesting correlation is -.34 (.05 < p <.10) between Level
II derivatives (i.e., very disguised) and the direct marker "cancer."
Just as we would expect, one kind of marker tends to compensate for
the other. If, for defensive or other reasons, a patient with cancer does not allow the disease to be coded directly, using the word
"cancer," then she tends to use more disguised derivatives to do the
job. The fact that we have a near-significant correlation between
these two sets of words tends to suggest that they have something in
common; and the fact that this correlation disappears when we move
to the control patients suggests that the underlying disease process
is the key.

In looking at the correlation between Level I markers and direct
markers, in both cancer and control groups, these tend to be zero,
suggesting that one set does not substitute for the other. These
findings may tell us something about the nature of displacement.
Level I derivatives are, by definition, quite close to the criterion,
relatively undisguised. If a patient, for defensive reasons, is
"searching" for another way to code the illness than the word "cancer," these data suggest that she will look for more disguise rather
than less, and this makes a great deal of clinical sense.

Now let's return to the analysis of marker words (t < 2.0) used by defended and afraid patients and ask to what extent they are words with multiple meanings. We counted the separate usages listed in Webster's Unabridged for each word, and found that defended patients' marker words had a slightly higher number of meanings on the average (9.4) than did the marker words for the afraid patients (6.5). In other words, polysema, or multiple meaning, may be an important characteristic of marker words for defended patients. The ambiguity of these words allows many meanings to be carried simultaneously, and a significant sense, carrying an important latent meaning, may be smuggled along on the back of a seemingly innocent marker. Clearly unambiguous words, on the other hand (like "cancer"), may be explicitly rejected by defended patients because there is, conversely, no chance for disguise. So we seem to see two stages of disguise at work among defended patients. In the first place, there is a preference for ambiguous words with many meanings. Secondly, these markers are lifted into the surface structure where they become tangential to the intended meaning of the speaker--needed to fill out a phrase or complete a cliché, but not vital to the communication of the speaker's conscious message.

. . .

In a recent book on language and psychoanalysis, Edelson (1975) has this to say about the way the analyst listens:

"The psychoanalyst is not necessarily focally aware of the speech of the analysand as an opaque object of attention, any more than is the athlete of his muscles' actions or the musician of his fingers' movements. Language is transparent; we hear through it to what is signified by it. We are focally aware of what we understand language to represent--its meaning or what is intended by its use. We are only subsidiarily aware of the multidimensional characteristics of linguistics objects, but, usually without realizing it, we depend on this subsidiary awareness for understanding the full import of these symbolic entities" (p. 27).

Our data on marker words begin to hint at just how precisely information is encoded in the specific words used by the patient, and how crucial is the level of defense in understanding the code. In the "good hours" of relatively undefended analytic patients, we experience their language as both transparent and evocative; we move readily from <u>what</u> the patient is saying to <u>how</u> he is saying it, from what Edelson calls the level of representation to the level of presentation. The redundancy is cumulative. What we learn from form is reinforced by content and vice versa, in a gratifying upward spiral of discovery. The code is clearly accessible, and the speech patterns are comparable to what we see in the afraid patients in our cancer study. Although not everything is on the surface in the sense that the patient does explicitly say to the doctor "I have cancer" (compare Weissman's studies of predilection for death in which the knowledge was actually articulated), the latent content of the disease process is brought clearly into the surface structure in the form of two unambiguous markers, "death" and "cancer."

Our defended patients give us a sample of a more normal hour where resistance is still operating, and disguise is the rule rather than the exception. Their best marker, the word "dark," is, without question, a prime attribute of cancer and a favorite of poets (see, for example, Sir Walter Raleigh: "In the dark and silent grave"; Shakespeare: "The motions of his spirit are dull as night/ And his affections dark as Erebus"; Tennyson: "Give us long rest or death, dark death or dreamful ease"; there are many other examples which I could name). But given only the single marker "dark," we would, as clinicians, have a more difficult job detecting the latent process. And if we were word-wise and computer-sensitive and isolated all 12 of the significant marker words in Table 2, we would still have a hard job zeroing in on cervical cancer as the unconscious idea. The very richness of the language is a handicap; if we try to follow every possible lead, we will never break the code.

We do something else instead. We analyze the resistance. We try to turn our defended patients into anxious patients by working on the denial, the displacement, the intellectualization, and all other interferences between the unconscious and the patient's speech. Our data on the cancer patients makes clear why this step is crucial. Once we analyze away some of the defenses, then the transformations become more transparent and the derivatives easier to master. Instead of having to decode such ambiguous displacements as "dark" and "disgusted" (see Table 2), we find ourselves dealing with "death" and "cancer," provided, that is, that we can sense their significantly higher frequency which, in the present sample of interviews, is no small task. But the principle remains the same, whether or not we can put it to use. Once we analyze the defense, the disguise begins to disappear: the unconscious begins to speak clearly (which is partly what we mean by insight); and, the patient can continue the analysis on his own, frequently saying as he leaves, "I feel as if I knew that all the time."

Of course, the patients in this study are not in analysis, but it begins to appear as if the rules governing natural language apply to a wide range of situations, and that what holds for the relation between words and defense in a sitting-up interview may well apply, with minor variations, to the analytic situation. Our corpus of natural language gives us the opportunity to make a number of natural experiments and find how transformations actually take place, how they are modified by defense, and how much of this process a sensitive interviewer can be aware of. Let me conclude by listing some directions we might want to take.

1. What are the transformation rules which turn a latent process, like cancer, into surface markers like "dark?" A thorough study of the context in which "dark" appears in our cancer patients, compared to our controls, should give us some clues. We would suspect, first, that the context would be innocent with respect to the patient's condition, in order to reinforce the disguise and make it less accessible as a marker to both patient and interviewer. Second, because the marker is overdetermined, we would expect that its usage might be a little strained or out of place, not quite as obvious as a slip of the tongue, but lying along the same dimension. Unfortunately, I doubt if we will be able to pick up the more obvious intrusions for the simple reason that they are no longer in the corpus, having been unintentionally edited out during the time the tape was being transcribed. It is a commonplace that secretaries abhor bad grammar, and as a result, the corpus has already been somewhat sanitized (or un-naturalized). Nevertheless, further study of context seems like a promising direction to take.

2. Can we watch the transformations at work? By that I mean, can we look at the transcript of the interview in a dynamic manner, and watch the patient defending herself against certain thoughts as they emerge? One clue that this kind of process can be studied comes from an analysis of displacement over time. As you know, one way in which isolation can be expressed is to separate in time the two parts of a concept which ordinarily belong together. "Death" alone is somewhat less forbidding for the patients in this sample, particularly when used to refer to someone else, than "death" in conjunction with "cancer." We looked first at the way our defended patients used the word "death"; significantly more often it is used as a displaced referent (e.g., "He died a natural death") by the defended patients than by the afraid patients (p $<.05$, Fisher exact test). Then we picked those patients who use both the words "death" and "cancer" at least once in the course of an interview, and measured the minimum distance (in lines of text) between the two markers. Defended patients allow more time to elapse between the two markers than do afraid patients; that is, defended patients separate the two markers by a larger number of words, increasing the amount of isolation (p $<.01$, one-tailed Mann-Whitney test). This is what we might expect clinically, but aren't you surprised at how systematically the process appears?

3. The data on displacement over time suggest that the defended patients are carefully monitoring, at some level of awareness, the specific words in the speech stream. Evidence for this monitoring also comes from the fact that clear markers, like "cancer," do not appear significantly more often in the defended cancer patients.

At the level of individual words, we seem to have a form of resistance which is quite specific, probably operating out of awareness, which seems to complement the more familiar process of over-determination. Listening clinically, we learn to expect obvious breaks in the speech stream such as short or long silences, incomplete sentences, and the like; less obvious is the systematic deletion of certain key words (except in those cases when the patient doesn't use proper names). We might describe these omissions as a preclinical form of denial that is operating all the time, primarily affecting the surface of the language. It would be interesting to study the point where the process begins. Suppose we look at the emergence of the marker word "cancer" in the course of the interviews of afraid patients, and compare it with the emergence in defended patients. Is there a clear difference in the two distributions? Is there an obvious point where the word begins to disappear, and does this point coincide with the emergence of the idea of death, as our data on displacement might suggest?

4. Lastly, I would like to make a few comments about the use of words as prodromal indicators. To what extent can we use speech samples of patients at risk as diagnostic measures of their physical condition? The striking emergence of "death" among our cancer patients together with the fact that it emerged when the patient was not fully conscious that she was harboring a cancer process (remember, the interviews were conducted before the biopsy results were made known, and there is no correlation between the patient's subjective concern and the diagnosis), suggest that it might be possible to develop an early warning system that would respond to differences in natural language. But the age-old question persists, how does the patient "know?"

One possible explanation comes from the research on stress. We know that heart disease is exacerbated in so-called Type A patients, patients who are clearly reacting to stress. Some animal experiments, using cancer-bearing mice, have shown how it is possible to facilitate or inhibit the emergence of the symptom by manipulating environmental stress: noise, handling, exposure, crowding, etc. It seems possible that both the marker word "death" and the presence of diagnosed cervical carcinoma are both correlated with a third factor-- a recent increase in stress. It affects the patient's hopelessness, as conveyed by the deep structure, enabling Schmale to make positive predictions of the outcome of the biopsy; it affects the surface structure, producing an increased frequency of the marker word "death" and it may well interfere with the operation of the normal immune mechanism which keeps spontaneous cell division under control. It remains to be seen whether language change can actually anticipate gross cellular irregularity. If it can, we may have a promising application of what has been, up to now, primarily basic research, and a welcome confrontation of a key principle of psychoanalytic theory--that the patient knows more than all of us.

REFERENCES

Becker, J. D. The phrasal lexicon. Theoretical issues in natural language processing. Workshop presented at M.I.T., June, 1975.

Bransford, J. D. & Franks, J. J. The abstraction of linguistic ideas. Cognitive Psychology, 1971, 2, 331-350.

Edelson, M. Language and interpretation in psychoanalysis. New Haven: Yale University Press, 1975.

Gill, M. M. Topography and systems in psychoanalytic theory. New York: International Universities Press, 1963.

Gray, P. Psychoanalytic technique and the ego's capacity for viewing intrapsychic activity. Journal of the American Psychoanalytic Association, 1973, 21, 474-494.

Howes, D. A word count of spoken English. Journal of Verbal Learning and Verbal Behavior, 1966, 5, 572-604.

Jenkins, J. J. Remember that old theory of memory? Well, forget it! American Psychologist, 1974, 29, 785-795.

Mosteller, F. & Wallace, D. L. Inference and disputed authorship: The Federalist. Reading, Mass.: Addison-Wesley, 1964.

Schmale, A. H., & Iker, H. P. The affect of hopelessness and the development of cancer. Psychosomatic Medicine, 1966, 28, 714-721.

Stone, P. J., Dunphy, D. C., Smith, M. S., & Ogilvie, D. The general inquirer: A computer approach to content analysis. Cambridge, Mass.: M.I.T. Press, 1966.

Weisman, A. & Hackett, T. P. Predilection to death. Psychosomatic Medicine, 1961, 23, 232-255.

TWO CLASSES OF CONCOMITANT CHANGE IN A PSYCHOTHERAPY[1]

Leonard M. Horowitz

Stanford University

Palo Alto, California

The work that I shall describe in this paper was conducted with colleagues at the Mt. Zion Psychiatric Clinic in San Francisco. I would especially like to acknowledge my debt to Harold Sampson, Ellen Siegelman, Joseph Weiss, and Shirley Goodfriend for their various major roles in the work described. The goal of our work has been to combine rigorous methodology with accurate clinical formulations so as to achieve a blend that is clinically sensible, methodologically sound, and heuristically useful.

Our work was based on one patient's verbal output during a psychoanalysis. This verbal output could be used to relate the patient's patterns of communicating with other people to underlying psychological structures. The patient's speech, which showed systematic changes over time, was related, through multiple convergent methods, to inferred psychological changes. Thus, by studying what the patient said over successive hours, we gained a clearer understanding of (a) the nature of her problem and (b) significant changes which were related to the solution of the problem.

To begin with, let us first consider two important classes of behavior that may be identified and examined in any psychoanalytic psychotherapy. One class contains those behaviors which are designed to bring the person <u>closer</u> to another person (Type C). These behaviors occur when a patient cooperates, collaborates, or concurs with another person, share thoughts and feelings, is intimate, warm, and loving.

---

[1] This study was supported in part by Grant MH 13914 of the National Institute of Mental Health.

In expressing these behaviors, the person is positively engaged
with another person. In contrast, other behaviors are designed
to produce a psychological distance or differentiation from the
other person (Type D), and the person is negatively engaged with
the other person. They occur when a patient defies another person,
disagrees with, distrusts, or disapproves of the other person, hates,
criticizes, or opposes the other person.[2] Ethologists have made a
similar distinction between cohesive behaviors, which bring organisms together, and dispersal behaviors which drive organisms apart
(Mussen & Rosenzweig, 1973, Chapter 28). The two types of behaviors
show a complex interplay throughout the phylogenetic scale, promoting the survival of both the individual and the species.

Corresponding C and D behaviors sometimes look like a pair of
polar opposites (e.g., defy vs. submit, hate vs. love, be different
from vs. be similar to). Indeed, in their clearest, most explicit
and overt forms, they are contradictory. However, mixtures of apparently contradictory behaviors can occur simultaneously. For example, a single behavior might simultaneously seem to fit both
categories--e.g., an affectionate pinch, a tease, a grudging compliment, or an unwilling compliance. The statement "My mother was
probably being honest for once" contains both a compliment and a
criticism.

A psychological "problem" is experienced when a person lacks
control in translating impulse into behavior. For example, he might
intend to express one impulse yet find himself expressing another
coexisting impulse. That is, on the one hand, he might find
himself unable to express an intended behavior directly and would
complain, for example, that he cannot cooperate or cannot fight
though he wants to. On the other hand, he might find himself expressing a behavior more intensely or more compulsively than he
wants to, complaining that he has to share intimacies or has to
defy though he does not want to; such behaviors would have an obligatory quality.

A successful therapy should help a person gain control over
each kind of behavior. He should acquire the capacity to experience
and express more directly both C and D behaviors. One goal of the
following studies is to objectify such improvements and to examine
the relationship between them.

---

[2] C and D behaviors always reflect an involvement with the other
person and thus differ from behaviors reflecting a simple avoidance
of the other person. Therefore, the distinction actually implies two
bases of classification, one telling whether the subject is involved
with another person, the other telling whether that involvement is
positive or negative.

STUDY 1:   TWO CONCOMITANT CHANGES

METHOD

This set of studies was based on a psychoanalytic case treated
by a psychoanalyst who was not familiar with the views expressed
here. Every session of the analysis was tape recorded with the
written consent of the patient. The analyst also took process
notes during each hour describing the content of the hour. As
the patient was talking, he was writing. His notes, however, did
not report any commentary or clinical inference; they only summarized
the patient's talk and his own interventions.

A group of clinical psychologists and psychoanalysts met weekly
to discuss the case. Drawing only upon the process notes of the
first 10 hours and information of the intake interview, they formulated the case and predicted a sequence of changes. The following
case description summarizes the main details of the case and the
group's formulation and clinical prediction.

Sometimes a person intends a behavioral double message, but
other times he does not. If he did not intend both C and D behaviors but they both occurred anyway, we would say that his behavior
exhibited poor control. In a psychotherapy like the one described
below, poorly controlled behaviors could be identified. When the
patient wanted to be affectionate, she found herself provoking.
When she wanted to demur, she found herself yielding. Her poor control was also accompanied by psychological distress.

Impulse vs. behavior. To clarify poorly controlled behaviors,
let us begin with a basic postulate of psychoanalytic (as well as
other) theories, namely that an impulse[3] precedes any nonreflexive
behavior. The distinction is analogous to the psycholinguist's
distinction between the underlying abstract representation of a
thought and the corresponding surface structure of verbal behavior;
one, an inferred private event, precedes the other, an observable
surface phenomenon. The impulse, an encoded representation, becomes decoded through a grammar that involves optional and obligatory rules and transformations; the defense mechanisms would thus
be viewed as a subset of transformations that occur during decoding
(cf. Suppes & Warren, 1975).

Just as the correspondence between the deep and the surface
structure of language is not necessarily one-to-one, the impulse is

---

3
The term impulse is meant to be neutral theoretically in the way that
the term underlying abstract representation is neutral. Thus, for
example, no energic connotations are intended.

not necessarily isomorphic to the behavior; different relationships can exist between them. Sometimes an impulse is directly expressed in behavior; at other times the behavior is simply inhibited; and, at still other times, the behavior is partly camouflaged by another behavior derived from another impulse. Thus, if a behavior exhibited both a C and a D component, we would assume that two different impulses, a C and a D impulse, both existed. An affectionate pinch, according to the postulate, would result from simultaneous impulses to hurt and to be close to the same person.

Case description and formulation. The patient, Mrs. C, was a prim, married schoolteacher in her late twenties who came to treatment complaining of sexual frigidity, difficulty experiencing pleasurable feelings, and low self-esteem. Her father was a professional man, and her mother was a housewife. She was the second of four children (an older sister, a younger sister, and a much younger brother). When the treatment began, Mrs. C had been married for less than two years. She considered her marriage successful though she felt that her sexual inadequacy created a major marital problem.

Mrs. C's parents were described as controlled people, undemonstrative of any affection. The mother, who was an organized and efficient woman, ran the house well. She was also very controlling, and the patient felt in danger of being "owned" by her. On the other hand, the mother was not able to defend herself very well. Once, for example, the patient hit the mother in the stomach, and the mother could not defend herself or correct the patient except by retiring to her bedroom in obvious discomfort, leaving the patient to feel guilty, helpless, and frightened. The patient thus came to feel capable of hurting other people, and guilty over aggression and assertiveness. Between the ages of five and eight, she had recurrent nightmares of something happening to her mother.

The father was also undemonstrative and easily embarrassed by other peoples' displays of affection. Although he was generally controlled, he sometimes lost control of his anger and had temper tantrums that revealed murderous rage; at times Mrs. C felt that he was capable of killing her. The father was also upset by crying women and became angry over masochistic displays from the patient.

In the period before the analysis began, Mrs. C was feeling beleaguered and upset. In situations that called for intimacy, she experienced intense ambivalence which left her feeling confused and in turmoil. The ambivalence resulted from numerous opposing tendencies: If she had an impulse to be sadistic, for example, she felt potentially guilty. Then, identifying with her mother, she would turn to masochistic feelings (feeling hurt, victimized, neglected,

unfavored) which served to camouflage sadistic impulses. These
feelings, however, were also unsatisfactory in that she felt that
they would upset other people as they had upset her father, who
sometimes lost control of his sadism. Thus, the patient could not
express either sadistic or masochistic impulses comfortably and
shifted between them, using each tendency to undo the other. The
result for her was turmoil and confusion, and she was sometimes
unable to focus her thoughts. She also felt vulnerable to criticism
since she was unable to defend herself against others.

Mrs. C's sexual frigidity may be related to her difficulties
with aggression: Since she chould not comfortably distance herself
from other people, sexual intimacy could be a problem in that she
did not have the means of ending the closeness when she wanted to.
Thus, an impairment in Type D behaviors could produce a corresponding impairment in Type C behaviors.

It was therefore hypothesized that during the treatment, Mrs.
C first had to develop a better capacity to defend herself against
other people (stubbornly resist other people without feeling guilty,
disagree with other people, etc.) in order to allow herself to get
closer to other people. It was hypothesized that as she acquired
a better capacity for Type D behavior, she would feel less vulnerable by Type C behavior and would express Type C behaviors more
freely.

The following procedure was designed to test this hypothesis.
It might be noted at this point that during the first 100 hours of
treatment (covering a period of approximately six months), Mrs. C
did achieve an increased, though limited, capacity to respond sex-
ally. She also became more able to free associate easily, to reveal symptoms and preoccupations, and to think and work more produc-
tively. She became more able to express and tolerate strong feelings,
and found herself exercising a better-modulated discipline over the
students in her class.

Procedure. The first step was to examine Mrs. C's ability to
comfortably express behaviors of Type D. A prominent subset of
Type D behaviors contained instances in which she blamed, criticized,
disagreed with, or opposed another person (the therapist or somcone
elsc). Three clinicians independently read the process notes of
the first 100 hours, looking for all passages in the notes that
described such behaviors (in the present or in the past, toward
the therapist or anyone else). These passages were generally recorded verbatim. However, a passage out of context was sometimes
ambiguous, so some editing was necessary to eliminate this ambiguity.
Then the three clinicians together reviewed all of the passages
that they had identified and retained the ones that they agreed
were instances of blaming, criticizing, disagreeing, or opposing.
Their resulting set contained 190 passages.

Then a 4-point rating scale was developed to assess the direct-ness of the behavior described in each passage. If the blame or criticism was only implied, or if it was expressed tentatively with extreme discomfort, the scale value was 1; as the behavior became more explicit and direct, the scale value increased. A rating of "2" meant that a Type D behavior was expressed but immediately un-done. Ratings of "3" and "4" meant that a Type D behavior was overtly expressed--"3" by telling a third party about it, and "4" by directly confronting the offending party. Examples of the dif-ferent scale values are shown in Table 1. Note that "3" was scored when the patient, speaking to the therapist, criticized a third per-son, while "4" was scored for a more direct behavior (e.g., criti-cizing the therapist directly). Each rating was also increased by .5 if the event occurred in the present tense (after the treatment began). Thus, the possible ratings were 1.0, 1.5, 2.0, . . ., 4.5.

The passages were divided into two subsets, and the passages of each subset were presented independently to four clinical psy-chologists who were naive about the case. Each passage appeared on a 3 x 5 inch index card, and the cards were presented one by one in random order. Explicit scoring rules were developed for rating the passages, and the judges followed these rules in rating each behavior.

A similar procedure was followed for identifying and rating the Type C behaviors. A prominent subset of these behaviors included behaviors in which the patient complimented someone, felt affection or compassion for someone, or wanted to be loved by someone. Two clinical psychologists read the process notes of the first 100 hours, looking for all passages in the notes that described such behaviors (in the past or in the present, toward the therapist or someone else). These passages, like the Type D passages, were recorded verbatim. As with the Type D passages, the clinicians reviewed the passages that they had identified and retained the ones that they could agree to be instances of Type C behaviors. The resulting set contained 106 passages.

A 4-point rating scale was also developed to assess the direct-ness of these behaviors. This scale was deliberately constructed to resemble the D scale in form. If the closeness was implied or ex-pressed with extreme uncertainty, unclarity, or discomfort, the scale value was 1. A rating of "2" denoted an expression of closeness with immediate undoing. As the behavior became more explicit and direct, the scale value increased: "3" indicated that the feeling of close-ness was expressed to a third party, and "4" indicated that it was expressed directly to the second party. The meanings of the differ-ent scale values are shown in Table 2, together with examples. Each rating was also increased by .5 if the event occurred in the present tense (after the treatment began). The possible ratings thus ranged from 1.0 to 4.5.

Table 1

The Rating Categories and Examples

Type D Behavior

Observed D Behavior	Example
I. Implied blame, criticism, disagreement:	(Hour 4) It is very hard for her to suddenly be stopped when I call the time. When she gets to talking, her feelings well up and it is hard for her to get them under control. So she feels somewhat upset.
II. Blame, criticism, disagreement, and then immediate undoing:	(Hour 41) Next her thoughts turned to the principal at school, and the essence of this was that he wanted the kids to be reading at an earlier stage. She thinks she disagrees with him on this, but then, maybe she's wrong.
III. Blame, criticism, disagreement of a third person:	(Hour 77) On Saturday her brother's friend and the friend's girlfriend were over, and her brother wanted them both to stay overnight, but her mother had answered no. She said she didn't have time to make the arrangements. Patient was very upset with this; she thought her mother should have been able to do it, and it led her to raise many questions about her mother's priorities.
IV. Direct confrontation of someone:	(Hour 99) She wanted sympathy from Bill, and his response was to want to have intercourse. Then she made up her mind that she simply wasn't going to and didn't.

These passages were also presented to a panel of four clinical psychologists who were naive about the case. Each passage appeared on a 3 x 5 inch index card, and the cards were presented one by one in random order. Explicit scoring rules were developed for rating the passages, and the judges followed these rules to rate each behavior.

Table 2

The Rating Categories and Examples

Type C Behavior

Observed C Behavior	Example
I. Implied feeling of closenss but confused, unclear, or dysphoric:	(Hour 2) She was also troubled with not getting any reactions from me. No interaction. She was afraid that maybe she needed approval.
II. Feeling close or affectionate with immediate undoing:	(Hour 6) She referred to a woman that she had to dinner and how nice and free this woman was and yet how she felt compelled to think of something critical.
III. Affection, admiration, or closeness told to a third person:	(Hour 59) This week she felt closer to Bill than she ever has, and she said there were times when she really wanted intercourse.
IV. Direct expression of affection, admiration, or closeness:	(Hour 94) When Bill came home last night, she was happy that he was home and she said so.

RESULTS

Type D behaviors. The 100 sessions were grouped into 10-session blocks denoted I, II, III, ..., X. The number of passages within each block were: I, 31; II, 13; III, 18; IV, 9; V, 35; VI, 13; VII, 13; VIII, 10; IX, 29; X, 19. The ratings of passages within each block were averaged, and the means ranged from 2.62 to 3.81. These means are reported in Figure 1, which shows the development of the Type D behavior across successive blocks of sessions.

In order to compare the frequencies of past and present events, the relative frequencies of 3.0's and 3.5's were compared. There were 101 passages with these ratings. For each block of 20 sessions, the relative frequency of 3.5's (present tense) was computed. For successive 20-session blocks, the values were: 6/24 = .25; 8/16 = .50; 17/26 = .65; 8/11 = .73; and 19/24 = .79. Thus, the patient increasingly came to criticize others for events in her current life. Events in the past tense were apparently less threatening for her and provided a convenient starting point for the therapy, but as the sessions progressed, she shifted her focus to her current life.

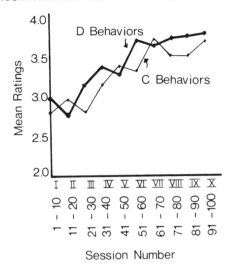

Figure 1. Mean Rating of Passages in Each Block of Hours.

Type C behaviors. The 106 Type C items were also grouped into
10-session blocks, with the following frequencies within each block:
Block I, 11; II, 9; III, 15; IV, 10; V, 9; VI, 12; VII, 14; VIII, 9;
IX, 5; X, 12. The ratings of the passages within each block were
then averaged, and the resulting means ranged from 2.67 to 3.75.
Figure 1 shows the development of the Type C behaviors across successive blocks of sessions.

The Type C behaviors in general were rated lower than the Type
D behaviors. The proportion of the Type C behaviors that were rated
1.0 to 2.5 was .33, while the corresponding proportion for Type D
behaviors was .19. These two proportions differed significantly;
a chi-square test of the frequencies yielded X^2 (1) = 6.47, p <.02.
There were also significantly fewer Type C passages than Type D
passages; X^2 (1) = 23.3, p <.001. Thus, during the first 100 hours,
Type C behaviors differed in two ways from Type D behaviors: Type
C behaviors were not expressed as frequently, and they were more often expressed indirectly (lower ratings).

Thus, it is clear that two types of changes occurred, but the
question still remains as to whether a change occurred in the patient's presenting complaint, sexual frigidity. Therefore, every
reference to the patient's sexual behavior was noted throughout the
100 hours. There were 18 such references (comprising a subset of
the 106 Type C passages), all occurring between Hours 28 and 100.
Each passage contained the word "intercourse" except one that contained the phrase "sexual interest." Here are some examples: From
Hour 33 (rated 2.5): "Sometimes when she is trying to make herself
have intercourse with Bill, she feels as though she wants to hurt him.

She just doesn't understand it. She'll go from feeling very warm to
feeling nothing toward him suddenly." From Hour 67 (rated 4.5):
"This weekend she and Bill had intercourse, and she was thinking how
different it can be when she's thinking about him and feeling close
to him and not all wrapped up in herself."

Seven passages occurred in the first 50 sessions, and 11 occurred in the last 50 sessions. The C rating assigned to each passage was noted. For those in the early block, six had ratings of
1.5 to 2.5, and one (in Hour 43) had a rating of 3.5 to 4.5. Of
the 11 passages in the later block, four had ratings of 1.5 to 2.5,
and seven had ratings of 3.5 to 4.5. The seven passages with high
ratings were mainly simple, direct statements that the patient had
had sexual intercourse. A Fisher exact test was performed to test
the significance of this difference; the chance probability of the
observed pattern or a more extreme one is .022.

Thus, the overall changes observed in the patient's Type C
behavior included changes in her reports of sexual behavior. Further evidence that these changes are not trivial will be examined
in Study 2.

STUDY 2:   THE RELATIONSHIP BETWEEN C AND D BEHAVIORS

The capacities to express Type C and Type D behaviors comfortably seem to be related, since a defect in D can produce a corresponding defect in C. That is, if a person does not have the capacity
to distance himself, then he may experience intimacy as unsafe, since
he would not be able to disengage himself from the closeness when he
wanted to and would thus run the danger of feeling oppressed or en-
trapped in an unacceptable relationship. On the other hand, once
he gained the capacity to distance himself, he could defend himself
better, and closeness would not be as threatening.

Thus, as a patient gains the capacity to express Type D behaviors comfortably, he should find himself better able to express Type
C behaviors. As he gains the capacity to fight, he should find himself more able to be intimate. In any block of therapy sessions in
which significant gains are observed in Type D behaviors, improvement should subsequently be observed in Type C behaviors. This hypothesis is examined below.

METHOD, RESULTS, AND DISCUSSION

In Figure 1 of Study 1, the C graph resembles the general form
of the D graph. In order to examine the relationship between the
graphs more closely, the positions of greatest increase along each
graph were noted. A "significant improvement" in either function is
defined as an increment from Block i to Block i+1 that exceeded .25.

Significant improvements in Type D behavior occurred three times--
from Block III to Block IV, from Block IV to Block V, and from Block
VI to Block VII. In each case, the significant improvement in the
Type C behavior followed a significant improvement in the Type D
behavior: An improvement in D occurred from II to III, an improvement in C occurred from III to IV. The chance probability that the
three Type C improvements occurred in those particular three positions is .012.

In addition, a "setback" in either function is defined as a de-
crement from Block i to Block i+1. A setback in the Type D behavior occurred three times--from Block I to Block II, from Block IV
to Block V, and from Block VI to Block VII. A setback also occurred
three times in the Type C behavior--from Block II to Block III, from
Block V to Block VI, and from Block VII to Block VIII. Thus, a setback in the Type C behavior always followed a setback in the Type D
behavior. The two graphs therefore took very similar courses, with
one displaced from the other by one block of sessions.

The data therefore suggest that the patient's progress in expressing Type C behaviors followed her progress in expressing Type
D behaviors. As she became progressively able to criticize, oppose,
and disagree with other people, she felt progressively less vulnerable; then, feeling less vulnerable, she could relax her defenses
and permit herself to feel close, affectionate, and compassionate
toward other people. If the two graphs had simply exhibited a correlation, other factors could account for their concomitant rise and
fall. But their displacement in time suggests that an advance in
one may have facilitated an advance in the other.

This inference must be made with reservations for three reasons.
First, the relationship may only describe an idiosyncrasy of one patient's progress and needs to be replicated on other cases. Second,
changes in Type C and Type D behaviors, as operationalized here, may
be trivial. That is, they may reflect changes that occur in any developing human relationship in the way the partners relate to each
other (talking more directly, less cautiously, less formally) and are
thus not necessarily therapeutic. For example, the C and D rating
scales were specifically designed to be formally alike, with "2,"
as one example, denoting undoing on each scale. Thus, it is possible
that whenever Mrs. C entered a new relationship with someone, she
would initially qualify with great caution any statements that she
made so as to present a balanced view on any subject; such a tendency
would involve statements that would get rated "2." Then, as she came
to know the other person better, she might drop this tendency and
become more direct. In that case, her conversation with any acquaintance over time would show increasingly fewer 2's. In fact, a decline
in 2's might be observed on other potential scales; e.g., a scale
describing her expression of narcissism (bragging, showing off, etc.).
Furthermore, as the 2's disappeared, the mean ratings would increase.

If this interpretation were correct, though, C and D changes should occur simultaneously, rather than one consistently lagging behind the other. Therefore, the lag between graphs would need to be explained. One way to explain it might be to add an assumption that the class of behavior which produces greater discomfort (intimacy for Mrs. C) shows a more gradual disappearance of 2's, causing the C graph to progress more slowly. Then we would expect both graphs to show a general improvement with one progressing more rapidly than the other. But then we would have to explain occasional setbacks in each graph. A setback might be viewed either as a random fluctuation in the data or due to occasional situational stresses. Neither view, however, would explain why a setback in the D graph is followed by a setback in the C graph. That is, these assumptions could not account for the orderly lag between setbacks. Nor would they account for Mrs. C's increased capacity to engage in sexual intercourse as the treatment progressed. Thus, the formal similarity between the two scales alone cannot account for the results in Figure 1.

Finally another kind of explanation might account for the observations of Figure 1. Suppose the direct expression of aggression is in some sense incompatible with the direct expression of intimacy, so that the relative prominence of one would imply a relative decline in the other. Then, as one graph rose from Block i to Block i+1, the other graph would fall. For example, in Figure 1, as the two graphs proceed from Block I to Block II, the C graph rises while the D graph falls, causing the graphs to cross. Then, proceeding to Block III, the C graph falls while the D graph rises, producing another crossing. Additional crossings occur as the graphs proceed to Blocks V, VI, VII, and VIII. This characterization of the data has the virtue of parsimony, but it does not explain why both graphs would show concomitant overall improvement. It also suggests that the frequency of Type D behaviors should be strongly and negatively related to the frequency of Type C behaviors. The correlation was negative, but it was not significant; $r = -0.33$, $p > .20$.

Thus, alternative hypotheses may account for some aspects of the data, and perhaps even accurately account for aspects of the therapeutic process. However, they do not adequately explain the lag between graphs or the overall improvement in each type of behavior. For this reason, it is tentatively concluded that improvement in Type D behavior, at least in this patient, permitted subsequent improvement in Type C behavior.

STUDY 3:   AN EXAMINATION OF MRS. C'S COMPLAINTS

Mrs. C's presenting complaint (sexual frigidity) reflected an inability to be intimate with her husband. In the course of 100 hours of treatment, however, she mentioned a large number of other problems which were not directly related to sexual frigidity but which clarify the nature of her distress. Many of these complaints were expressed in the form "I can't (do something)" or "I have to (do something)," revealing inhibitions and compulsions. A given complaint was often idiosyncratic, but, as the following study shows, a large subset of these complaints could be classified according to the C and D categories. Since the presenting complaint was sexual frigidity, it was hypothesized that a large number of complaints would reveal more general problems over Type C behavior. In addition, however, it was hypothesized that many complaints would also reflect problems over Type D behavior.

METHOD, RESULTS AND DISCUSSION

Ten readers read through the process notes of the 100 sessions searching for all complaints about behavioral problems that contained the words "can't" and "has to" (or near-synonyms like "finds it hard to"). At least two readers read the material of every session as a way of locating all such statements. The readers identified 248 complaints involving "can't" and 103 complaints involving "has to," making a total of 351 complaints. Some examples are shown in Table 3.

The statements were divided into four sets, three containing "can't" complaints and one containing "has to" complaints. The statements within a set were randomly ordered and presented to a group of 20 judges (10 graduate students and 10 clinicians in each group). Each judge was asked to read each statement and consider the behavior that was mentioned, placing it into one of four categories which were labeled "Type C," "Type D," "Ambiguous," or "Irrelevant." Type C and Type D behaviors were defined for the judge, and examples of each were supplied. The judge was told to classify the behavior as Type C or Type D if it was unambiguously one or the other. If the behavior was probably C or D but ambiguous as to which, he was to categorize the item as Ambiguous. Finally, if the behavior seemed unrelated to the C and D categories (because it was not interpersonal or because it was neutral with respect to the other person), he was to classify the item as Irrelevant.

The judges' categorizations of a given complaint were tabulated to show how many judges placed that complaint in each of the four categories. Each complaint was then classified according to the distribution of judges' responses. A statement was considered a Type C complaint if 14 or more judges classified it as Type C; similarly for the other categories. Using this 14-or-more criterion, 60 complaints were of Type C, 56 were of Type D, 0 were Ambiguous, and 22 were Irrelevant. The remaining items did not meet the 14-or-more criterion--e.g., one statement was classified as Type C by 12 judges and as Irrelevant by 8 judges.

Of the 138 statements that did meet the criterion, only 22 (less than 16%) were judged Irrelevant to the C and D categories. The complaints of Type C and Type D were then examined further to determine

Table 3

Examples of Mrs. C's Complaints

Can't C

She couldn't look at her assistant while thanking her.
She can't believe her husband when he says he loves her.
She can't praise her assistant.
She finds it difficult to relate to the boys she teaches at school.
She couldn't handle boys her age who were interested in her; she
    always managed to do something that got rid of them.
She finds it hard to call faculty members at school by their first
    name.

Has to C

She feels compelled to tell her supervisor when she has a good idea.
It would be nice not to have to care whether her parents care,
    but she does.
She feels she has to please the therapist.

Can't D

She wishes she could walk off and leave people, but she can't.
She is questioning some of the teaching methods, and she just
    can't bring herself to tell the supervisor.
She wanted to be abrupt, but couldn't.
She finds it hard to confront her father the way an acquaintance
    of hers once did to her own father.
They have a cleaning man now, and she finds it very difficult to
    give him direction.

Has to D

She just has to fight against her husband.
When a child at school bristles, she feels she just has to be
    obeyed.
She recalled how nice this woman was and yet how she felt com-
    pelled to think of something critical.
She felt compelled to argue very strongly.
She went through a period in high school and college when she
    just had to be nasty to her mother.
She has a compulsion to do anything that will make people not
    like her.

how many were of the "can't" form and how many were of the "has to"
form. The resulting data are shown in Table 4. The highest frequency
was for complaints of the form "Can't C," a form which corresponds to
the presenting complaint, sexual frigidity. It should be noted, however, that very few of these "Can't C" complaints were specifically

Table 4

Frequencies of Different

Types of Complaints

	Type C	Type D	Total
Can't	51	24	75
Has to	9	32	41
	60	56	116

sexual in content (see the examples cited in Table 3). They concerned various people--the patient's husband, therapist, pupils,
assistant--and they involved various forms of closeness--giving
unilaterally to other people (praising, helping, reassuring, comforting, disclosing personal information) as well as exchanging
(relating to other people, trusting, believing, returning love,
feeling close to or relaxed with).

The X^2 computed for Table 4 was 20.7, $p < .001$. Thus, the proportion of "can't" items among the Type C complaints (.85) differed
significantly from the proportion of "can't" items among the Type D
complaints (.43). Whereas Type C complaints were typically of the
"can't" form, Type D complaints were more evenly divided between the
two. The frequency of "can't" and "has to" among the Type D complaints did not differ significantly; $X^2 = 0.88$ $p > .25$.

However, the two forms of Type D complaints did differ as to
the person mentioned. Complaints of the "can't" form often concerned
people in authority (the patient's parents, her supervisor, the
school principal) while those of the "has to" form often concerned
peers and subordinates (her colleagues, siblings, pupils, assistant).
The proportion of "Can't D" complaints involving authority figures
was .50, while that proportion for "Has to D" complaints was .09.
The corresponding proportions of complaints involving peers and subordinates were, respectively, .29 and .66. The value of X^2 computed
on the matrix of frequencies was 9.85, $p < .005$.

Various Type D behaviors were cited as posing problems. Some
involved assertiveness (getting her own way, sticking to her views,
developing her own teaching method, making demands on other people,
disagreeing with other people), while others involved aggression

(expressing anger, being nasty to people, criticizing other people, opposing other people).

The data thus show that Mrs. C experienced a conflict over expressing or not expressing behaviors of both types. At other times her "solution" was to inhibit the behavior altogether (Can't C, Can't D), but at other times her solution was to express the behavior in an obligatory way (Has to C, Has to D). The data of Table 4 show that both kinds of solutions occurred for Type D behaviors, revealing the two sides of a conflict. But behaviors of Type C were handled less flexibly; these behaviors were more uniformly inhibited (Can't C). This lesser flexibility of the Type C behavior further suggests that the problem over Type C behavior was more severe, a fact which again may be related to the lag in Mrs. C's progress on Type C behaviors.

STUDY 4:   THE ORDERLY EMERGENCE OF THEMES

A patient's goal in treatment is to solve personal problems. Mrs. C, for example, was initially unable to engage in sexual activity comfortably, and her primary goal was to overcome this disability. Throughout the treatment, Mrs. C seemed to adopt specific strategies (intentionally or fortuitously) to achieve her overall goal. As one strategy, for example, she was sometimes silent. When the therapist comfortably accepted her silence, she subsequently seemed to identify problems more clearly and then showed behavioral change. On the other hand, when the therapist was intolerant or uncomfortable (e.g., reminded her of the "basic rule"), the therapeutic work seemed to decline.

Strategies can be generated by patients to help them attain their overall goal. As one strategy, for example, the patient might engage the therapist in some interaction which, if handled correctly by the therapist, would produce a therapeutic benefit (e.g., reduce the patient's guilt over some feeling, cognition, or behavior). Many such strategies occur throughout a treatment.

It is assumed that these strategies are always designed to maximize the solution of the patient's personal problems. However, there is also one important constraint upon the patient's behavior in executing the strategy; namely, that his own discomfort (e.g., guilt, sadness, anxiety, feeling of vulnerability) must be kept below some level 0. If the patient's discomfort were to exceed 0, he would have to take some corrective step to reduce the discomfort, if possible. For example, if he felt intolerably guilty over having possibly hurt the therapist, he might take steps to restore the therapist's self-esteem and thus feel less guilty.

Thus, a given strategy could only work if it kept the patient's discomfort below 0. Furthermore, when a strategy does work and the patient successfully achieves the subgoal, his discomfort drops; through generalization, the discomfort is also reduced for related cognitions, behaviors, and feelings not yet mastered. Then, the patient would be able to undertake further therapeutic strategies that formerly would have been too threatening.

Mrs. C's primary treatment goal was to feel intimate with her husband. According to Study 2, to achieve this eventual goal, she first needed to be able to criticize her husband more comfortably. Criticizing her husband, of course, would have initially produced discomfort exceeding 0, so she had to work first on criticizing less threatening objects, like casual acquaintances. Thus, a hierarchy would exist of subgoals plus strategies for attaining them.

In gaining control over her Type D behaviors, then, Mrs. C should first express aggression toward relatively innocuous people (e.g., people she only knew casually or people temporally removed from her current life). Later, as she mastered easier tasks, she could express aggression toward increasingly significant objects. The result would be a relatively well-ordered progression of objects throughout the first 100 hours. This hypothesis is tested below.

METHOD, RESULTS, AND DISCUSSION

Each Type D passage that was rated 3.0 or more was sorted according to the object of the blame, criticism, disagreement, or opposition. The most frequently cited objects were the therapist, her parents, and her husband. The various objects were sorted into five categories: (a) the therapist; (b) her husband; (c) other relatives; (d) her colleagues and others at school; and (e) various casual acquaintances, as shown in Table 5.

A frequency count was made of each object, and Table 5 shows how often each category occurred for each 20-session block. The highest frequency for each category is denoted by an asterisk.

The patient's relatives were the primary target of the Type D behaviors in the first block of sessions; these passages were mainly rated 3.0. Thus, the therapy opened with the patient criticizing her relatives for events from her earlier life.

Her family continued to be a primary target of criticism throughout the hours, but in the middle block of hours, two other targets became a primary focus of criticism--various casual acquaintances (e.g., a local grocer, the manager of an art gallery, a girl in the waiting room) and the therapist. Objects in both categories were primarily attacked for behavior in her current life--the analyst directly (primarily 4.5) and the casual acquaintances indirectly (primarily 3.5). Both categories represented bolder instances of

Table 5

Frequency of Occurrence of Different Objects of
Criticism, Blame, and Opposition

	Session					
	1-20	21-40	41-60	61-80	81-100	Total
All relatives (except hus- band) (Mainly 3.0)	23*	12	18	6	11	70
Casual acquaintances (Mainly 3.5)	2	1	6*	4	5	18
Therapist (Mainly 4.5)	1	1	11*	5	11*	29
Husband (Mainly 4.5)	2	4	1	3	8*	18
Colleagues + others at school (Mainly 3.5)	1	3	2	2	10*	18
						153

*The highest frequency for that object.

Type D behaviors than her initial criticisms since they concerned
her current life. They are, however, relatively nonthreatening
objects of attack--the analyst, because the patient has tested out
his reactions and discovered that he is tolerant of criticism and
opposition; and the casual acquaintances, because of their relative
unimportance in the patient's life.

In the last block of hours, the patient came to criticize and
oppose two further targets in her current life; namely, her husband
and her colleagues at school. These strategies are even bolder
steps, of course, and perhaps are only possible because of the
earlier therapeutic work.

The transitions in Table 5 thus show a shift from the past to the present tense, and a shift from less threatening to more threatening individuals. The shifts are mediated by Type D behaviors directed at the analyst, who was tolerant, undefensive, and objectively investigatory. As Mrs. C became able to criticize him, she could apparently then work on criticizing her husband and thus eventually feel closer to him.

The mechanism by which this process works can be viewed in terms of the principle of generalization: Initially Mrs. C felt uncomfortable criticizing because she believed that her criticism hurt the other person, causing her to feel guilty. When she criticized the therapist, however, she observed from his reaction that he was not hurt and her guilt was reduced. Her reduced guilt then generalized to other potential objects of criticism, so she could now experiment with other such objects. Concomitant experiments in everyday life probably helped reduce her guilt further. For similar reasons, the objects of Mrs. C's criticism can be hierarchically ordered as to the initial discomfort they produced. Criticizing her husband was especially threatening because of its potentially noxious consequence for her marriage and would have initially produced discomfort exceeding 0. Thus, Mrs. C had to work first on criticizing a less threatening object, like the therapist, or still less threatening objects, like casual acquaintances. The data in Table 5 show that Mrs. C came to criticize increasingly threatening objects as the treatment progressed.

In order to determine whether a parallel process also occurred with Type C behaviors, the same procedure was applied to the 71 passages reporting Type C behaviors that had been rated 3.0 or more. The objects of these behaviors were also classified into the same five categories. There were fewer passages of Type C, so the frequencies are substantially less stable. The frequencies are reported in Table 6.

The progression of objects superficially parallels that shown in Table 5. The earliest Type C behaviors often focused on the patient's relatives and casual acquaintances. In the middle hours, she focused more on the therapist, and in later hours, on her husband and colleagues at school. Thus, in general, intimacy and distance were expressed toward the same class of objects in a given block of hours.

One object of particular interest, of course, was the patient's husband. There were 18 Type C behaviors directed at her husband throughout the 100 hours (Table 6), and 18 Type D behaviors directed at him (Table 5). The main difference between the C and D behaviors, however, was that the D behaviors by the end of the 100 hours were primarily 4.5 (direct confrontation), while the Type C behaviors were primarily 3.5 (comments to the therapist about warm and tender feelings toward her husband). This result further shows the lag in the

Table 6

Frequency of Occurrence of Different Objects of
Affection, Compliment, and Compassion

	Session					
	1-20	21-40	41-60	61-80	81-100	Total
All relatives (except husband) (Mainly 3.0 and 3.5)	6*	0	5	4	4	19
Casual acquaintances (Mainly 3.0)	3	4*	4*	0	1	12
Therapist (Mainly 4.5)	1	4	3	5*	2	15
Husband (Mainly 3.5)	1	1	4	7*	5	18
Colleagues + others at school (Mainly 3.5)	1	1	1	1	3*	7
						71

*The highest frequency for that object.

patient's progress in expressing Type C behavior during the 100
hours.

GENERAL DISCUSSION

The present work has examined several explicit hypotheses about
the nature of Mrs. C's psychopathology and therapeutic progress as
inferred from her verbal behavior. One major result showed that
Mrs. C's difficulty in expressing Type C behavior was related to her
difficulty in expressing Type D behavior; thus, the way to solve one
specifiable set of problems involved the simultaneous treatment of
another set.

Another major result of the present study showed that the <u>order</u> in which objects of C and D behaviors emerged followed a regularity which seemed to be largely under the patient's control. The therapist's comments undoubtedly contributed to this regularity, but they were probably not the major determinant. For if they were, the mechanism for producing this regularity would have to be very subtle since it would have to explain (a) how the therapist through his own comments became a major object of contradictory behaviors (sometimes C, sometimes D), and (b) how the therapist's comments managed to produce a smooth transition across time (i) from objects of the past to objects of the present, and (ii) from less significant objects to more significant ones, with the therapist himself as the mediating object.

One early theme in Mrs. C's therapy consisted of her criticizing her parents for events of the past. This kind of theme often occurs early in a treatment as the patient spontaneously produces data from the past. It is possible that Mrs. C saw as one demand characteristic of therapy that she criticize her parents for events of the past, but in our view, she was not only producing personal data but was also serving very specific therapeutic ends by beginning the treatment in this way. Her criticisms allowed her to test the therapist's reaction to one very mild form of Type D behavior and assure herself of the safety of future strategies. This low-level criticizing can be viewed as an early test of a therapist.

Horowitz, et al. (1975) have previously discussed the idea of a test in the following way: Before a patient can adopt the various strategies that will help him achieve his subgoals during a therapy, he needs to assure himself that it is safe to do so. Safety depends, in part, on the therapist's reactions at critical times, so during a therapy the patient continually tests the therapist and evaluates his reactions. One possible way for the therapist to pass a test which the patient poses is to remain neutral. The term "neutral" is not the ideal term, but it will be used until a better term is found. The important requirement is that the therapist's intervention show a sensitivity to opposing horns of the patient's dilemma and avoid communicating messages that are undesirable with respect to any aspect of the conflict (cf. Bateson, et al., 1956). For example, a therapist can sometimes achieve this effect by objectively investigating the issues which underlie a conflict without taking a stand that favors either side of the conflict. Through his questions and comments, a therapist might help a patient articulate the conflict without committing himself (the therapist) to one stand or the other. In that sense, he would remain neutral. Similarly, a therapist would not condemn or criticize a patient, placate him, or act hurt, angry, or guilty. When the therapist passes such a test, the patient is expected to feel safer, and feeling sufficiently safe, he can then use the strategy in question.

Thus, as one major sequence in a therapy, a test is performed, the therapist passes the test, and the patient feels secure enough to take a bolder step toward achieving his subgoal.

Not all patients would be able to begin a therapy by criticizing their parents for events of the past, however. For some patients, the early history has been so painful that early memories would arouse distress exceeding 0. In that case, the patient would have to find some less threatening opening strategy. Thus, the particular order in which themes emerge depends upon case-specific details.

The choice of strategy would also depend upon the patient's particular problems, subgoals, and major treatment goal. Mrs. C, for example, initially experienced discomfort in criticizing, blaming, and opposing other people, but she had somewhat less difficulty saying "no" to certain requests. For example, she initially handled her intimacy problem by refusing her husband intercourse. Other patients, however, would be less able to say "no" (behaviorally or symbolically) and as a result, might show more severe impairments in the capacity to disbelieve, distrust, disagree, be silent, refuse sex, etc.—in a word, to be autonomous. In that case, the early phase of treatment would have to focus more on the patient's discomfort over a different subset of D behaviors. Thus, Type C and Type D behaviors, as abstract families of behavior, are universally significant in a treatment, but the subset of interest in a particular patient is undoubtedly case-specific.

REFERENCES

Bateson, G., Jackson, D. D., Haley, J., & Weakland, J. H. Toward a theory of schizophrenia. Behavioral Science, 1956, 1, 251-264.

Horowitz, L., Sampson, H., Siegelman, A., Wolfson, A., & Weiss, J. On the identification of warded off mental contents. Journal of Abnormal Psychology, 1975, 84, 545-558.

Mussen, P., & Rosenzweig, M. R. Psychology, an introduction. Lexington, Massachusetts: D. C. Heath, 1973.

Smith, M. J. When I say no, I feel guilty. New York: Bantam Books, 1975.

Suppes, P., & Warren, H. On the generation and classification of defense mechanisms. International Journal of Psychoanalysis, 1975, 56, 405-414.

ISSUES POSED BY SECTION 6

Jacob A. Arlow

State University of New York, Downstate Medical Center

Brooklyn, New York 11203

My contribution to this symposium comes from my position as a
practicing psychoanalyst who has more than a passing interest in problems of validation of interpretation and methodology of research.
As a form of therapy, psychoanalysis represents a special type of
communication. The analyst is a participant-observer in a dynamic
process. He is concerned that the process should eventuate in a
definite way, namely, in an acceptable resolution of the patient's
unconscious conflicts and in the restoration of the patient's mental
health, whatever that may mean. To a certain extent, the analyst is
a compromised observer in the sense that he is not completely neutral.
Accordingly, the psychoanalyst has a compelling interest in validating
conclusions drawn from this special form of communication.

The approach the analyst uses and his frame of reference, especially the strictures of the psychoanalytic situation, afford him a
unique set of observations difficult, if not impossible, to duplicate
by other methods of investigation. It also provides the analyst with
a unique set of problems relating to interpretation and validation.
This brings the analyst into closer rapport with the other disciplines
represented at this conference, in the sense that he is aware of the
extent to which he shares problems of a similar nature with them.
Each of the modes of investigation discussed today has its advantages
and its disadvantages, so that communication among ourselves represents an important step in our mutual scientific enrichment. It is
clear from what we have heard to this point that we face an imperative need to complement each other's work and conclusions, utilizing
what we learn from our respective disciplines, and noting honestly
those problems that our special tools do not enable us to solve. We
need each other's help.

This sets the stage for my discussion of the three papers that have just been presented. I am grateful to fortuitous circumstances which caused me to read the papers in a different order from the way they were presented today. I read Dr. Spence's paper, then Dr. Horowitz's and finally Dr. Luborsky's. I discovered that all of them, from different vantage points, in one way or another were dealing with the same problem, namely, the problem of method. Basically, they all try to do the same thing, i.e., to reduce the rich and complicated data of the therapeutic interaction into units which are definable and manageable for purposes of study. Their goal was to establish conditions which would enable them to quantify the experience in ways that could yield valid and comparable conclusions. Both Dr. Shapiro and Dr. Rubinstein have discussed the nature of the difficulties involved in the two different disciplines and the pitfalls in the path of using proximate consensus as a measure for reliability of conclusions. In the end we are faced with the problem of validation.

If we examine the methods used in the three presentations under discussion, we see that these papers can be ranged in increasing order of complexity from the point of view of the nature of the unit of the data of observation involved. Dr. Spence tackles the problem from what might be called the smallest possible unit, namely, the word and its meaning. A basic approach of word meaning and word content enables Dr. Spence to reduce the experience of his observations into terms that are more easily quantifiable. However, once these solid observations are placed against the background of the theoretical assumptions, the problems involved in reaching reliable conclusions become much more complicated. The concept of defense centered around the opposing trends of repression and abreaction. Other mechanisms of defense such as isolation, denial, and projection did not figure in the discussion. In general, these mechanisms of defense present very special problems. What is striking about all three of them is the fact that derivatives of what is being warded-off appear in consciousness. If one concentrates solely on the mechanisms of repression and the phenomenon of abreaction, as Dr. Spence did, one has to reduce the conceptualization of the dynamic process into a quantitative, economic, hydrostatic model in which only what is repressed exerts the dynamic thrust that causes elements to appear in consciousness. The simple quantitative relationship that Dr. Spence suggests does not rule out alternative possibilities for interpreting the data. In spite of this, as I will attempt to show, there is a great deal of value in using this method because much can be learned from concentrating on the smallest unit of the word in the broader context of the psychoanalytic situation. There are rich and exciting possibilities in following Dr. Spence's approach.

Dr. Horowitz dealt with units of a more complex nature. He concentrated on the element of categories of interaction, which introduced the possibility of even more variables in the range of explanation.

Finally, Dr. Luborsky presented a global approach to the interpretation of the data of observation in the therapeutic interaction.
He emphasized a core conflictual relationship which perforce involves
elaborate ramifications of method. In spite of the complexity of
his formulations, it may perhaps offer a greater yield of results
than one could obtain by using methods involving simpler units of
data. What is striking about the implications of research in the
psychoanalytic situation is the fact that the investigation of a
simple word unit, analytically pursued, sometimes enables us to validate conclusions about broader, more complex ways of organizing the
data, either in the form of the core conflictual relationship that
Dr. Luborsky suggests, or the concept of persistent, unconscious
fantasy that I have discussed elsewhere (Arlow, 1969a, 1969b).

The basis for these observations grows out of certain fundamental
assumptions of psychoanalysis, the idea of the dynamic continuity of
mental life and of the persistence of unconscious conflicts usually
organized in the form of persistent fantasies. These serve to create
the mental set or the context which indicates how one perceives, selects, interprets, and responds to stimuli, especially stimuli emanating from other individuals during communication at all levels. To
illustrate what I mean, let us borrow the striking vignette which Dr.
Spence gave us. He said that if you ask someone, "Do you have your
watch on?"--and the person says "Yes," this is an irrelevant and occasionally frustrating and irritating answer. However, it may be an
entirely appropriate answer. If the mother of a young man going off
to school for the first time, asks, "Do you have your handkerchief?";
"Do you have your umbrella?"; "Do you have your lunch money?"; "Do
you have your watch on?"--the appropriate answer to each of these
questions is "Yes." This only illustrates that communication takes
place along lines of continuity, with meanings and expectations determined by context and contiguity.

The specific advantage of the psychoanalytic situation is its
ability to establish standard conditions that enable the observer to
exploit to the fullest those added meanings that come from the special
temporal and textual configurations of data. When we break down the
data of observation into smaller and smaller units, we perforce take
them out of the continuity of the therapeutic dynamic. In doing so,
we introduce an artifact in our method, and minimize the opportunity
to take advantage of that most important aspect of the therapeutic
interaction, namely, the unconscious dimension of the experience.
This is unfortunate because in context, as I suggested earlier, the
study of the small unit may have far-reaching implications. This
derives from the fact that so much of perception, behavior, and communication is metaphorical in nature. Even the simplest metaphorical
expressions used in the therapeutic context can be analyzed and understood as outcroppings of unconscious fantasy. The analysis of specific details of language used for graphic purposes demonstrates the
ubiquitous influence of psychic determinism (Sharpe, 1940; Greenson,

1953; Arlow, 1969a). If some mode of study could be envisioned which
would enable the observer to link the simple word units of metaphorical significance with the inferrable context of meaning, we would
have a most useful instrument for studying communication in the therapeutic relationship. As it stands, we are constantly beset by the
temptation to substitute phenomenology for a genuine grasp of the
deeper nature of communication.

Much of the difficulty lies in the fact that the therapeutic interaction is an oral interaction. Reading the record is not the same
as hearing the actual experience. Even an oral report of the interaction may have more impact than reading the record. This fact has
been demonstrated in many independent studies in different ways. For
example, Dr. Edelheit presented segments of tape recordings of sessions to different groups. The consensus of the different listeners
was of high order. When he took the same material to other groups and
presented the data in written form, the consensus was very low. As
in dramatic performances, reading the record of a therapeutic interaction leaves open the possibility of interpretation by the reader in
terms of inflection, accent, emphasis, etc. In spite of this, using
different readers with different groups regularly brings out a more
intuitive and accurate grasp of the therapeutic interaction than that
which comes from reading a written text. In my own teaching, I have
used such material. When the protocols were read in advance, the dis-
parity of interpretation was very high. When the material was read in
class, consensus was much greater. However, when I had the members
of the class read the same protocol several times by themselves, I
found that their interpretations came closer to the understanding of
the analyst who was conducting the treatment. In this respect, my
observations confirmed the usefulness of Dr. Luborsky's method of
having his observers read segments of a section, again and again, until it takes on meaning.

A good part of communication in the therapeutic relationship
transcends meanings conveyed by the verbal text alone. Much of what
is communicated remains unverbalized and is transmitted by mode of
behavior and by other means of expression. Behavior in the therapeutic situation is more than nonverbal communication. Many forms of
action can be understood as motor metaphors, i.e., motor counterparts
of figures of speech employing such mechanisms as hyperbole, symbolic
representation, allusion, pars pro toto expression, etc. Communicatio
in the therapeutic situation occurs in the context of a definite pattern of empathic interaction (Beres and Arlow, 1974). For this to be
possible, an affective atmosphere must characterize the interaction
between the two principals. This affective tone reflects the empathic
relationship between the two, and depends on the mutual identification
which takes place over a period of time as a result of the patient's
sharing his confidences and experiences with the therapist. It is
very important to understand how this relationship arises. In the
way the patient communicates his material, one can discern all the

mechanisms and techniques characteristic of creative, aesthetic productions. The patient unconsciously prefigures or arranges his communications in such a way as to arouse in the therapist an awareness
of derivatives of unconscious fantasy. In this way, it may be said
that the patient acts upon the therapist in the same way as the poet
acts upon his audience. The combination of form and substance evokes
in the therapist feelings and thoughts which are derivatives of an
unconscious fantasy of his own, corresponding to that of the patient's.
They may not be identical in form and detail, but they are related to
identical themes and substance. The feelings and thoughts aroused in
the therapist serve as clues or guideposts indicating the direction
for further therapeutic communication. This process can be seen most
clearly when treatment is progressing favorably, i.e., patient and
therapist are in empathic accord. When this occurs, the therapist
can rely upon his ability to understand the almost infinite number
of items presented to him, and to organize them into meaningful concepts, because when he is in empathic accord with his patient, he can
rely on his powers of intuition, i.e., on his ability to organize the
data of observation outside of conscious awareness.

This is only the first half of the process of interpreting communication in the therapeutic situation; this is the aesthetic part
of the interaction, and while it represents the base from which interpretations may occur in the mind of the therapist, of itself it
is not a sufficient base to justify or validate the correctness of
interpretation. Here, the second part of the therapist's task begins,
and this part is a disciplined one. For the interpretation to be
valid and meaningful, the intuitively-derived conclusion must be
subjected to a cognitive matching with the material, to a conscious
organization of the evidence into meaningful relationships. There
are definite criteria by which this process is accomplished. These
are, first and foremost, contiguity in context, followed by similarity and dissimilarity, repetition, coherence, convergence and consistency. The therapist's response cannot be considered on a par with
objective data, and intuition alone cannot validate interpretation.

From the foregoing, we can appreciate some of the difficulties
in interpreting form or surface structures out of their dynamic context. The analysis of word content and meaning, or of the significance of crucial interactions or relationships can be misleading when
we consider that the process of defense may transform the significance
of these elements through the use of such mechanisms as representation
by the opposite, denial, or projection. In the actual therapeutic experience, it is by no means an easy task to distinguish form from content or content from form in the patient's communications. To illustrate this point, I frequently cite the experience of a patient who
began her session by speaking slowly, promising to discuss a dream,
finding reasons why she should not present it, then intellectualizing
at great length about whether the dream was a defense, a resistance

to the investigation of our problem, a combination of both or a further expression of the difficulties which had been under consideration. She returns to her intention to tell the dream, but finds reasons for not doing so at the particular moment. She thinks she could
be responding in this way because of what she had learned recently in
her treatment, but then again, she is not sure that this is so. The
patient continued in this vein for most of the session, finally describing a portion of the dream, apologizing for not giving all of
it, explaining that she could not complete the presentation of the
dream, and returning to the kind of communication reported earlier
in the session. When I used this material for teaching purposes, I
asked the class to describe their own affective responses to the material. After a momentary silence, what usually followed was a spontaneous, contagious, outburst of laughter as the individuals in the
group sensed their relief upon discovering that the other members of
the group had felt the same sense of boredom, irritation, and impa-
tience which they had experienced individually. They had all felt
frustrated. To continue with the report: it took several sessions
for this patient finally to get around to completing the presentation of her dream. The content of the dream expressed the wish to
frustrate the therapist, making him feel incompetent and impotent to
deal with her resistances. But this idea had already been communicated in the first ten or fifteen minutes of the session by the form of
her presentation. The analysis of the form was as sure a guide to
the content the patient meant to communicate as the analysis of the
dream could have been. Actually, by the time the total dream was
presented, the dream was superfluous for either purposes of communication or interpretation.

Some words can communicate feeling and affect independent of the
meaning that the word form conveys. The presentation by Dr. Spence
and earlier studies conducted by Dr. Dahl, using computers to analyze
verbal elements in therapeutic communication, brought to my mind observations I had made about some special linguistic features in the
therapeutic interaction. Certain words have sound qualities that
affect the listener and influence his mood even when he is unaware of
the fact. For example, over the years I have come to recognize how
patients, in situations of frustration or mounting aggression, would
articulate their mood by introducing some verbal productions with
the sound "a-a-a-sh--." I used to regard this expression as a trun-
cated form of a suppressed intention to say the words, "ah shit."
After a while, in a number of instances of the same affective quality,
i.e., frustration and mounting aggression, my ear caught the "a-a-a-sh"
sound not as an expletive, but as part of the significant verb in the
patient's productions. Under such circumstances, the patient would
use such verbs as smash, dash, bash, crash, hash, slash, mash, etc.
The "a-s-h" sound had a certain affective connotation to which I became sensitized. It seemed to suggest aggressive intent of a moderate quality, continued over some period of time. When I concentrated
on the quality of the sound of the central verbs used to convey the

patient's thoughts in such circumstances, it seemed to me that as the patient's feelings became more intense, i.e., with rising frustration and increasing aggression, the quality of the sounds of the verbs used changed to smack, hack, whack, crack, etc. These verbs, partly by virtue of their sound, suggested more violent forms of aggression than in the earlier "a-s-h" group, but aggression of a more circumscribed type limited in time to one or two acts of violence. Rangell (1954), in a study of poise and the significance of the snout area, noted a mixture of unpleasant feelings of a pejorative nature implying envy and hostility in the sm, sn, schm, or shm sounds--a concept which brought together such words as smug, schmuck, shmo, snob, schnook, etc.

Most of the time, the working analyst makes such observations en passant, but cannot, in a systematic way, pursue the implications of his observations. It is even possible that if he were able to review the record of communication in the therapeutic relationship, many more such findings could be brought to light. Unfortunately, the nature of the therapeutic process does not afford the luxury of such leisurely investigation. Here is a project for further investigation which I will offer to Drs. Dahl, Spence, Luborsky, and Horowitz. The computer could be very useful in such a study, which could bring to light not only the relationships between certain word sounds and the meanings they convey, but also the ability of such sounds to influence empathic processes in the therapist. I might also add that there may be some implications for the study of linguistics. I was surprised to learn that all the verbs with the a-c-k sounds that I mentioned above were derived from Middle German, from words which ultimately had a common meaning, namely, to break or to destroy.

The unconscious selection of words with a definitive, affective sound quality that can be observed in the therapeutic communication, seems to me to be closely related to the use of alliteration in poetry. These sounds have certain affective connotations which are built into the surface structure of words, and I assume that different linguistic experiences attach special meanings to various sound combinations. Except for the satirical ones, few lullabies in the English language are rich in k, g, and d sounds. On the other hand, a very definite mood is created by the r and the s sound, as in the opening lines of Masefield's "Spanish Waters."

> Spanish waters, Spanish waters
> You are ringing in my ears
> Like a slow, sweet piece of music
> In the grey, forgotten years.

Could we find similar uses to evoke mood in therapeutic communication by studying the patterns of utilization of sounds in the record of therapy? In this regard, Dr. Spence's experimental design, concentrating on word meaning, could probably be expanded to include the

affective tone transmitted by the sound combinations. I was struck
particularly by his concentration on the word "dark." Apart from
the metaphoric possibilities that such a word may suggest, the very
sound itself, the sharp ending of the word on the harsh k sound suggests the possibility of exploring similar words with anxiety-produc-
ing, ominous implications, from the point of view of the sound patterns they contain and the affective tone they transmit. As I suggested earlier, Dr. Spence's approach concentrating on the simplest
unit of communication--the word--offers many possibilities for investigations which could lead in several different directions.

     The subtleties involved in investigating how mood and meaning
are conveyed in the therapeutic situation are enormous. The influence of specific combinations of sound, just mentioned, is only one
of many factors that remain to be studied. All this points to one
major danger that arises in the study of the therapeutic interaction
from the analysis, statistical or otherwise, of samples of the record.
The danger one may fall into, I call the "phenomenological error."
It consists of assigning meaning of a deeper, i.e., unconscious, or
genetic significance on the basis of the surface phenomenon, in keeping with preconceived categories of judgment. Such categorization is
unavoidable when statistical sorting and evaluation are employed, but
such categorization, unless rigidly limited in keeping with the research design, may be fraught with error. For example, in a study of
eroticism, frequency of intercourse and/or number of partners, carefully tabulated, may be entirely misleading when derived from the experience of a typical Don Juan patient who is either fending off unconscious homosexual inclinations and/or using sexuality as a vehicle
for hostility against women. Another example illustrates misleading
conclusions regarding the genesis of forms of behavior. In the case
of overeating, the so-called oral disturbance may or may not be connected with fixations or traumas originating in the so-called oral
phase. Overeating may represent regressive-defensive distortions,
or even direct expression of conflict-laden fantasies from later
periods. It seems to me that much of the uncertainty concerning re-
constructions made in child analysis, especially by the Kleinians,
arises from this phenomenological error.

     Dr. Luborsky's attempt to delineate a core conflict, I think, is
well-founded and has far-reaching implications. The main transference
theme in any analysis is only one manifestation of such a core conflic
The methodology Dr. Luborsky has proposed is, in my opinion, reproduc-
ible and corresponds with experiences that I have had in studying a
comparable concept, namely, the central position of the persistent
unconscious fantasy not only in the productions that appear in the
therapeutic situation, but also in the manner in which the individual
perceives, apprehends, interprets, and responds to the data of external stimulation. I believe that Dr. Luborsky's concept of the
core conflict expresses, in different terms, the relationship of phenomena which are derivative in nature--derivative from the unconscious
fantasy-life of the individual.

Here, I would like to offer another project for joint study.
There are many sessions of a very rich quality in the therapeutic
experience, which lend themselves for study by a strictly formal approach. It could be very illuminating to list and categorize all
the action verbs and objects of the verbs that appear in a particular session, and to repeat such studies in various samples in the
course of progress of treatment. I think the results would confirm
Dr. Luborsky's concept of the core conflict, as I have been able to
validate the concept of the persistent unconscious fantasy. The results are so striking that sometimes one is tempted to define neurosis
in terms of a broken-down computer, namely, whatever you feed into it,
the same sort of thing comes out. The patient misperceives, misunder-
stands, and misresponds to present reality in terms of the persistent
conflicts of the past. Evidence of derivatives of the persistent mis-
perception and misresponding to reality can be found not only in the
transference, but in dreams, slips of the tongue, current symptomatology, and recalled fantasies from earlier in life. Dr. Luborsky
has grasped a good portion of this experience in his concept of the
core relationship. By the same token, Dr. Horowitz's approach emphasizing certain special types of relationships, and Dr. Spence's concentration on specific words and content--all of these I consider
valuable instrumentalities for widening and deepening the investiga-
tive approach to different phenomena which, in the long run I believe,
find a common point of origin in some basic organizing fantasy. Some
of these approaches may lead us more quickly than others to the nature
of this fantasy; while others may explicate the process by which defensive distortions, metaphor, identification, and object relations
influence the final clinical appearance of the data. In any event,
however, all the methods proposed in the three papers presented here,
offer a promise to quantify and objectify our experience and to reduce
the data to manageable units that can be employed to test hypotheses
proffered by the various disciplines. All of this suggests a collaboration between the experimenter and the clinician that must eventuate
in the mutual enrichment of both.

REFERENCES

Arlow, J. A. Unconscious fantasy and disturbances of conscious ex-
    perience. Psychoanalytic Quarterly, 1969, Vol. 38, 1-27. (a)

Arlow, J. A. Fantasy, memory and reality testing. Psychoanalytic
    Quarterly, 1969, Vol. 38, 28-51. (b)

Beres, D. & Arlow, J. A. Fantasy and identification in empathy.
    Psychoanalytic Quarterly, 1974, Vol. 43, 26-50.

Greenson, R. On boredom. Journal of the American Psychoanalytic As-
    sociation, 1953, Vol. 1, 7-21.

Rangell, L. Psychology of poise with a special elaboration of the
  psychic significance of the snout or peri oral region. _Interna-
  tional Journal of Psychoanalysis_, 1950, Vol. 35, 313-332.

Sharpe, E. Psychophysical problems revealed in language: an examination of metaphor. _International Journal of Psychoanalysis_,
  1940, Vol. 21, 201-213.

EPILOGUE

In concluding this book with a set of papers
which focus upon the delineation of meaning and
intentionality in the verbal dialogue, we come
full circle upon our beginnings. We have seen how
"Life in the dialogue" entails the continuing
struggle with the processes of engagement–disengagement, fusion and differentiation, self and
object—in short, the effort to establish a unique
sort of "intimate separation" between one and the
other; a separation which enables the difficult
task of communicating. We have traveled the path
from the automatic, built in self- and object-
regulating strategies of the newborn and preverbal infant, to the highly complex, never fully
conscious, communicative structures of the adult
striving to improve and master his relations to
himself and others. It is this view of the communicative process as a struggle for mastery which
characterizes the psychoanalytic contribution to
a theory of communication. Hopefully, this view
will enrich such a theory and provide a new, more
complete perspective on the study of communicative processes.

INDEX